The Self-Care Advisor

The Self-Care Advisor

The essential home health guide for you and your family

Time Inc Health

Printed in the United States of America

This book is not intended to replace common sense or a doctor's advice. Given the differences of age, gender, and medical history, only your doctor can render a definitive diagnosis and recommend treatment for you and your family. The *Self-Care Advisor* is as accurate as its publisher, authors, and medical consultants can make it; nevertheless, they disclaim all liability and cannot be held responsible for any problems that may arise from its use.

Second edition
First printing: October 1996

ISBN: 0-9644119-2-X

Medical Advisors

C. Everett Koop, M.D.
Former United States Surgeon General
Medical Director, Time Life Medical

Florence Comite, M.D.
Founder, Women's Health at Yale
Associate Professor, Internal Medicine,
Pediatrics, Obstetrics and Gynecology
Yale University School of Medicine
Deputy Medical Director, Time Life Medical

Chairmen of the Advisory Board

David Chernof, M.D., F.A.C.P.
Associate Clinical Professor of Medicine (Hematology/Oncology), University of California Los Angeles Medical Center; former Senior Medical Director, Blue Cross of California

Ronald J. Pion, M.D.
Clinical Professor (Obstetrics and Gynecology), University of California Los Angeles Medical Center; Chairman and CEO, Lynx Worldwide, Inc.

Ernie Chaney, M.D.
Professor of Family and Community Medicine, University of Kansas School of Medicine–Wichita

Gregory Gray, M.D., Ph.D.
Chairman, Department of Psychiatry, Charles R. Drew University of Medicine and Science; Director, Augustus F. Hawkins Comprehensive Community Mental Health Center

Margaret Hammerschlag, M.D.
Professor of Pediatrics and Medicine, State University of New York, Health Sciences Center, Brooklyn

Stephen Hanauer, M.D.
Professor of Medicine and Clinical Pharmacology, University of Chicago Medical Center

John Heckenlively, M.D.
Professor of Ophthalmology, Jules Stein Eye Institute, University of California Los Angeles Medical Center

Ron Kaufman, M.D., F.A.C.P., F.A.C.R.
Associate Professor of Medicine (Rheumatology), University of Southern California School of Medicine; Chief of Staff, Los Angeles County–University of Southern California Medical Center

Denis Kollar, M.D.
Emergency physician, Queen of the Valley Hospital, West Covina, California; Chairman, American Emergency Physicians Medical Group

John M. Luce, M.D.
Professor of Medicine and Anesthesiology, University of California San Francisco

Stephen N. Rous, M.D., F.A.C.S., F.A.A.P.
Professor of Surgery, Urology Department, Dartmouth Medical School; Chief of Urology, Veterans Affairs Medical Center, White River Junction, Vermont

Rowena Sobczyk, M.D.
Director, After Hours, Meridian Medical Group (Prucare), Atlanta, Georgia

Michael A. Weber, M.D.
Chairman, Department of Medicine, The Brookdale University Hospital and Medical Center; Professor of Medicine, State University of New York, Health Sciences Center, Brooklyn

Barry W. Wolcott, M.D.
Associate Professor of Military and Emergency Medicine, Uniformed Services University of the Health Sciences, Bethesda, Maryland; Vice President for Medical Affairs, Informed Access Systems

Gayle E. Woodson, M.D.
Professor of Otolaryngology, University of Tennessee, Memphis College of Medicine

If you don't take care of
your body, where will you live?

~Aaron Goode, age 10

Contents

If you don't find what you're looking for here, turn to the index, which begins on page 326.

If you don't find what you're looking for here, turn to the index, which begins on page 326.

If you don't find what you're looking for here, turn to the index, which begins on page 326.

How This Book Can Help

The most useful rule for taking care of your health may be one you seldom hear: Remember who's in charge. The important day-to-day decisions about your own health and vitality are made by one person—you.

Many people go to the doctor when they don't need to. Many do the reverse and don't go when they *do* need to. The *Self-Care Advisor* steers you clear of both extremes, showing what you can do to take care of yourself and your family and when it's time to call your doctor.

This book covers more than 300 of the most common health concerns in the United States. It is arranged much the way a human body is: If you know where you hurt, you can turn to that section in the table of contents. If you miss what you're looking for there, you'll find it in the comprehensive index that starts on page 326. You'll also find basic emergency and first-aid techniques at the front of the book, and a unique guide to healthy living on pages 297 to 325.

Most sections include quick-reference charts. A chart may provide a ready answer to your question about a symptom; it may direct you to an entry elsewhere in the book; or it may suggest calling your doctor.

If the book directs you to a doctor, you may need to call for advice only, or for both advice and an appointment. If you need to see the doctor right away, the book will say so: "Call for a prompt appointment."

When you need emergency help, you may see "Call 911 or go to an emergency room **right away.**" When the problem could be fatal, the advice is simply "Call 911," because it's safer to wait for paramedics to arrive than to drive to a hospital; the medics have training and equipment that most of us don't possess.

Some areas of the country don't have 911 service. If yours doesn't, you should find your local emergency number in the front of the phone book. Post it on your telephones. Use 911 only when you're fairly certain you need it; your health insurance might not cover an ambulance trip for a nonemergency. Use the same guideline for going to an emergency room; in some, you may find yourself facing a longer wait than you would in a doctor's office.

Thanks to our board of medical advisors and to the many other doctors who helped with the *Self-Care Advisor,* you can trust the information it contains. Of course, if your doctor's advice conflicts with advice you find in the book, listen to your doctor; he or she should know your medical history and specific needs. In the end, though, it is *your* health. There's nothing like being a full, informed partner in the choices that you and your family will be making. We hope this book will become a trusted friend along the way and that it helps you enjoy a long and healthy life.

Emergencies & First Aid

In this section, you'll find situations that can be life-threatening and will call for fast action. Read it before you need it, so you're prepared to act without panic.

Make a special point of reading "Life-Saving Skills" on pages 14 to 25. This is a guide to the basic life-support techniques you would need for many accidents and injuries—the ABCs, CPR, the recovery position, and handling severe bleeding, choking, and shock. You don't have to memorize the details. If you're at least familiar with the methods, you may be able to keep someone alive.

First-aid instructions begin on page 26. Common injuries and problems appear in alphabetical order.

Emergency and first-aid advice is sometimes updated. Check with your local chapter of the American Red Cross or American Heart Association every year or so to learn of any changes. Better yet, take one of the CPR or first-aid courses offered by the American Red Cross, the American Heart Association, or your local fire or rescue department.

It's easy to set yourself up with the basic tools for a first-aid kit. They're listed on page 23.

About calling for help: You'll be advised at times to call 911. If your area doesn't have 911 service, you should find your local emergency number in the front of the telephone book. Take time now to write that local emergency number below, and also to post it on your telephones.

My local emergency number

Life-Saving Skills

When it's a matter of life and death, you'll need to know some basic emergency techniques. Don't waste time worrying about doing every step perfectly. Just do the best you can.

SIGNS OF A LIFE IN DANGER

- Severe bleeding.
- No breathing.
- No heartbeat or pulse.
- Choking: The person can't get air.
- Shock: Irregular pulse and breathing, cold skin. The person may be unconscious.

WHAT TO DO

The American Red Cross suggests 3 basic steps for any emergency:

Check the scene and the person.
Call 911 or your local emergency number.
Care for the person.

- Check the scene for things that could be a danger to the person or to you—fire, flood, traffic, spilled chemicals, or other threats. Don't be a dead hero. If danger is extreme, wait for professionals—police, firefighters, paramedics—to deal with it.
- Check the person. Try to find out what's wrong. Is it a life-threatening emergency? Don't move a badly injured person unless he or she is about to be hurt even worse by something on the scene. In that case, move the person and yourself out of harm's way before starting treatment.
- Call for help. Shout if you're alone with the person. If the person isn't breathing or has no heartbeat, phone 911 or send someone to do it. Don't start emergency treatment until you have called 911.
- Call on bystanders. See if anyone nearby has had more first-aid or CPR training than you have. Ask them to help.
- Care for the person. Treat the most serious problem first. Look for a medical alert tag on the person. If you find one, do what it says.
- Care for yourself. Protect yourself from a stranger's blood and other body fluids. Wear gloves if you have them. Put cloth or plastic between the person's body fluids and yourself, especially if you have open cuts or scrapes. While giving care, don't touch your mouth, nose, or eyes, or eat or drink anything. Wash your hands, or use alcohol wipes, right after giving first aid.

CHECKING THE ABCs

Airway. Open it. Gently tilt the person's head back and lift the chin. This will get air to the lungs through the nose and mouth. Caution: If you suspect a head, neck, or back injury, do not tilt the head. Moving it could cause further injury (see page 38).

Breathing. Look, listen, and feel for it. Look to see if the person's chest is rising and falling. Listen and feel for exhaled breath by putting your ear to the person's mouth.

Circulation. Check for a pulse. Using 2 fingers, feel for a pulse on either side of the neck slightly under the jaw, between the front of the throat and the long muscle on the side of the neck. For an infant (under 1 year), use 2 fingers to feel for a pulse on the inside of the arm between the armpit and the elbow. Listen for a heartbeat by putting your ear to the person's chest.

Severe Bleeding

SIGNS AND SYMPTOMS

- Spurting or gushing blood.
- Bleeding that won't stop.

Heavy bleeding that spurts or won't stop can quickly threaten a person's life.

WHAT TO DO

- Call 911 or go to an emergency room **right away.**
- Press right on the wound with a sterile dressing or the cleanest cloth you have—or your hand if you have no cloth. If a cloth becomes soaked with blood, don't remove it. Put a new cloth on top of it, and keep pressing. **Caution:** If an object is stuck in the wound, press around it, not on top of it. Don't press on an **eye injury** (see page 34) or an open **fracture** (see page 37).
- Make the person as comfortable as possible. Raise the place that's bleeding higher than the heart, if you can, to reduce blood flow. **Caution:** If you suspect a **head, neck, or back injury** (see page 38), don't move the person. You might cause further injury.
- If the person is bleeding around a broken bone, don't wash or probe the wound. Just stop the bleeding with a clean cloth (see **fractures and dislocations,** page 37). **Caution:** Don't try to remove anything stuck in the wound, especially in a chest or back wound.
- If the bleeding spurts or gushes—or if slower bleeding doesn't stop after 5 minutes—find a pressure point where an artery can be squeezed shut (see box at right).
- When the bleeding stops, don't remove the cloths you've been using. Wrap the wound in a bandage or more cloths. If something is stuck in the wound, wrap around it, not over it.
- If the person is unconscious, check the **ABCs** (see box on page 14): Lift the chin to open the airway, then check for breathing and pulse. Watch for signs of **shock** (see page 24): weak and rapid pulse, shallow breathing, cold skin, confusion, loss of consciousness.
- If the person is not breathing or has no pulse, start **CPR** (see page 16).

WHEN BLEEDING WON'T STOP

When nothing else works, pressing on an artery may stop the bleeding. Pressure points are places where an artery can be squeezed shut. Use a pressure point between the wound and the heart.

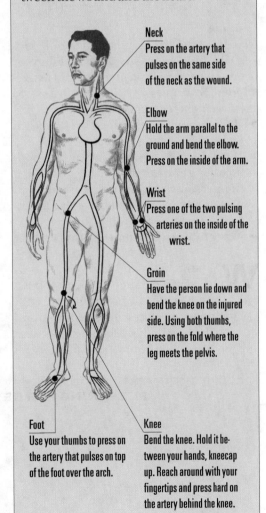

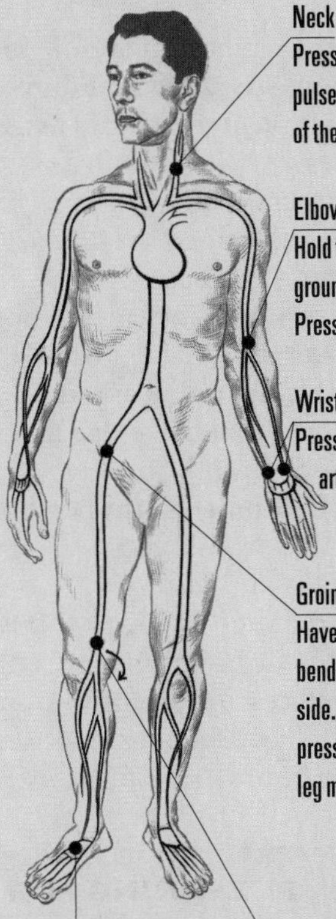

Neck
Press on the artery that pulses on the same side of the neck as the wound.
Elbow
Hold the arm parallel to the ground and bend the elbow. Press on the inside of the arm.
Wrist
Press one of the two pulsing arteries on the inside of the wrist.
Groin
Have the person lie down and bend the knee on the injured side. Using both thumbs, press on the fold where the leg meets the pelvis.
Foot
Use your thumbs to press on the artery that pulses on top of the foot over the arch.
Knee
Bend the knee. Hold it between your hands, kneecap up. Reach around with your fingertips and press hard on the artery behind the knee.

Rescue Breathing and CPR

Cardiopulmonary resuscitation for adults and children over 8

SIGNS AND SYMPTOMS

- No breathing: Chest doesn't move.
- No pulse or heartbeat.
- Pale or bluish skin.
- Loss of consciousness.

Cautions:
CPR can cause serious injury, including broken ribs and damage to the liver, lungs, or heart. The information here is meant as a reminder for people with CPR training, not as a replacement for that training.

- ➤ If you haven't been trained in CPR, ask if anyone else at the scene has.
- ➤ Don't do chest compressions unless both breathing and heartbeat have stopped. If the person still has a pulse, chest compressions can cause an irregular heartbeat. Use rescue breathing only.
- ➤ Never practice CPR on a healthy person.

When the heart and lungs stop working, brain damage or death follows within minutes. Rescue breathing and CPR (a combination of rescue breathing and chest compressions) keep feeding blood and oxygen to the brain until the person can breathe alone, or until medical help arrives.

The American Red Cross and many rescue organizations train people in CPR. Think about taking a course so you'll be prepared for emergencies.

WHAT TO DO

For an adult or a child over 8 (for an **infant,** see page 18; for a **child 1 to 8,** see page 19):

- ➤ Check the **ABCs** (see box on page 14): Lift the chin to open the airway, then check for breathing and pulse. See if the person's chest rises. Put your ear to his or her mouth to listen and feel for breathing for about 5 seconds.
- ➤ If the person is not breathing, call 911 **right away.**
- ➤ Lay the person down, face up. Kneel alongside, halfway between the head and chest. **Caution:** If you suspect **choking,** see page 20. If you suspect a **head, neck, or back injury,** see page 38. Moving the person may cause further injury.
- ➤ Tilt the head back and lift the chin to open the airway.
- ➤ If the person is still not breathing, start rescue breathing.

Rescue breathing

- ➤ Pinch the person's nose shut. Put your mouth over his or her mouth and seal your lips tightly against the skin.
- ➤ Breathe slowly and gently into the mouth for 1½ to 2 seconds, watching for the person's chest to rise.
- ➤ Remove your mouth and let the chest fall. Repeat with a second breath. **Caution:**

PREPARING FOR RESCUE BREATHING

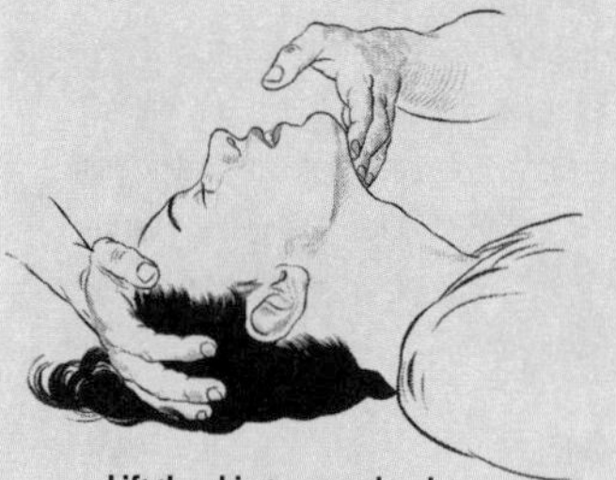
Lift the chin to open the airway.

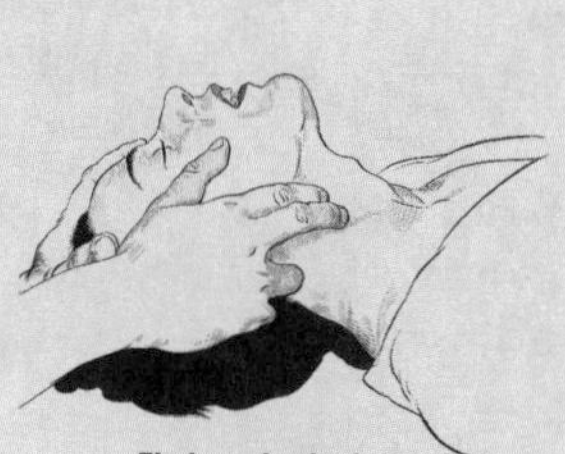
Find a pulse in the neck.

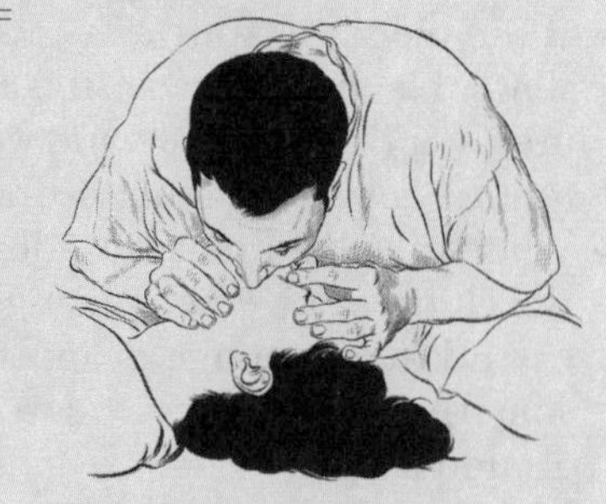
Pinch the nose shut. Breathe into the mouth.

Breathe just hard enough and long enough to make the chest rise. If you breathe too hard, air can be forced into the stomach, and that can cause vomiting.

- If the chest does not rise, tilt the head farther back. Give 2 breaths again.
- Check for a heartbeat. Using 2 fingers, feel for a pulse on either side of the neck slightly under the jaw, between the front of the throat and the long muscle on the side of the neck.
- If you feel a pulse, continue rescue breathing at the rate of 1 breath every 5 seconds. Check the pulse every 12 breaths. Time breaths like this: Count slowly, "One thousand one, one thousand two, one thousand three"; on "one thousand four" take a breath; breathe into the person on "one thousand five," and so on.
- Continue until the person can breathe alone, or until medical help arrives.
- If you feel no pulse or heartbeat, get ready to do chest compressions.

Chest compressions

Caution: Before you start, be sure you feel no heartbeat. If the person has a pulse, chest compressions are not needed, and they can cause an irregular heartbeat. Use rescue breathing only.

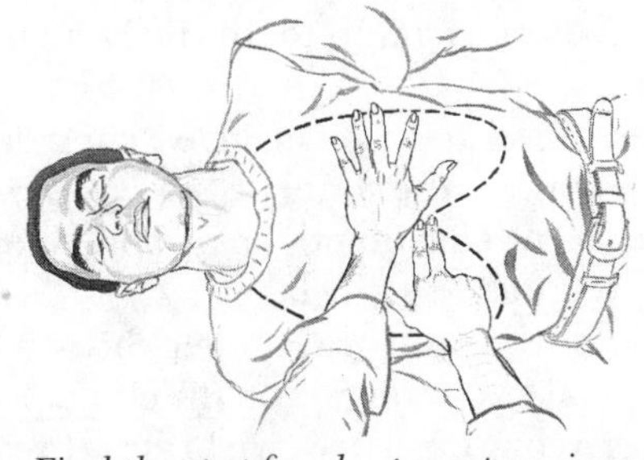

Find the spot for chest compressions.

- Kneel beside the person. Put your hands on the person's breastbone, keeping your shoulders right above your hands.
- Use the index and middle finger of one hand to touch the notch where the ribs meet the breastbone.
- Put the heel of your other hand above this notch, on the midline of the breastbone on the side closer to the person's head.

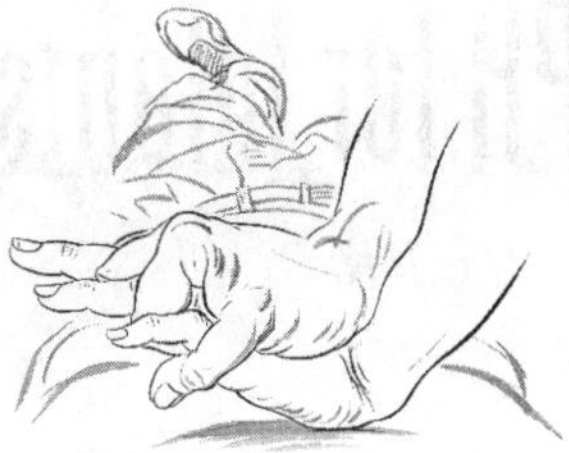

Push with the heel of your bottom hand.

- Now lift your first hand and put it on top of the second. Interlace the fingers of both hands and tilt them up so that only the heel of your bottom hand remains on the person's chest. Keep your arms straight and your elbows locked.

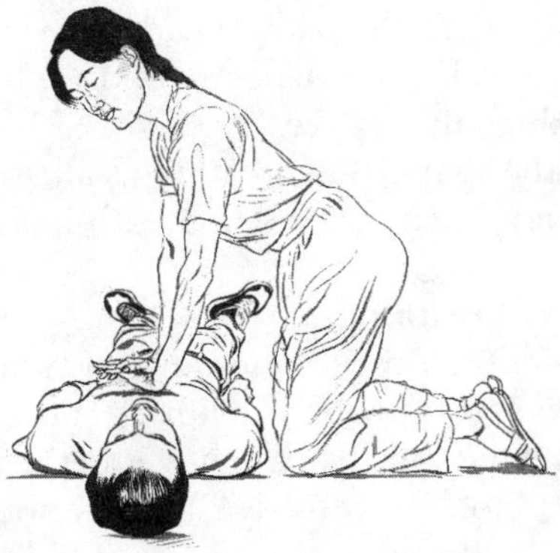

Kneel so you can push straight down with your elbows locked.

- Push straight down, depressing the breastbone 1½ to 2 inches.
- Release the pressure so the chest rises, but don't take your hands off the chest.
- Give 15 compressions, pushing straight down on the count of "*one* and *two* and *three* and *four*. . . ." Use short thrusts.
- Alternate with rescue breathing—give 2 breaths, then 15 chest compressions, then 2 more breaths, 15 more chest compressions, and so on. Repeat the series 4 times. Then check for a pulse.
- Continue the cycle until the person regains a pulse and can breathe on his or her own, or until medical help arrives. **If you feel a pulse, stop chest compressions and do rescue breathing only, until the person can breathe alone.**

CPR for Infants

Up to age 1

Caution: CPR can cause serious injury. Babies are small and tender, so be gentle.

WHAT TO DO

- Check the **ABCs** (see box on page 14): Open the airway, look at the chest for breathing, check for circulation (a pulse).
- Lay the infant face up on a firm surface. Gently tilt the head back to open the airway. Don't tilt a baby's head back very far.

Caution: If you suspect choking, turn to **choking infant,** page 22.

- If the infant is not breathing, call 911 **right away.** Then start rescue breathing.

Rescue breathing

- Lift the chin with one hand and seal your lips over the baby's mouth and nose.
- Breathe slowly and gently into the infant for 1 to 1½ seconds, just hard enough to make the chest rise. An infant's lungs are small and don't need much air.

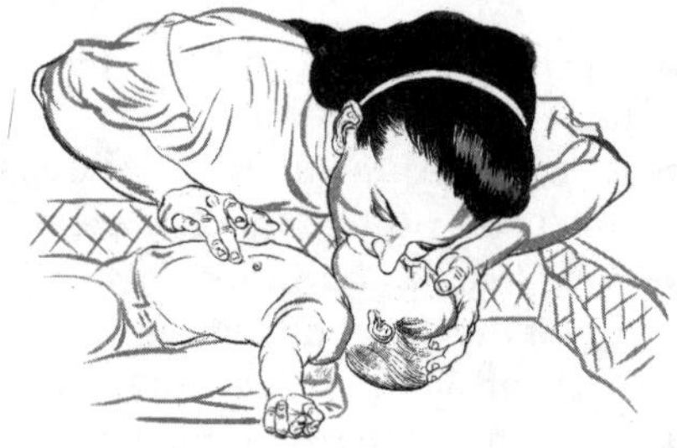

Breathe into the baby's nose and mouth.

- Remove your mouth and turn your head to watch the chest fall. Repeat with a second soft breath.
- Check for a pulse. Using 2 fingers, feel on the inside of the upper arm, halfway between the armpit and the elbow, for 5 to 10 seconds. Also, put your ear to the chest to listen for a heartbeat.
- If the infant has a pulse but still is not breathing, keep giving rescue breathing.
- Give 1 breath about every 3 seconds. Time them like this: Breathe into the baby as you count "a thousand and one," pause and take a breath at "a thousand and two," then breathe into the baby at "a thousand and three," and so on.
- If breath doesn't go in, see **choking infant** (page 22).
- Check for a pulse every 20 breaths, which is about 1 minute.
- If the infant has no pulse after you've felt for it for 5 to 10 seconds, start chest compressions.

Chest compressions

Caution: Before you start, be sure you feel no heartbeat. If the baby has a pulse, chest compressions are not needed, and they can cause an irregular heartbeat. Use rescue breathing only.

- Place the infant on his or her back on a firm surface.

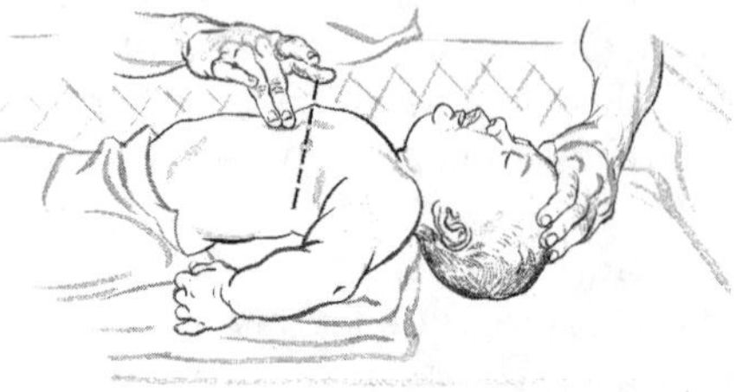

Press in the middle of the baby's breastbone.

- Put 2 fingers on the breastbone just below an imaginary line between the nipples. Use your free hand to tilt the head back gently.
- Pressing straight down, give 5 chest compressions on the count of *"one, two, three,"* and so on. The infant's breastbone should depress just ½ to 1 inch.
- Release the pressure between thrusts, but don't take your fingers off the chest.
- After 5 compressions, give 1 rescue breath. Then do 5 more compressions and another rescue breath. Repeat the cycle 20 times. Then check for a pulse. Continue until the infant regains a pulse and begins to breathe on his or her own. **As soon as you know the infant has a pulse, stop chest compressions.**

CPR for Children

Ages 1 to 8

CPR for children uses less force and faster rescue breathing and compressions than adult CPR. For children over 8, see page 16.

WHAT TO DO

- Lay the child face up on a firm surface. Check the **ABCs** (see box on page 14): Gently tilt the head back and lift the chin to open the airway, and check for breathing and pulse. Don't tip the head back very far. **Caution:** If you suspect choking, turn to **choking,** page 20.
- If the child is not breathing, call 911 **right away.** Then begin rescue breathing.

Rescue breathing

- Pinch the child's nose shut. Seal your lips over his or her mouth. Breathe slowly and gently into the child's mouth for 1 to 1½ seconds, with just enough force to make the chest rise.
- Remove your mouth and let the chest fall. Repeat with a second breath.
- If the child is still not breathing, give 1 breath every 3 seconds. Time them like this: Breathe into the child as you count "a thousand and one," take a breath on "a thousand and two," breathe into the child on "a thousand and three," and so on.
- Check for a pulse every 20 breaths, which is about 1 minute: Using 2 fingers, gently feel for a pulse on the side of the neck just under the jaw. Put your ear to the chest to listen for a heartbeat.
- If the child has a pulse but still is not breathing, keep giving rescue breaths.
- If you are sure the child has no pulse after you've felt for it for 5 to 10 seconds, get ready for chest compressions. **Caution:** Before you start, be sure you feel no heartbeat. If the child has a pulse, chest compressions are not needed, and they can cause an irregular heartbeat. Use rescue breathing only.

Chest compressions

- Kneel next to the child so your shoulders are directly over the chest. Tilt the child's head back with one hand. With your other hand, find the notch where the ribs meet the bottom of the breastbone (the midline).
- Put the heel of that hand on the midline of the child's breastbone. Keep your arm straight and elbow locked.
- Push straight down with the heel of your hand just hard enough to depress the breastbone 1½ to 2 inches. Compressions take about 3 seconds.
- Release the pressure so the chest rises, but don't take your hand off the chest.
- Give 5 chest compressions on the count of *"one* and *two* and *three* and *four* and *five."*
- After giving 5 compressions, give 1 rescue breath. Repeat the cycle of 5 compressions and 1 breath 20 times, which is about 1 minute. Then check for a pulse. Continue until the child regains a pulse and can breathe alone or until medical help arrives. **As soon as you know the child has a pulse, stop chest compressions.**

KEEP CHILDREN SAFE

Some safeguards can limit the chances that you'll need to perform CPR for a child. Take these steps:

- Put safety covers or tape over electrical outlets.
- Store electrical appliances away from the sink, tub, and toilet.
- Never leave a child alone in the bathtub, at a pool, or near any body of water. Keep toilet seat lids down. Cover kiddie pools.
- Prevent choking: Keep buttons, coins, and other small objects out of reach. Don't give children toys that have small loose pieces.
- Prevent strangling: Keep shade and drapery pulls, and plastic bags, out of children's reach.

Choking: Adult

SIGNS AND SYMPTOMS

- High-pitched wheezing.
- Clutching at the neck, bulging eyes.
- Inability to speak, cough forcefully, or breathe.
- Bluish face.
- Seizure or loss of consciousness.

WHAT TO DO

- Watch carefully. Encourage the person to cough. Let him or her try to cough up the object. It's possible to breathe with a partly blocked airway: If a person can cough forcefully or talk, he or she is getting enough air.
- Call 911 **right away** if the person can't speak, cough forcefully, or breathe, or if he or she is making a high-pitched wheezing sound.
- If the person can't get any air at all, give abdominal thrusts (the **Heimlich maneuver**—see box below).

If the person loses consciousness:

- Lay the person face up on a firm surface.
- Check and sweep the mouth: Hold the tongue and lift the chin. Looking into the mouth, slip a finger along the inside of the cheek and across the back of the mouth and out to remove objects and fluids. **Caution:** Do not try to remove anything unless you can see and grasp it.
- Tilt the head back and lift the chin to open the airway.
- Put your ear to the person's mouth to listen and feel for breathing.
- If the person is unconscious and not able to breathe, it is more important to get air in than to get the object out. Begin rescue breathing.
- Pinch the person's nose shut with one hand. Seal your mouth tightly over his or her mouth. Breathe long enough and hard enough to make the chest rise. Remove your mouth and watch for the chest to fall. Repeat the breath.
- If the chest does not move: Tilt the head farther back and give 2 more breaths.
- If chest still does not rise, give 5 abdominal thrusts: Straddle the person. Put the heel of one of your hands in the middle of

THE HEIMLICH MANEUVER

- Stand behind the person. Wrap your arms around his or her waist.
- Make a fist with one hand, and put the thumb side against the middle of the abdomen—just below the ribs but above the navel. Grab the fist with your other hand.
- Give up to 5 quick, forceful thrusts inward and upward into the abdomen. Pause, then repeat until the blockage comes out or medical help arrives. See the instructions above for what to do if the person loses consciousness.

Caution: If the person is pregnant or fat, give thrusts higher on the chest, against the center of the breastbone.

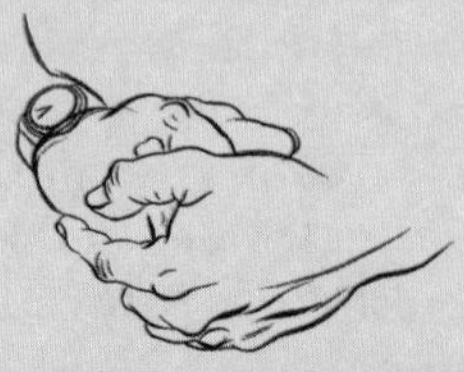

Grab your fist with your other hand.

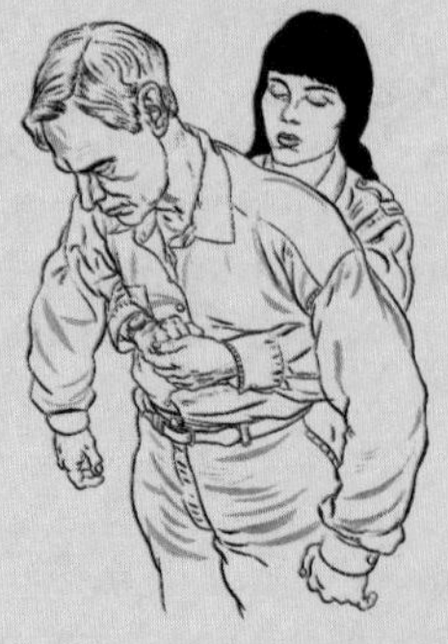

Hug the person and pull up into the abdomen.

HOW TO AVOID CHOKING

Thousands of people die from choking every year—mostly babies and older people. To limit chances of choking:

- Cut food into small pieces.
- Chew food until it is soft before you swallow it.
- If you wear dentures, take small bites, chew slowly, and try to eat soft foods—dentures make it harder to sense when food is soft enough to be swallowed easily.
- Don't give babies or small children small, hard, or firm pieces of food—such as hot dogs or carrot chunks—that can stick in the throat.
- Don't eat on the run—haste can make you bolt chunks of food. Sit down and take time to enjoy your meal.
- Don't laugh or talk excitedly while you're eating—talk between bites, after you've swallowed.
- Don't drink a lot of alcohol and eat—it dims your ability to tell when food is chewed and dulls the nerves that signal your body to swallow.

the abdomen just below the ribs and above the navel. Put the other hand on top. Give up to 5 quick thrusts upward and into the abdomen, aiming toward the person's head.

- Check the mouth again. Tilt the head and give 2 breaths.
- If the chest still does not rise, repeat the 5 thrusts, mouth sweep, and 2 breaths. Continue until the blockage comes out, the person begins breathing, or medical help arrives.

If you are choking and alone:

- Give yourself abdominal thrusts with your fist: Put a fist in the middle of your abdomen below the ribs and above your navel. Use your other hand to thrust the fist up and into your abdomen until the object pops out.
- Or use a chair back, railing, or other firm object: Bend forward over it, and press your abdomen against it firmly until the object comes out. **Caution:** Don't lean on a sharp edge that could hurt you.

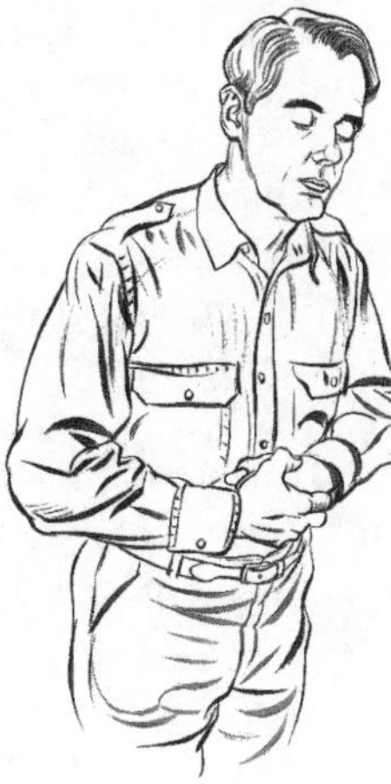

Pull your fist up hard into your abdomen or ...

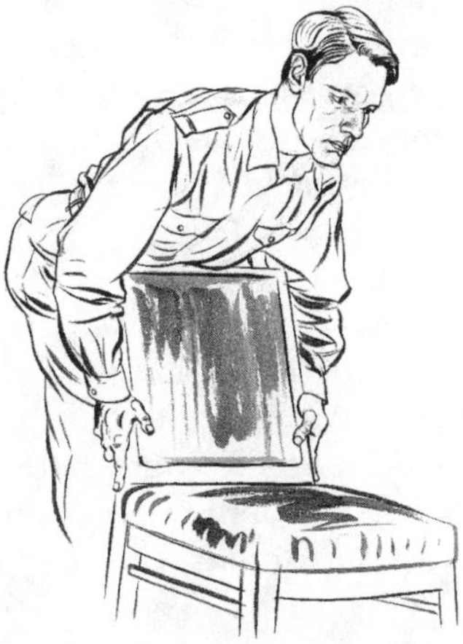

...use a chair back to give yourself abdominal thrusts.

- If you can see and grasp the object stuck in your throat, try to pull it out. **Caution:** Don't try to grab an object you can't see. You might force it farther down your windpipe.
- Even if you get the object unstuck, call your doctor for advice or go to an emergency room. You could have problems from the choking or the first aid.

Choking: Infant

Up to age 1

SIGNS AND SYMPTOMS

- Gagging or coughing that doesn't stop, or gets weak.
- High-pitched wheezing cough.
- Unable to cry, cough, or breathe.
- Loss of consciousness.

Choking is a serious threat to babies. They can choke on foods or fluids, or on small objects they put in their mouths. Don't give small, hard food that can stick in the airway. Don't leave small objects and coins where an infant can find them. Check with your fingers if you suspect an infant has something in his or her mouth.

WHAT TO DO

- If the infant can cough or cry, watch him or her carefully.
- Call 911 **right away** if the infant can't stop coughing, can't cry or cough forcefully, makes a high-pitched wheezing sound, or stops breathing. **Then:**
- Give 5 back blows: Lay the infant face down on your forearm so the head is lower than the chest. Support the head with your hand. With the heel of the other hand, strike the back 5 times between the shoulder blades. **Caution:** Babies are small and tender, so take extra care to be gentle.

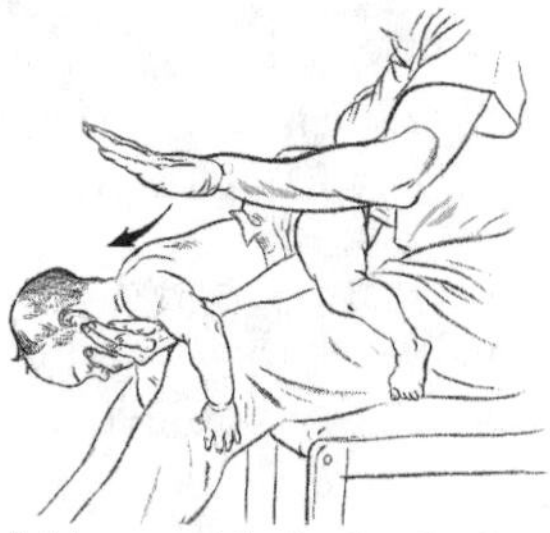

Give back blows with the heel of your hand.

- If the object doesn't pop out, give chest thrusts: Turn the infant face up, keeping the head lower than the rest of the body. Put 2 or 3 fingers in the center of the breastbone. Give 5 thrusts about 1 inch deep.

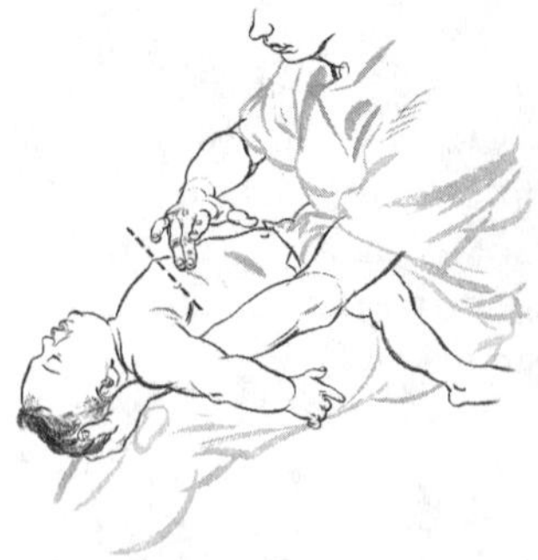

If back blows don't work, give thrusts in the center of the breastbone.

- Alternate 5 blows and 5 thrusts until the object comes out, or the infant starts to breathe or cough. Stop as soon as the baby can breathe, cough, or cry.

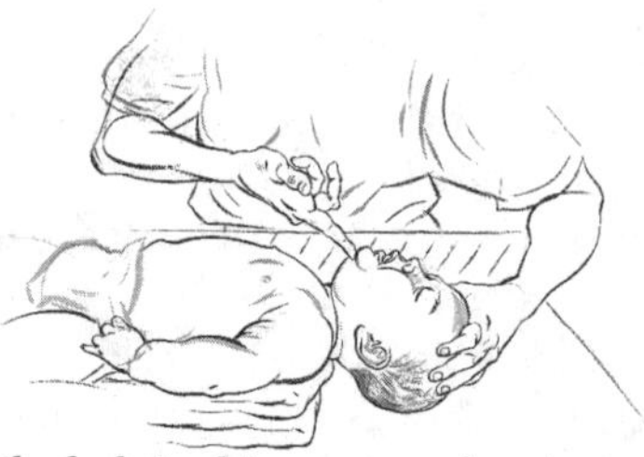

Lift the baby's chin to open the airway.

- If the infant is unconscious and not breathing, begin rescue breathing. The goal now is to get air in, not to get the object out.
- Put the baby on his or her back. Tilt the head back and seal your lips tightly over the baby's nose and mouth. Give 2 breaths. Breathe just long enough and hard enough to make the chest rise.
- If the air will not go in, tilt the head farther back and try 2 more breaths. Give 5 back blows, 5 chest thrusts, and check the airway.
- Look into the mouth and sweep the inside with your little finger to remove any objects or fluids. Gently tilt the head back.
- If you can see an object and can reach it, try to remove it with your finger. **Caution:** Be careful not to push it farther down the throat. Don't try to remove anything you can't see.
- If the chest still does not rise, keep repeating 5 back blows, 5 chest thrusts, a check for objects in the mouth, and 2 breaths until help arrives or the object pops out.

YOUR HOME PHARMACY

A well-stocked home medicine chest has what you need for most minor ailments and injuries, when you need it. It can save you the stress of trying to find an open drugstore at 2 A.M. The following list covers ills from sprained ankles to the flu. Remember that all medicines should be stored in a cool, dry spot and out of the reach of children.

For headaches, colds, and coughs:
Acetaminophen (adult and children's strength)—for pain and fever
Aspirin—not for children (see box on **Reye's syndrome,** page 96)
Ibuprofen—for swelling and cramps
Antihistamine—for allergies
Decongestant—for clogged nose and sinuses
Expectorant—for thick coughs
Cough suppressant
For poisoning:
Activated charcoal—to absorb poison
Ipecac—to make someone vomit
For digestion problems:
Antacid—for indigestion, heartburn
Antidiarrhea medicine
Disposable enema
Laxative (bulk-forming)
For skin:
Calamine lotion—for skin irritations
Foot powder—for athlete's foot
Petroleum jelly—for dry lips and skin
Sunscreen (SPF 15 or above)
Witch hazel—for itching
Basic supplies:
Adhesive tape, 1 inch wide
Adhesive bandages, assorted sizes
Elastic bandage (3 inches wide)
Cotton swabs and balls
Antibiotic ointment
Hydrogen peroxide
Rubbing alcohol
Scissors
Thermometer
Tweezers
Eye cup
Eye drops

A BASIC FIRST-AID KIT

Every household should have at least one well-equipped first-aid kit with an emergency handbook. Every member of the family should know where it is. Keep another kit in your car. You can buy a first-aid kit or make your own. Either way, be sure that it includes these items:
Emergency phone numbers
Gauze pads and rolls, assorted sizes
Adhesive tape, 1 and 2 inches wide
Assorted small adhesive bandages
Triangular bandage
Chemical cold pack
Small and large plastic bags
Disposable gloves
Antiseptic wipes or towelettes
Flashlight and extra batteries
Safety pins
Scissors and tweezers
Thermal blanket
Syrup of ipecac, small bottle
Antiseptic ointment
Activated charcoal

Source: American Red Cross

ABOUT CALLING 911 . . .

Don't hang up too soon.
When you call, be sure to give the address. Give the phone number you're calling from. Say what's wrong. Tell what happened. Say how many are hurt or sick. Give your name. And don't hang up until the emergency dispatcher does.

Don't cry wolf.
Your local emergency number is for just one thing—emergencies that threaten human life. Use it when you need it, but don't misuse it. About 40 percent of 911 calls are for nonemergencies, and they tie up help that someone else needs.

Shock

How to spot it, how to treat it

Shock is the body's reaction to a sudden, severe loss of blood from a wound or illness. Blood pressure drops, robbing organs and tissues of vital blood and oxygen. Shock can be caused by **severe bleeding** (see page 15), dehydration, heart disorders, an allergic reaction (**shock from allergy,** see this page), an infection such as **blood poisoning** (see page 31), or **toxic shock syndrome** (see page 248). It can be fatal if not treated right away, so it calls for emergency care as soon as you see it.

SIGNS AND SYMPTOMS

From blood loss, dehydration, heart disorders:
- Weak, rapid, or irregular heartbeat.
- Cold, damp, pale, or bluish skin.
- Shortness of breath or rapid, shallow breathing.
- Dilated (widened) pupils.
- Intense thirst.
- Confusion, dizziness, or feeling faint.
- Loss of consciousness.

From internal bleeding:
Same as blood loss, plus:
- Coughing up or vomiting blood.
- Bleeding from the rectum or vagina.
- Blood in the urine, or abnormally heavy menstrual flow.
- Swelling, hardness, tenderness, or bruising in abdomen or other areas.
- Wounds or other signs of a blow to the head, chest, or abdomen.

WHAT TO DO

For most types of shock:
➤ Call 911 **right away,** or send someone for help.

Caution: If you suspect a fractured pelvis or a **head, neck, or back injury** (see page 38), do not move the person unless you must. You may do further damage.

➤ Check the **ABCs** (see page 14): Lift the chin to open the airway, and check for breathing and pulse.

➤ If the person is not breathing or has no pulse or heartbeat, begin **CPR** (page 16).

➤ Lay the person on his or her back, with feet propped up 12 inches so blood can flow toward the brain.

➤ Find the cause of shock. Look for injuries: If you see a bleeding wound, press on it. If you find a **fracture or dislocation,** keep it from moving (see page 37). If the person has been stung by an insect or is having **shock from allergy,** see below.

➤ Keep the person warm. Loosen tight clothing, and cover him or her with blankets or clothes. If the ground is cold, put blankets or newspapers underneath the person as well.

➤ Check the **ABCs** often. If the person begins to vomit or to bleed from the mouth or nose, turn the head to the side to keep the airway open.

➤ Keep the person calm and still.

Cautions:

➤ Don't give anything to eat or drink.

➤ Don't put a pillow or padding under the head—it might cause further damage to an injured head or neck, and might bend the neck so that breathing becomes hard.

➤ Don't use an electric blanket or other form of direct heat.

Shock From Allergy

Some people get a severe allergic reaction to bee stings, bites from other insects, or certain foods or drugs. This is called anaphylactic shock. The reaction is often immediate. It can be fatal if the throat swells shut, blocking the airway.

If you know you have strong allergic reactions, you may want to keep on hand an emergency kit with an antihistamine and a shot of epinephrine. Ask your doctor. It's a

RECOVERY POSITION

An unconscious but still breathing person should be put in the recovery position to keep the airway open. **Caution:** Don't put someone in this position if you suspect a **head, neck, or back injury** (see page 38). In that case, moving the person could cause further damage.

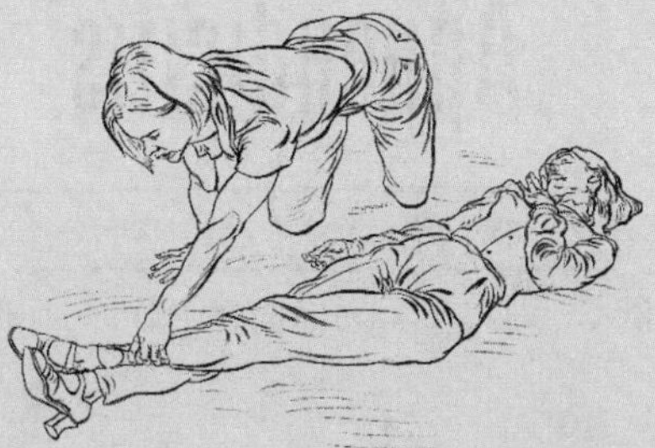

1. Kneel beside the person. Turn the head toward you. Tuck the arm closest to you under the person's body, keeping it straight. Put the other arm across the chest, and cross the far ankle over the one nearest to you.

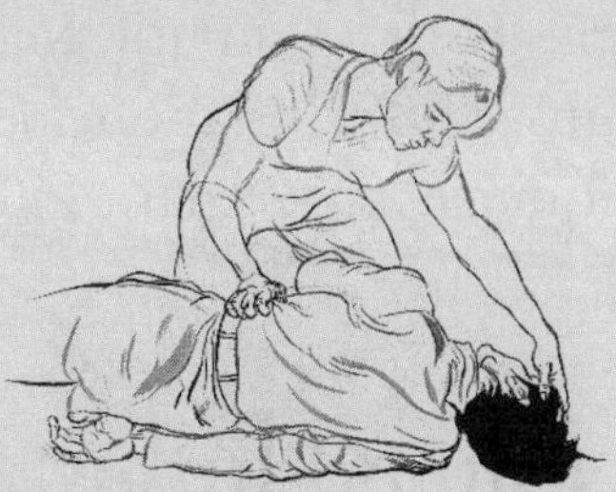

2. Support the head with one hand. Grip the person's clothes at the far hip with the other hand and pull the person gently over onto his or her side. Support the person's body with your knees as it rolls.

3. Carefully tilt the chin back to open the airway. Then bend the top arm and knee to prop up the body and make breathing easier. Make sure the bottom arm is out from under the body, lying straight beside it.

Check often to see that the person is breathing and has a heartbeat.

good idea to carry the kit to picnics, hikes, and outdoor events.

SIGNS AND SYMPTOMS

- Hot, reddened skin on the face and other places.
- Intense itching, or hives.
- Rapid swelling of face or tongue.
- Speeded-up heart rate.
- Wheezing and trouble breathing.
- Dizziness.
- Abdominal cramps, nausea, and sometimes vomiting.
- Loss of consciousness.

WHAT TO DO

Call 911 **right away,** and treat the person as for other types of shock.

- Try to find the source of the reaction. If it's a bee sting and you see a stinger, scrape it off or pluck it out as quickly as you can. Don't waste time looking for a credit card or knife to scrape with. A stinger keeps injecting venom after it's torn off the insect, and even a slight delay means you'll get a bigger dose.
- Some people who know they have severe allergic reactions carry an emergency kit. Help the person take the medication, usually a shot of epinephrine. Follow the instructions in the kit. **Caution:** Don't give epinephrine to an older person or one who has heart trouble.
- Get the person to an emergency room as soon as possible after giving an epinephrine shot. He or she may have side effects.
- If the person stops breathing or does not have a pulse, begin **CPR** (see page 16).

First Aid

Here is advice on how to handle the most common injuries and illnesses, in alphabetical order. Many of these problems call for techniques covered in "Life-Saving Skills," on pages 14 to 25.

Animal Bites

WHAT TO DO

➤ Press directly on the wound until the bleeding stops, using a clean cloth (or, if you have to, your hand). Hold the edges of the flesh together (see **cuts, scrapes, and wounds,** page 30).
➤ If the bite is minor, clean it well with soap and water. Then put on antibiotic ointment and a bandage.
➤ If the bite is deep, don't clean the wound after you stop the bleeding. Call your doctor for a prompt appointment. A deep bite may need stitches and could become infected. You may need a tetanus shot or rabies treatment.
➤ If possible (whether the animal is wild or a pet), have your local animal control center confine the animal and check it for rabies. Unvaccinated pets—along with stray cats and dogs, and wild animals such as raccoons, bats, foxes, and skunks—may carry rabies. Rabies infection is rare but can be fatal if not treated.
➤ Report any wild animal bites to your doctor and local health department or animal control center.

Cautions:

➤ Don't go near an animal that is drooling or foaming at the mouth, acting strangely, or biting for no reason. It may be rabid. Call your doctor and local health department or animal control center.
➤ Watch for signs of infection in a bite wound: redness, pain, swelling, tenderness, pus, hot skin, fever. Call your doctor for advice if you see these signs.

Appendicitis

SIGNS AND SYMPTOMS

- Pain in the abdomen. It may start in the upper part, then move in a few hours to the lower right. The pain often gets worse until it becomes sharp and severe.
- Vomiting, nausea, or loss of appetite.
- Constipation or, less often, diarrhea.
- Low fever.

An inflamed and infected appendix (appendicitis) can rupture after 24 hours and spread infection to nearby organs. To prevent this, a surgeon removes the appendix before it ruptures.

Pain in the abdomen may also signal **food poisoning** (see page 36), **gallstones** (see page 125), **kidney stones** (see page 138), a urinary tract infection (see **painful urination,** page 140), or an intestinal blockage (see **abdominal pain** chart, page 119).

WHAT TO DO

➤ If abdominal pain lasts for more than 4 hours, call a doctor for emergency advice. If you can't get one, call 911 or go to an emergency room.
➤ Keep the person quiet and as comfortable as possible.
➤ Watch the symptoms for 4 to 12 hours, looking out for severe pain in the lower right abdomen.

Cautions:

➤ If the person is constipated, don't give

him or her laxatives. They can indirectly cause the appendix to rupture.
- ➤ Don't use an electric blanket or apply direct heat to the abdomen.
- ➤ Painkillers or antibiotics can mask symptoms, so don't give them if you suspect appendicitis.

Bee and Wasp Stings

SIGNS AND SYMPTOMS

Minor stings:
- ■ Pain that lasts for several hours.
- ■ Redness, swelling, and itching or burning at the sting site.

Allergic reactions to stings:
- ■ Severe itching or hives.
- ■ Dizziness.
- ■ Reddish rash.
- ■ Cramping.
- ■ Trouble breathing.
- ■ Swelling of the eyes, lips, tongue, or throat.
- ■ Fever.
- ■ Drowsiness or loss of consciousness.
- ■ **Shock from allergy** (see page 24).

WHAT TO DO

All stings:
- ➤ If you see a stinger, scrape it off or pluck it out as quickly as you can. Don't waste time looking for a credit card or knife to scrape with. A stinger keeps injecting venom after it's torn off the insect, and even a slight delay means you'll get a bigger dose.
- ➤ Wash the area with soap and water.
- ➤ Apply a cold compress.

Allergic reactions to stings:
- ➤ Call 911 or go to an emergency room **right away.**
- ➤ Watch for the symptoms of **shock from allergy** (see page 24), such as wheezing or severe trouble breathing, rapid heartbeat, nausea, or loss of consciousness.
- ➤ If you have an emergency kit with epinephrine to counter allergic reactions, give the drug. **Caution:** Don't give epinephrine to an older person or one who has a heart condition.
- ➤ If needed, begin **CPR** (see page 16).
- ➤ If you know you are allergic to insect bites, wear a medical alert tag and ask your doctor about an emergency kit with a shot of epinephrine. It's a good idea to carry the kit to picnics, hikes, and outdoor sports events.

Blow to the Abdomen

SIGNS AND SYMPTOMS

- ■ Hard or tender abdomen.
- ■ Vomiting, nausea, or loss of appetite.
- ■ Bleeding from the rectum or vagina, or blood in the urine.
- ■ Cold, clammy skin.
- ■ Weak, rapid pulse.
- ■ Uneven (rapid or slow) breathing.
- ■ Confusion or memory loss.

Watch for signs of abdominal injuries after any accident. A blow to the abdomen may lead to **shock** from internal bleeding (see page 24), a life-threatening condition.

WHAT TO DO

- ➤ Call 911 or go to an emergency room **right away.**
- ➤ Check the **ABCs** (see box on page 14): Lift the chin to open the airway, then check for breathing and pulse.
- ➤ If you see signs of **shock,** follow the instructions on page 24.
- ➤ If the person is not breathing or has no pulse, begin **CPR** (see page 16).
- ➤ While waiting for medical help, lay the person down with the feet higher than the heart. Keep him or her warm with a blanket, and loosen any tight clothing. **Caution:** Do not give the person anything to eat or drink.

Burns

SIGNS AND SYMPTOMS

- Red marks, dry white marks, or charring.
- Pain.
- Blistering.
- Swelling.

Burns are ranked as first-, second-, third-, or fourth-degree, depending on their depth (not the area they cover or how painful they are). **First-degree burns** sear only the outer layer of the skin, but can be very painful. **Second-degree burns** injure both the outer and inner layers of skin and often produce blisters, swelling, and severe pain. **Third-degree burns**—charred or white skin—are painless because they burn down through all the layers of the skin, including the nerve endings. **Fourth-degree burns** go through all the layers of skin to the tissues and organs below.

WHAT TO DO

- ➤ Move the person away from the burn source. If his or her clothing is on fire, lay the person on the ground and smother the flames with a blanket, coat, or any other handy cloth. Or tell the person to lie down and roll over slowly. **Caution:** If you suspect a **head, neck, or back injury** (see page 38), don't move the person unless you absolutely have to. Moving may cause further injury.
- ➤ Call 911 or go to an emergency room **right away** if the burns cover more than one body part; if they involve the face, hands, feet, or genitals; or if they appear to be third- or fourth-degree.
- ➤ If the person is unconscious, check the **ABCs** (see box on page 14): Lift the chin to open the airway, then check for breathing and pulse. If the person is not breathing or has no pulse, begin **CPR** (see page 16).
- ➤ Take off clothing or jewelry in the burned area before swelling begins. **Cautions:** Don't pull away any clothing stuck to burned skin. Don't blow on burned skin.

BURNS FROM CHEMICALS

Signs and Symptoms

- Blisters or burn marks.
- Headache or stomach pain.
- Trouble breathing.
- Seizures or dizziness.
- Loss of consciousness.

What to Do

- ➤ Move the person away from the chemical.
- ➤ Brush off any dry chemicals. Protect your hands with gloves or clothing when doing so.
- ➤ Run water over the injured area for at least 15 minutes to dilute the chemical. Use plenty of water. If you know what caused the burn, read the label on the packaging for the maker's emergency instructions, or call a doctor **right away.**
- ➤ If the burn is in the eye, pour water over the open eye from the inside corner to the outside (see **eye injuries,** page 34). Go to an emergency room **right away.**
- ➤ Take off the person's jewelry and any clothing that may have touched the chemical.
- ➤ Cover the burn with a dry sterile bandage.
- ➤ Call a doctor for an emergency appointment. If you can't get one, call 911 or go to an emergency room.
- ➤ If the person is unconscious, check the **ABCs** (see box on page 14): Lift the chin to open the airway, then check for breathing and pulse.
- ➤ If the person is not breathing or has no pulse or heartbeat, call 911 and begin **CPR** (see page 16).

- If the burned area is smaller than the size of the person's chest, cover it loosely with a cloth that has been soaked in cool water and wrung out, or hold the burned area under cool running water or in a bowl of cool water for about 10 minutes, or until the pain stops or decreases.
- If the burn is larger than the size of the person's chest, don't put water on it (this could lead to hypothermia). Cover the burned skin loosely with a clean, dry cloth. If fluid oozes through the cloth, put another cloth over it.
- To reduce swelling, raise the burned area higher than the person's heart.
- Unless the person is vomiting or unconscious, you may give small sips of water.
- If the person is unconscious but still breathing, support the head and roll him or her onto the side, into the **recovery position** (see page 25).

Cautions:

- Do not put the person in the recovery position if you suspect a **head, neck, or back injury** (see page 38), or if the burn is on the chest or elsewhere on the front of the body.
- Don't put ice, ointments, lotions, butter, or baking soda on the burn.
- Don't break any blisters.
- Don't use adhesive tape or bandages, or cotton balls. They stick to the skin.

Chest Pain

SIGNS AND SYMPTOMS

- Dull, sharp, crushing, stabbing, or severe burning pain, or pressure or tightness in the chest. Pain may spread to the jaw, neck, back, or arms, especially the left arm.

See the **chest pain** chart (page 107). Depending on the type of pain and other symptoms, chest pain could signal a number of ailments, including **heart attack** (see page 39), angina, a collapsed lung, pleurisy (inflammation of the sac around the lungs), an injured rib or a pulled chest muscle, an **ulcer** (see page 136), **heartburn** (see page 127), or **anxiety** (see page 210). Never ignore chest pain that lasts longer than a few minutes.

WHAT TO DO

- If you suspect a **heart attack** (see page 39), call 911 **right away.**

Childbirth

Emergency

SIGNS AND SYMPTOMS

- Contractions of the uterus 2 to 3 minutes apart.
- A liquid discharge from the woman's vagina.
- An overwhelming urge by the woman to push, or to move her bowels.
- Feeling or seeing the baby's head between the woman's legs.

Caution: Childbirth is a natural process, even when it comes unexpectedly at home or on the way to the hospital. If you are in labor or with someone who is about to give birth, don't try to stop the process or delay delivery. Stay calm and call for help.

WHAT TO DO

Before delivery:

- Call a doctor for emergency instructions. If you can't get one, call 911 or go to an emergency room **right away.**
- If you have no time to get to a hospital and medical help hasn't yet arrived, prepare a place—with a plastic sheet and clean linens and pillows, if possible—for mother and child.
- Collect clean towels, sheets, or other cloths. Sterilize scissors or a knife and a few feet of string by plunging them into boiling water.
- Keep the woman warm. Make her com-

fortable. Help her take off her clothes from the waist down.

- Remove your jewelry and wristwatch. Wash your hands well with soap and hot water. Scrub under your nails.
- Stay calm. Help the woman take slow, deep, calming breaths.
- Try to get a medical person—at a fire, police, or rescue department or a hospital—on the phone to talk you through the delivery.

During delivery:

- You will see some bloody fluid and other discharge. Watch for the baby's head to appear in the opening to the vagina. This means birth is about to happen. Have a clean towel or cloth to wrap the baby in as soon as the baby comes out.
- Be ready to support the baby's head as it comes through the vagina. The baby's shoulders and body should follow on the next contractions. **Caution:** Don't pull on the baby's head. Support it gently as the shoulders slide out.
- When the head emerges, see if the umbilical cord is wrapped around the baby's neck. If it is, use 2 fingers to gently ease it over the baby's head.
- There may be a gush of fluid as the baby's body slides out, and the baby will be very slippery. Have the clean cloth or towel ready to grasp the baby.
- If the baby doesn't come out headfirst, don't try to pull the baby out. Support the body as best you can, and get medical help **right away.**

After delivery:

- The baby may still be wrapped in a bag of fluids (the amniotic sac). If so, rip the sac open with your fingers. Gently clear it away from the baby's mouth and nose.
- Hold the newborn with his or her head lower than the body. Turn the head to the side, so that fluids will drain from the baby's mouth and nose.
- If the baby doesn't start breathing within 30 seconds, keep the head lower than the body. Gently tap the soles of the baby's feet, and then rub the baby's back.
- If the baby is still not breathing, begin **infant rescue breathing** (see page 18). Use only very gentle puffs of air.
- If the baby is breathing, wipe the nose and mouth gently with a clean cloth or towel. Don't wash the baby.
- Give the baby to the mother and encourage her to nurse right away. The baby's sucking helps release a hormone that makes the uterus contract and prevents further bleeding.
- Don't cut the umbilical cord, and don't pull on it. It is attached to the placenta, or afterbirth, which will come out 10 to 20 minutes after the baby does.
- If medical help is nearby, wrap the baby, umbilical cord, and placenta together. If the mother and baby can't get prompt medical treatment, you may need to cut the cord.

If you need to cut the cord:

- Wait until the umbilical cord stops pulsating, at least 5 minutes. Use the string you sterilized to tie off the cord at least 7 inches from the baby's navel. Make a second tie about 3 inches beyond that, closer to the mother. Be sure both ties are tight.
- Use sterilized scissors or a sterilized knife to cut the cord between the two knots.
- Wait for the placenta to come out. There will be some bleeding from the vagina. Be sure to save the placenta. Handle it with care. Put it in a plastic bag so a doctor can look at it later.
- Keep the mother and baby together and warm until they get medical treatment.

Cuts, Scrapes, and Wounds

Life is full of scrapes, cuts, and punctures. Scrapes can hurt, but they usually bleed only a little. Cuts can bleed heavily. Puncture wounds may not bleed much, unless they rupture major blood vessels or organs, but they can get infected.

WHAT TO DO

➤ Call for emergency medical advice if a wound is deeper than one-quarter inch and longer than 1 inch; if it has jagged edges; or if bleeding doesn't stop after 5 minutes. If you can't get a doctor, go to an emergency room.

Severe bleeding:

➤ Call 911 or go to an emergency room **right away** (see **when bleeding won't stop,** page 15).

Head wound:

➤ If the injury is more than a minor bump or surface cut, call 911 **right away.**

➤ Do not move the person unless you absolutely must; this can cause further injury (see **head, neck, and back injuries,** page 38).

➤ If a head wound is bleeding but not deep, cover the wound with a clean bandage or cloth. Press directly on the wound. If a cloth becomes soaked with blood, don't remove it. Put another cloth on top of it, and keep pressing.

➤ Put a cold compress over the wound to ease pain and swelling.

➤ Keep the person calm and still until medical help arrives.

➤ Watch the person for 24 hours for signs of serious injury—confusion, unusual drowsiness, bleeding from the ears or nose, or loss of movement on one side of the body.

Eye or eyelid cut:

➤ Cover both eyes lightly with bandages. **Caution:** Don't apply direct pressure to a bleeding eye.

➤ Call a doctor for an emergency appointment. If you can't get one, call 911 or go to an emergency room.

Minor bleeding, a puncture wound, or a scrape:

➤ Clean the wound with soap and water.

➤ Cover the wound with a bandage to stop the bleeding and prevent infection. If you are using an elastic bandage, be sure it's not so tight that it cuts off internal blood flow. Make sure you can slip a finger between the bandage and the skin.

➤ For deep puncture wounds, call your doctor for emergency advice.

➤ Watch for signs of infection: redness, pus, swelling, pain, and fever. If the wound becomes infected, call a doctor for advice.

➤ Make sure the person has a current vaccination against tetanus.

BLOOD POISONING

Blood poisoning (septicemia) is the term for a bacterial infection in the blood. This may spread from a wound, appendicitis, a burn, a urinary tract or lung infection, dental work, or injecting street drugs. The bloodstream then carries the infection to other parts of the body.

Signs and Symptoms

- Chills and fever.
- Headache.
- Fatigue or confusion.
- Nausea, diarrhea, or lost appetite.
- Warm, flushed skin.
- Increased heart rate.

What to Do

➤ Call a doctor for emergency advice. If you can't get one, call 911 or go to an emergency room. You may need antibiotics.

➤ Watch for signs of septic shock, a common side effect of blood poisoning with some of the following symptoms: rapid pulse and breathing, temperature below normal, fainting, and possibly confusion or coma. If symptoms appear, call 911 **right away.** If you are waiting for medical help to arrive, see **shock,** page 24.

Drowning

SIGNS AND SYMPTOMS

- Pale or bluish skin, especially the lips.
- Cold body.
- Loss of consciousness.
- No breathing.

Drowning occurs when water blocks the air supply to the lungs. Big bodies of water aren't the only places it happens. People also drown at home—in bathtubs, backyard pools, and whirlpool baths. Toddlers can drown in pails and toilets. Knowledge of rescue breathing and CPR can save a life.

WHAT TO DO

In the water:

➤ If you see a person floating facedown in the water or having trouble swimming, tell any nearby lifeguard or emergency worker and call 911 **right away.**

➤ If you are in the water with a drowning person who has stopped breathing, begin the rescue breathing phase of **CPR** (see page 16), if possible. Tilt the head back, pinch the nostrils closed, and breathe into the mouth. As you pause between breaths, move toward land. **Caution:** Don't try rescue breathing in the water unless you can safely stand up in it, or unless you are a very strong swimmer.

Out of the water:

➤ If a person has been pulled from the water unconscious, check the **ABCs** (see box on page 14): Lift the chin to open the airway, then check for breathing and pulse. If the person is not breathing or does not have a pulse or heartbeat, begin **CPR** (see page 16). If the person is a child or an infant, see page 19 or 18.

➤ People who have almost drowned often cough up water and food during rescue breathing. Turn the head to the side from time to time to allow water and vomit to drain from the mouth, and sweep out the mouth with your finger.

➤ If the person is on land and unconscious but breathing, support the head and roll him or her onto the side into the **recovery position** (see box on page 25) to keep the airway open. **Caution:** Don't move the person into the recovery position if you suspect a **head, neck, or back injury** (see page 38)—such as from a diving accident.

➤ Remove wet clothing, and cover the person with a coat, blanket, or dry clothes.

➤ Help the person rest quietly until medical help arrives.

Caution: In cold water or icy conditions, watch for symptoms of **hypothermia** (shivering, uncoordinated movements, drowsiness, loss of consciousness). See page 41.

Ear Emergencies

SIGNS AND SYMPTOMS

- Earache.
- Muffled or lost hearing; ringing in the ear.
- Swelling or redness.
- Blood or other fluids draining from the ear.
- Dizziness, nausea, or vomiting.

While an earache may signal an ear emergency, it is also a sign of less serious problems, ranging from an **ear infection** (see page 73) to a blockage from **earwax** (see page 74). If you have a long-lasting earache, call your doctor for advice.

WHAT TO DO

If blood or fluids are draining from the ear:

➤ If you suspect a head injury, call 911 or go to an emergency room **right away.**

➤ Cover the ear loosely with a clean cloth. Tape it in place. Don't try to clean the ear.

➤ Lay the person face up while waiting for medical help. **Caution:** If you suspect a **head, neck, or back injury** (see page 38), don't move the person; this could cause permanent injury.

If an eardrum has burst:

- ➤ If a person suddenly has pain, ringing, or buzzing in the ear; trouble hearing; or discharge (including pus or blood), an eardrum may be ruptured. Call a doctor for a prompt appointment.
- ➤ To prevent infection, cover the ear with a dry sterile pad.
- ➤ Give an over-the-counter pain reliever such as acetaminophen or aspirin. Never give aspirin to a child under 12 who has chicken pox, flu, a cold, or any other illness you suspect of being caused by a virus (see box on **Reye's syndrome,** page 96).

If a foreign object is in the ear:

- ➤ Shake it out: Have the person tilt his or her head so that the sore ear faces down. Straighten the ear canal by gently pulling the top part of the ear up and back, then shake the head. **Caution:** Don't shake an infant or a young child.
- ➤ If nothing comes out, look for the object in the ear. If you can see it, use a pair of tweezers carefully to try to remove it. Don't try to remove a live insect or hard object.
- ➤ If you can't see it, don't try to take it out. Go to a doctor or an emergency room.

If a live insect is in the ear:

- ➤ Try floating the insect out by pouring a small amount of warm (not hot) oil—baby, mineral, or olive—into the ear. This may also ease pain.
- ➤ To apply oil: Have the person tilt the head so the sore ear is up. Gently open the ear by pulling it upward and back. Slowly pour in the warm oil and watch for the insect to float out.

Cautions:

- ➤ Don't push on anything in the ear or push anything into the ear.
- ➤ Don't try to remove any hard, smooth object such as a BB or bead.
- ➤ Don't work on the ear if the person (above all a child) won't hold still.
- ➤ Never strike anyone on the head to try to clear an ear.

Electric Shock

SIGNS AND SYMPTOMS

- Deep, charred, or small burns on the mouth or other parts of the body.
- Tingling sensation.
- Sudden dizziness or headache.
- Muscle pains.
- Loss of consciousness, which may include no breath or heartbeat.

WHAT TO DO

- ➤ Remove the source of electricity as quickly and safely as possible. **Caution:** Don't touch the person until the current is off or gone. Don't use appliance switches—they may not work. Unplug the appliance or turn off main power switches.
- ➤ If you can't turn the current off, get the person away from it. **Caution:** Don't use your hands or anything metal or wet. Insulate yourself by standing on a rubber mat, newspapers or books, something wooden, or a pile of clothing or linens. Use a dry, nonconducting object to separate the person from the current: a stick, a wooden chair or small table, or a rope.
- ➤ When you can touch the person safely, check the **ABC**s (see box on page 14): Lift the chin to open the airway, then check for breathing and pulse.
- ➤ Look for injuries, especially burns. If you see either one, call 911 **right away. Caution:** Electrical burns are often deeper and more serious than they appear.
- ➤ Give first aid for **burns** (see page 28).
- ➤ Cover the person and make him or her as comfortable as possible.
- ➤ If the person might have been struck by lightning, call 911 **right away.** It's all right to touch a lightning victim and begin first aid—the electricity is gone.
- ➤ For other electric shocks, call a doctor for emergency advice. If you can't get one, call 911 or go to an emergency room, even if the person seems unharmed.

If someone has been shocked by a downed electrical wire:

- ➤ Stay at least 20 feet away from high-voltage current.
- ➤ Call 911, then call the power company to have the current turned off.
- ➤ If the person is inside a car or truck and is conscious, tell him or her to stay there unless there is a fire or other immediate danger. If the person must leave the car, tell him or her not to touch the car and the ground at the same time. Have the person jump clear of the vehicle.
- ➤ As soon as the power is off or the person is clear of the current, begin first aid.

Cautions:

- ➤ Don't touch any electrical wire, car, or person in contact with a live wire.

Eye Injuries

SIGNS AND SYMPTOMS

- ■ Bruise or cut on the eye.
- ■ Pain.
- ■ Bloodshot eye.
- ■ Itching, dryness, or tears in the eye.
- ■ Blinking, or trouble keeping the eye open.
- ■ Sensitivity to light.
- ■ Trouble seeing.
- ■ Headache.
- ■ Different-size pupils.

WHAT TO DO

Foreign object in the eye:

- ➤ Call 911 or go to an emergency room **right away.**

Cautions:

- ➤ If the object is stuck in the eye, don't try to take it out.
- ➤ Don't touch the object; keep the person's hands away from the eye.
- ➤ If a large object such as a pencil is in the eye, tape a paper cone or cup over it to support the object. For a long object, punch a hole in the bottom of the cup. Cover the person's other eye with a clean cloth; this will help keep the injured eye from moving.
- ➤ For a small object, tie a clean cloth over both eyes for the trip to the emergency room.

Bleeding in the eye:

- ➤ If the eye is bleeding, cover both eyes with a clean cloth and raise the person's head above the heart. Then call 911 or go to an emergency room **right away. Caution:** Don't try to move the person if you suspect a **head, neck, or back injury** (see page 38). You may cause further injury.

Foreign objects not embedded in the eye:

- ➤ If the person is wearing contact lenses and can safely remove them, he or she should do so. The object may come out with the contact lens.
- ➤ If that doesn't work, clean your hands with soap and water, then ask the person to sit in good light and look up as you gently pull down the lower eyelid. Look inside the eye and the lower eyelid. If the object is there, pull the upper lid gently over the lower. The tears that follow may wash out the object.
- ➤ If tears don't wash the object out, flush the eye with running water—either from a cup or the tap. The person can also try opening his or her eyes underwater in a bowl of fresh tap water.

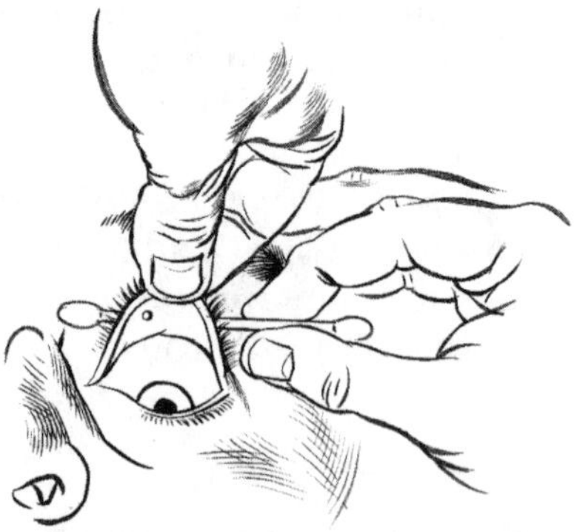

How to fold back the upper eyelid

- ➤ If you can't see the object in the lower lid or eye, ask the person to look down. Put a cotton swab or wooden matchstick lengthwise against the upper lid. Then pull up gently on the upper lashes and lid and fold the lid over the stick. You may now be

able to see the object. Use running water to wash it out, or take it out using the edge of a clean, soft, damp cloth or cotton swab.
- Wash the eye gently with cool water.
- If you can't find or remove the object, or you do remove it but the person is still in pain or can't see, tie a clean cloth over both eyes and go to an emergency room.

Cautions:
- If the object is on the colored part of the eye or on the pupil, don't try to remove it with anything but cool running water.
- Keep the person's hands away from the eye—rubbing can scratch the surface of the eye.

Scratched eyeball:
- Wash your hands. A scratched eyeball can become infected.
- Rinse the eye with cool, clean water for 5 to 15 minutes. The water should run from the inside corner of the eye to the outside. Hold the eyelid open to make sure the water gets under it.
- Cover both eyes with a clean cloth, and tie it loosely in place.
- Go to an emergency room.

Chemicals in the eye:
- Ask the person to remove contact lenses, if any. Then flush the eye for 15 to 20 minutes: Hold the eye open under running water from a faucet or cup. Let the water run from the inside to the outside corner of the eye. Make sure water gets under the lids. Keep the injured eye lowest, so chemicals don't run into the other eye.
- If both eyes are injured, let water run from the inside to the outside corners of both. Make sure water gets under the lids. **Cautions:** Don't put anything but water in the eye. Keep the person's hands away from the eyes.
- Tie a clean cloth over both eyes.
- Call 911 or go to an emergency room **right away**. Tell emergency nurses and doctors as much as you can about the chemicals involved.

Fainting and Loss of Consciousness

SIGNS AND SYMPTOMS

Just before fainting:
- Light-headedness, dizziness, weakness, or yawning.
- Pale, cold, or clammy skin.
- Sweat on the face, neck, or hands.

Prolonged loss of consciousness:
- Lack of awareness or no response for several minutes.

A moment of **fainting**—partial or brief loss of consciousness usually caused by a short-term drop in blood flow to the brain—is seldom harmful. **Loss of consciousness** for more than a minute or two, however, may mean something more serious: concussion, stroke, or other brain damage; abnormal heart rhythm or heart attack; major blood loss; a lack of oxygen in the blood; diabetic coma; epilepsy; or drug reaction. To find out whether someone is unconscious, tap the person on the shoulder and ask, "Are you okay?"

WHAT TO DO

Cautions:
- Don't try to revive someone by shaking, slapping, or dousing with cold water.
- Don't put a pillow under the person's head—this can bend the neck and block the airway.
- Don't give anything to eat or drink (including alcohol) until the person is fully conscious. If you know the person is diabetic, however, try giving sips of juice or soda (not sugarless).

Someone about to faint:
- Keep the person from falling, then help him or her to lie down.
- Raise the legs 8 to 12 inches, so that blood can flow to the brain.

- Use a cool, damp cloth to wipe the forehead.
- Loosen clothing that seems tight, above all at the neck or waist.

Someone who has already fainted:
- If you find an unconscious person and don't know the cause, look for a medical alert tag or an injury.
- Lay the person on his or her back. Raise the legs 8 to 12 inches. **Caution:** If you suspect a **head, neck, or back injury,** see page 38. Moving the person may cause further injury.
- Check the **ABCs** (see box on page 14): Lift the chin to open the airway, then check for breathing and pulse. If the person is not breathing or has no heartbeat, call 911 and begin **CPR** (see page 16).
- Loosen any tight clothing, above all at the neck or waist.
- If the person has fallen, check for injuries. Look especially for head wounds. If any, call a doctor for emergency advice. If you can't get one, call 911 or go to an emergency room.
- If the person is vomiting, turn the head to the side so the airway isn't blocked.

Lost consciousness (more than a minute):
- If the person is injured, move him or her only to avoid further injury. **Caution:** Don't try to move the person if you suspect a **head, neck, or back injury** (see page 38). You may cause further injury.
- Call 911.
- Check the **ABCs** (see box on page 14): Lift the chin to open the airway, then check for breathing and pulse. Begin **CPR** (see page 16) if the person isn't breathing or has no heartbeat or pulse.
- Keep the airway open: Roll the person onto his or her side while supporting the head. This is the **recovery position** (see box on page 25). **Caution:** Don't place a person in the recovery position if you suspect a head, neck, or back injury.
- Keep the person warm.
- Use a cool, damp cloth to wipe the forehead.
- Check for a medical alert tag that says whether the person has diabetes, epilepsy, or drug allergies. Tell medical people about it. (See page 43 for treatment of epileptic **seizures;** see page 24 for **shock from allergy.**)

Food Poisoning

SIGNS AND SYMPTOMS

Bacterial:
- Fever.
- Many stools or diarrhea (often severe or explosive), which may be bloody.
- Severe pain and cramping in the abdomen.
- Vomiting.

Botulism:
- Nausea, vomiting, diarrhea.
- Drooping eyelids or blurry vision.
- Dry mouth, trouble swallowing.
- Trouble breathing.
- Muscle weakness or paralysis.

Viral:
- Diarrhea, abdominal cramps, and vomiting.

Chemical:
- Diarrhea and vomiting.
- Sweating.
- Dizziness.
- Confusion.
- Tearing eyes.
- Drooling.
- Stomach pain.

Spoiled or contaminated food can lead to food poisoning. The most common type is **bacterial,** most often passed along by human hands during kitchen work or found in undercooked or unrefrigerated food. **Botulism** is a rare but severe form. It's caused by bacterial poisons that form when foods such as vegetables or fruits are incorrectly preserved or canned at home. **Viruses** that get into food and **chemical toxins** in certain foods—such as some mushrooms, moldy peanuts, and potato sprouts—can also cause food poisoning.

WHAT TO DO

- Call 911 or go to an emergency room **right away** if you see or feel symptoms of botulism (muscle weakness, trouble swallowing and breathing, blurred vision) or chemical food poisoning (vomiting, diarrhea, mental confusion, stomach pain). These can be fatal.
- If vomiting and diarrhea are severe, call your doctor for a prompt appointment. You may need treatment for dehydration (see **diarrhea,** page 122, and **nausea and vomiting,** page 133).
- Don't take antidiarrhea medicines if you suspect food poisoning. You should allow vomiting and diarrhea to flush the toxins out of your system. Don't eat solid food during periods of vomiting and diarrhea.
- As soon as you can keep fluids in your stomach, drink clear liquids such as water, sports drinks, or noncaffeinated tea for about 12 hours to replace fluids you've lost. Liquids should be room temperature, not cold. Sip the drinks; don't gulp. Next, eat bland foods for about 24 hours. Good choices include cooked cereals, rice, bread, and broth.

Fractures and Dislocations

SIGNS AND SYMPTOMS

- Pain.
- Body part is distorted.
- Bruised or discolored skin.
- Swelling.
- A bone is showing.
- Numbness.
- Lost function around injury.

Fractures are breaks, cracks, or chips in a bone. When the skin is not broken, it's called a closed fracture. When a bone breaks through the skin, it's called an open fracture. Open fractures are more dangerous, because they may lead to severe bleeding or infection. **Dislocations** happen when bones are moved from their normal place at a joint, so the joint stops working. Dislocated joints often appear deformed.

WHAT TO DO

Caution:
Don't move the person if you suspect a **head, neck, or back injury** (see page 38). You may cause further injury.

- Call 911 or go to an emergency room **right away** if the person shows symptoms of **shock** or **internal bleeding** (see page 24).
- Call 911 if he or she is unconscious or can't be moved. Check the **ABCs** (see page 14).
- Begin **CPR** (see page 16) if the person is not breathing or has no heartbeat.
- Unless you have to, don't move the person if you suspect an injured pelvis—this may also mean an injury to the low back. Keep the person still.
- Check for other injuries. If the person has an open fracture, stop the bleeding: Tie a clean cloth over the wound and press on it. Don't wash or probe the injury (see **cuts, scrapes, and wounds,** page 30).
- Apply a cold compress for 10 to 30 minutes, leave it off for 30 to 45 minutes, and repeat (see **R-I-C-E,** page 200).
- If the person is mobile and conscious, no matter whether you think a bone is broken or simply dislocated, call a doctor for a prompt appointment. If you can't get one, go to the nearest emergency room.

Cautions:

- If you aren't sure whether a bone is broken, treat it as though it were.
- Don't try to move a bone or joint that appears distorted.

To immobilize an injured finger or toe:

- Put a small piece of cloth or a cotton ball between the injured finger or toe and one that isn't hurt. Tape them together. Raise the finger or toe above the person's heart.

To immobilize a forearm, wrist, or hand:

- Supporting the injured area, place the forearm on the person's stomach. Put the injured arm, wrist, or hand on a magazine or newspaper padded with towels. Then fold the paper and padding around the arm to form a splint. Tie the splint in place on either side of the injury. The splint should go beyond the joints around the injury.

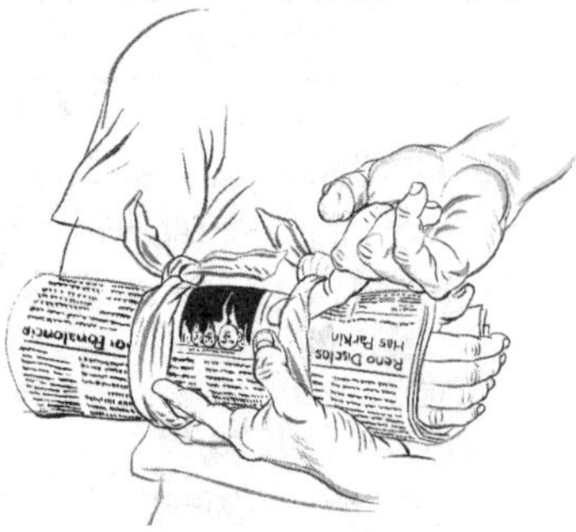

A splint made from newspaper

➤ To make a sling, fold a large cloth (a towel or shirt) into a triangle. Ease the wide part under the injured arm, with any extra cloth at the elbow. Tie the ends around the neck. Pin the extra cloth around the elbow. **Caution:** A sling should be snug, but not so tight that it cuts off blood flow.

To immobilize the lower leg:

➤ To make a splint using boards: Find 2 boards—broomsticks also work well—one the length of the person's leg from hip to heel, the other from groin to heel. Pad the boards with blankets or pillows, then tie them on either side of the leg at the groin, thigh, knee, and ankle.

➤ To make a splint using a blanket: Roll the blanket and place it lengthwise between the person's legs, then tie the legs together at the groin, thighs, knees, and ankles.

To immobilize the upper leg or hip:

Hip fractures cause bruising, swelling, tenderness, or deformity in the hip, and severe pain when the person tries to walk. **Caution:** Unless you have to move the person, don't splint a broken upper leg or hip.

➤ If you do have to use a splint: Find 2 boards, one long enough to reach from the person's armpit to the heel, the other from the groin to the heel. Pad them and tie them in place at the chest, waist, groin, thigh, knee, and ankle. But don't place a tie directly over the break.

Head, Neck, and Back Injuries

SIGNS AND SYMPTOMS

Head injury:

- Head wound, which may bleed heavily or show up as a lump or bruise.
- Blood or other fluid that drains from the mouth, nose, or ears, even with no direct injury to that area.
- Nausea, vomiting, or headache.
- Bruises around the eyes.
- Slurred speech or trouble breathing.
- Vision changes.
- Dizziness, confusion, seizures, or loss of consciousness.

Neck or back injuries:

- Severe pain.
- Trouble moving.
- Tingling in arms or legs.
- Lost control over bowel or bladder.
- Unusual posture of head, neck, or back.
- Unconsciousness.

Be especially alert for head, neck, and back injuries after vehicle accidents, jumping, falling, or diving accidents, and gunshot wounds to the head or chest. Multiple wounds, a broken helmet, or unconsciousness after physical trauma are other signs. People with head, neck, and back injuries need special care to avoid permanent paralysis. It's important to figure out the kind of injury.

WHAT TO DO

Don't move the injured person unless it's really necessary, as in the case of a fire, an explosion, or other life-and-death situation. Moving someone with a head, neck, or back injury could cause permanent spinal cord damage and even paralysis. If you must move someone, make sure the head, neck, and back are in a line and well supported. Don't turn the head sharply to straighten it.

- Call 911 **right away.**
- Keep a conscious person still and calm. This can be vital. Talk to him or her, and give emotional support.
- If the person is unconscious, check the **ABCs** (see box on page 14). Begin **CPR** (see page 16) if he or she isn't breathing or has no heartbeat or pulse. **Caution:** Don't move the neck unless you must to keep the airway open. If you need to place the person face up for CPR, do so very carefully, supporting the head, neck, and back together. Make sure they're in a straight line. Get someone to help.
- Treat any injuries such as **cuts, scrapes, or wounds** (see page 30), or **fractures and dislocations** (see page 37).
- Keep the person warm and as comfortable as you can until help arrives. Loosen tight clothing and cover him or her with a blanket, coat, or other clothing.
- Don't give anything to eat or drink.
- To help keep the person's head and spine still, gently place your hands on either side of the head to hold it in line with the body. **Caution:** Don't turn the head or pull on it to straighten it. Don't put a pillow under the head—bending the neck might block the airway.
- A person with a head injury may vomit without warning and choke. So watch carefully while waiting for help.
- If the person chokes, vomits, or loses consciousness, sweep the airway clear with your fingers. If you have to turn the person on his or her side, do so very carefully, supporting the head, neck, and back together. Make sure they're in a straight line. Get someone to help.

Cautions:

- Gently cradle the person's head and neck to keep them in line.
- Don't place the person in the recovery position described on page 25.

Heart Attack

SIGNS AND SYMPTOMS

- Crushing or squeezing chest pain or tightness that lasts 5 to 10 minutes and doesn't ease with rest. It often starts in the center of the chest, then spreads to the jaw, neck, back, or arms (most often the left arm).
- Shortness of breath.
- Fear or anxiety.
- Dizziness.
- Sweating.
- Nausea or vomiting.
- Pale or bluish lips, skin, or fingernails.
- Uneven heartbeat, or none.
- Unconsciousness.

WHAT TO DO

- Call 911 **right away.**
- If the person is unconscious, check the **ABCs** (see box on page 14): Lift the chin to open the airway, then check for breathing and pulse. Begin **CPR** (see page 16) if the person isn't breathing or has no heartbeat or pulse. **Caution:** Don't try to move the person if you suspect a **head, neck, or back injury** (see page 38). You may cause further injury.
- Loosen tight clothing.
- Keep the person as warm and comfortable as you can until help arrives.
- If the person has lost consciousness but is breathing and has a heartbeat, support the head and roll him or her into the **recovery position** (see page 25). **Caution:** Don't try to revive the person by shaking or slapping; don't throw cold water on the person.
- If the person is conscious, a sitting or partially sitting position may make breathing easier. Offer comfort. If the person has heart medication, help him or her take it, following label instructions.
- Give the person an aspirin to chew. It can help dissolve a blood clot causing the at-

tack. **Cautions:** Don't give aspirin if the person already takes it. If you can, also give the person up to 3 nitroglycerin pills to dissolve under the tongue, 5 minutes apart. Don't give any other medicine, or anything to eat or drink.
- Watch the person's breathing and pulse until medical help comes. If breathing or pulse stops, begin CPR.

Heat Stroke and Heat Exhaustion

SIGNS AND SYMPTOMS

Heat stroke:
- Temperature above 104 degrees.
- Hot, dry skin.
- Rapid breathing and pulse.
- Confusion, unconsciousness, or seizures.

Heat exhaustion:
- Rapid pulse.
- Clammy skin.
- Heavy sweating.
- Headache.
- Vomiting, nausea, or both.
- Stomach cramps; cramps in the arms and legs.
- Dizziness.

People get **heat stroke,** which needs emergency treatment, when they have been working or playing in a hot place for a long time. During heat stroke, the body's temperature rises to dangerous levels because its normal cooling system becomes overloaded and stops working. Then a person may lose consciousness or have seizures.

Heat exhaustion often happens when people work or exercise in hot weather and don't drink enough fluids. Then the body can't make enough sweat to cool itself. Heat exhaustion is less serious than heat stroke but may lead to it. Both are more common in the very young and the old.

WHAT TO DO

Heat stroke:
- Call 911 or go to an emergency room **right away.**
- Move the person to a cooler place as quickly as you can.
- Remove the person's clothing.
- Sponge or splash cool water on the person, or wrap him or her in wet towels or sheets. Put cool, wet cloths on the forehead.
- Fan the person—use your hand, a piece of paper, a fan, or a hair dryer set on cool.

Cautions:
- Don't use an alcohol rub.
- Don't give food or drink.

Heat exhaustion:
- Move the person to a cooler place as quickly as you can.
- Have the person sit or lie down if he or she is conscious. Raise the feet and loosen tight clothing. Remove any sweat-soaked clothing.
- Sponge or splash cool water on the person, or wrap him or her in wet towels or sheets. Put cool, wet cloths on the forehead.
- Fan the person—use your hand, a piece of paper, a fan, or a hair dryer set on cool.
- If the person is conscious and can swallow and breathe, give him or her a rehydration drink you can make: Mix 1 quart water with ½ teaspoon table salt, ½ teaspoon baking soda, 4 teaspoons cream of tartar, and 3 to 4 tablespoons sugar. **Caution:** Don't give to children under 12.
- If you can't make a rehydration drink, give sports drinks or fruit juices diluted with equal amounts of water.
- Be sure to give water or drinks in small sips. The person should drink until his or her urine is clear.
- If you take these steps and the person doesn't begin to improve, call 911 or go to an emergency room **right away.**

Cautions:
- Don't use an alcohol rub.
- Don't force the person to drink. Never give drinks with alcohol or caffeine (many soft drinks are loaded with caffeine).

Hypothermia and Frostbite

SIGNS AND SYMPTOMS

Hypothermia:
- Shivering.
- Loss of coordination; clumsiness.
- Weakness, sleepiness, or unconsciousness.

Frostbite:
- Cold, numb skin.
- Blue or white skin; blackened, waxy, or hard skin.
- Lost use of the injured part.

Hypothermia occurs when body temperature falls much lower than normal. If not treated, it can lead to loss of consciousness, cardiac arrest, and death. It can occur in mild weather if a person becomes wet and exhausted.

Older people can get hypothermia in cool temperatures, even inside a building. With age, the body becomes less able to maintain an even temperature and to sense cold.

If you suspect someone's temperature has dropped too far, check it with a thermometer. If you don't have one, feel the skin over the abdomen—it's a better gauge than the hands or feet. If it feels cold, the person may be in danger.

Frostbite, caused by long exposure to cold, freezes the skin and damages deeper tissues.

WHAT TO DO

Call 911 or go to an emergency room **right away,** if you can.

➤ If the person has symptoms of both hypothermia and frostbite, treat the hypothermia first while you wait for medical help.

Hypothermia:

➤ Check the **ABCs** (see box on page 14): Lift the chin to open the airway, then check for breathing and a pulse. Start rescue breathing if needed, and chest compressions if you can't find a pulse or heartbeat (see **CPR,** page 16). **Note:** People with hypothermia sometimes have slow, weak pulses; take extra time to check for one.

➤ Guide or carry the person to shelter.

➤ Change the person's clothing if it is wet.

➤ Slowly warm the person. Begin by covering his or her head and neck. Use your own body heat, blankets, or aluminum foil. Put warm compresses (cloths soaked in warm water) on the person's chest, neck, and groin. **Caution:** Don't use direct heat such as an electric blanket. Warming should be gradual. Don't rub the hands or feet roughly.

➤ If the person is conscious, offer sips of a warmed, sweet beverage; don't give any drinks with alcohol.

Frostbite:

➤ Get the person to shelter.

➤ Loosen tight clothing; remove any jewelry.

➤ If the person's hands or feet are frostbitten, soak them for 20 minutes in a bowl of water warmed to no more than 105 degrees (it should feel comfortably warm, not hot, to healthy skin). Stir the water gently; add warm water as it cools. Cover other areas of frostbite for 30 minutes or more with cloths soaked in warm water. As needed, resoak the cloths to keep them warm.

➤ If you don't have warm water, use blankets, newspapers, or your own body to warm the frostbitten skin.

➤ Dry the damaged area gently when it is soft and warm, and feeling and color have returned. Put clean, dry cloths over the injured area; put dry cloths between frostbitten fingers. Keep the area warm with more dry cloths.

Cautions:

➤ Don't use direct heat such as electric blankets or a campfire.

➤ Don't massage frostbitten skin.

➤ Don't let the person smoke, or drink anything with alcohol.

➤ Don't thaw frozen skin if it could freeze again before help arrives; refreezing can make the injury worse.

Nose Problems

SIGNS AND SYMPTOMS

Severe nosebleed:
- Bleeding from the nose or down the back of the throat.
- Gagging or choking.

Objects in the nose:
- Irritation or itching in the nose.
- Trouble breathing through one or both nostrils.
- Bleeding or smelly flow from a nostril.

WHAT TO DO

Severe nosebleed:
- ➤ Call a doctor for advice if blood is streaming down the back of the throat; if a nosebleed doesn't stop after 30 minutes; or if you suspect a **head, neck, or back injury** (see page 38). If you can't reach a doctor, call 911 or go to an emergency room.
- ➤ Have the person sit down and lean slightly forward.
- ➤ Pinch the nostrils shut for 5 to 10 minutes while the person leans forward. This may help keep blood from running down the throat and reduce the risk of vomiting.
- ➤ If the nosebleed continues after 10 minutes, have the person gently blow out excess blood. Do this only once.
- ➤ Pinch the nostrils shut for another 5 minutes. If the bleeding continues, put a small roll of cloth or tissue just inside the bleeding nostril. (Don't push the packing too far in—it should be easy to pull out.) Pinch the nostrils shut again.
- ➤ After the bleeding stops, hold a cold compress (a cloth soaked in cold water and wrung out) over the person's nose and face for about 10 minutes. Keep the person seated.
- ➤ After 30 minutes to an hour, take out the packing.
- ➤ To prevent drying or more bleeding, dab petroleum jelly inside the nostril.

Cautions:
- ➤ For 12 hours after the bleeding stops, the person shouldn't bend over, or blow or pick the nose.
- ➤ Watch for signs of a broken nose—it might be misshapen or bent, or you may see pain, swelling, or bruising around the eyes. Hold a cold compress or ice pack on the nose. Go to an emergency room.

Objects in the nose:
- ➤ First, ask the person to press a finger against the unblocked nostril and blow—this might help expel the object.
- ➤ If that doesn't work, sniffing pepper might help by causing a sneeze. Tell the person to inhale very lightly.
- ➤ If nothing works, go to an emergency room. **Caution:** Don't use tweezers or other tools to try to remove the object.

Poisoning

SIGNS AND SYMPTOMS

- Headache or stomachache.
- Dizziness or seizures.
- Chills and fever.
- Trouble seeing.
- Odd-smelling breath.
- Pale or bluish skin; burn marks.
- Vomiting, nausea, or both.
- Trouble breathing.
- Sleepiness, unconsciousness.

WHAT TO DO

- ➤ If the person has inhaled a poison gas such as chlorine, or carbon monoxide from car exhaust or a faulty heater, get him or her to fresh air as fast as you can. **Caution:** Avoid the fumes yourself. Get someone to help you.
- ➤ If the person has lost consciousness, call 911 and check the **ABCs** (see box on page 14): Lift the chin to open the airway, then check for breathing and a pulse.
- ➤ If the person has lost consciousness but is breathing, roll him or her into the **recovery position** (see box on page 25). **Caution:** Don't try to move the person if you

suspect a **head, neck, or back injury** (see page 38). You may cause further injury.

Caution: A person who has been poisoned may show few symptoms or symptoms not listed here, so you should search for clues. Try to find out what the poison is. If the person is conscious, ask what he or she inhaled or swallowed. Sniff for strange odors. Check stoves and heaters. Look around for medicines or chemicals; for detergents, air fresheners, or other household items; and for parts of plants the person may have swallowed.

POISONOUS HOUSEHOLD SUBSTANCES

Here are some common household items that are poisonous:

Alcohol	Mothballs
Antifreeze	Oven cleaner
Deodorizers	Paint
Detergents	Paint remover
Disinfectants	Paint thinner
Fuels	Pesticides
Herbicides	Tobacco
Household cleaners	Turpentine

Besides these items, many prescription and over-the-counter drugs are poisonous if you mix them with alcohol or take big doses.

POISONOUS PLANTS

A number of common garden plants and house plants are poisonous. So are many plant parts—seeds, berries, nuts, and bulbs—if swallowed. Call your local Poison Control Center if you have any questions about plants around your home. Some common plants to watch out for are:

Castor bean	Philodendron
Foxglove	Poison hemlock
Jimsonweed	Water hemlock
Oleander	

- Call your local Poison Control Center. Tell the person at the center what you think may be the cause of the poisoning. Listen to instructions.

Cautions:

- Don't try to make the person vomit unless you're told to.
- Don't give the person anything to eat or drink unless you're told to.
- Don't rely on poison-remedy directions from product labels.

Seizures

SIGNS AND SYMPTOMS

- Tingling feelings.
- Muscle spasms, twitching, stiffening, thrashing.
- Drooling.
- Fixed stare, or eyes rolled back.
- Lost bowel or bladder control.
- Sleepiness, confusion, loss of consciousness.

Seizures are seldom fatal, though they can be alarming. Causes include epilepsy, diabetes, heat stroke, fever (in children), electric shock, poisoning, brain injury, drug or alcohol abuse, and abruptly stopping heavy use of alcohol or other drugs.

WHAT TO DO

- If someone with you feels a seizure about to start or begins to lose balance, guide him or her to a safe spot. Check for a medical alert tag and any recent injury.
- Call 911 if this is the person's first seizure; if another seizure starts within a few minutes; if the seizure lasts more than about 3 minutes; if the person has diabetes, is pregnant, has been injured, or doesn't regain consciousness after the seizure ends.
- If the person stays unconscious for more than a few minutes after the muscles relax, check the **ABCs** (see box on page 14): Lift the chin to open the airway, then check for breathing and a pulse. If you can't find a

heartbeat or pulse. If the person isn't breathing, dial 911 **right away** and begin **CPR** (see page 16). **Caution:** Don't try to move the person if you suspect a **head, neck, or back injury** (see page 38). You may cause further injury.

- During a seizure, guard the person against self-injury: Take off eyeglasses; push away or pad anything hard nearby, such as furniture. Don't try to restrain the person unless it looks as if he or she is about to be injured.
- Lay the person on his or her side to keep vomit from getting into the lungs. Put something soft under the person's head to protect it.
- Don't put your hands near or in the person's mouth. Don't try to hold the person's tongue or put anything in his or her mouth. Jaws clamping down can inflict a bad bite.
- Loosen tight clothing.
- When the seizure is over, help the person get comfortable. Offer reassurance. The person may be confused or drowsy, and may fall asleep.
- Stay with the person until he or she is completely conscious and safe or until medical help arrives.

Shortness of Breath

SIGNS AND SYMPTOMS

- Breathlessness or labored breathing, even with little or no physical activity.
- Dizziness or light-headedness.
- See the **breathing problems and coughs** chart, page 87.

WHAT TO DO

- Help the person get comfortable. Sitting up can aid breathing.
- Offer reassurance. Shortness of breath can lead to panic, which can make breathing even harder.
- If the person can answer questions (even with gestures), try to find out the cause of the breathing trouble.
- If the person also has chest pain (which may be crushing, burning, or tight, and may spread to the jaw, neck, shoulder, or left arm), nausea, and dizziness, the person may be having a **heart attack** (see page 39). Call 911 **right away.**
- If the person is wheezing, coughing, or feels tight through the chest, he or she may be having an **asthma** attack (see page 89). If this is the first attack or if it is more serious than other attacks, call 911 or go to an emergency room **right away.** Help the person take any prescribed asthma medication.
- If the person also has a fever over 100 degrees or is coughing, he or she may have **acute bronchitis** (see page 91) or **pneumonia** (see page 98). Call a doctor for advice and an appointment. Give a pain reliever for fever, and a cough medicine. Never give aspirin to a child under 12 who has chicken pox, flu, a cold, or any other illness you suspect of being caused by a virus; see box on **Reye's syndrome,** page 96.
- If the person is also wheezing and coughin up mucus, he or she may have **chronic bronchitis** or **emphysema** (see page 92). The person may already be under a doctor's care.
- If the person has been worried about something, the symptoms may be related to **stress** (see page 222) or **anxiety** (see page 210).

Snakebites

SIGNS AND SYMPTOMS

Rattlesnake, cottonmouth, and copperhead bites:

- Pain that increases at the bitten spot.
- Rapid changes in skin color and swelling at the bitten spot.
- Twitching skin.

- Sweating, dizziness, nausea.
- Shock; convulsions.

Coral snake bites:

- Pain at the bitten spot.
- Sleepiness.
- Trouble seeing or speaking.
- Tremors, seizures, or delirium.

Four types of poisonous snakes live in the United States: rattlesnakes, cottonmouths (also called water moccasins), copperheads, and coral snakes. It's important to know which type bit you, so the hospital can give the right antivenin.

Rattlesnakes, cottonmouths, and copperheads have triangular heads, rather than the slimmer heads of other snakes. They all have long fangs, and their bites leave marks that are much alike—2 rows of marks, each topped by a fang wound. Copperheads and rattlesnakes shake their tails in warning, but copperheads don't have rattles. Cottonmouths, when angry, open their mouths to show the white lining that gives them their name. Coral snakes have red, black, and white or yellow rings, and black muzzles.

Snakebites seldom kill. The few deaths that occur are mostly from rattlesnakes. Coral snakes are the most poisonous, but they don't bite many people.

WHAT TO DO

If you're not certain a bite was made by a poisonous snake, act as if it were. Begin first aid:

- If the person has lost consciousness, check the **ABCs** (see box on page 14): Gently lift the chin to open the airway. Then check for breathing and a pulse. Start rescue breathing if needed, and chest compressions if you can't find a heartbeat or pulse (see **CPR,** page 16). Call 911 or go to an emergency room **right away** if you can. Tell the people there what kind of snake bit the person, if you know.
- If the person is conscious, keep him or her still and calm. If you can, lay the person down so the bite is below the level of the heart—blood from the bite, and any venom, will flow more slowly to the heart.
- Remove any tight clothing or jewelry near the bite.
- If the bite was on an arm or leg and you know the snake was poisonous, and that it will take more than 30 minutes to get help, tie a light tourniquet above the bite.
- If you have to kill the snake, try not to damage the head; it will help with identification. Stay away from the snake.

Cautions:

- Don't make cuts near the bite. Don't try to suck out venom with a snakebite kit or your mouth—these measures don't help.
- Don't put a cold compress or ice on the bite.
- Don't let the person walk. Carry the person if he or she has to be moved.

Spider Bites and Scorpion Stings

SIGNS AND SYMPTOMS

- Bite mark, sting mark, swelling, or blister at the bitten spot.
- Pain in the bite or sting area, or in the stomach.
- Nausea, vomiting, chills, or fever.
- Trouble breathing or swallowing.
- Severe sweating and excess saliva.

Two types of poisonous spiders live in the United States: the black widow and the brown recluse (fiddleback). Their bites are especially dangerous to children, seniors, and anyone who is ill. The black widow has a red spot on its abdomen and leaves only a faint red bite mark. The brown recluse has a brown, violin-shaped marking on its back; watch for a blister, swelling, and bull's-eye-shaped bite.

Scorpions have poisonous stingers in their long, upturned "tails," but only a few of the species found in the United States inflict fatal stings.

WHAT TO DO

- Wash the wound with soap and water.
- Apply an ice pack or cold compress.
- Call your doctor for emergency advice. If you can't get one, call 911 or go to an emergency room.
- If possible, bring the spider or scorpion to the doctor's office or emergency room.

Caution: Watch for signs of **shock from allergy** (see page 24). If they appear, call 911 **right away.**

Sprains and Strains

SIGNS AND SYMPTOMS

- Pain.
- Swelling.
- Bruising.

A **sprain** is a tear or stretch in a ligament, the tough band of tissue that connects the bones of a joint. Sprains are common in the ankles, knees, wrists, and fingers. A **strain** (often called a "pulled muscle") is a tear or stretch in a muscle or tendon, the band of tissue that attaches a muscle to bone. **Strains** often occur in the neck, back, thigh, and calf.

WHAT TO DO

- Treat a severe sprain or strain (marked by swelling and intense pain) as though it were a **fracture** (see page 37), and call a doctor for a prompt appointment.
- If the sprain or strain seems mild, apply a cold pack—a plastic bag of ice cubes or a package of frozen vegetables wrapped in a damp cloth—several times a day for up to 3 days. Leave it on no more than 10 to 30 minutes at a time. Leave it off 30 to 45 minutes between applications. Use moderate pressure. This should reduce the pain and swelling.
- Keep the injured area raised above the heart, if possible, to reduce fluid buildup and swelling.
- Put on an elastic bandage to support the sprained or strained area. Wrap the bandage in an upward spiral, starting several inches below the injured area. You may wrap the bandage over the ice pack temporarily. **Caution:** Don't wrap the bandage too tightly.
- If a sling is needed, see **fractures and dislocations,** page 37.
- Don't put any weight on the strain or sprain for 1 to 3 days.

Stroke

SIGNS AND SYMPTOMS

- Abrupt weakness or numbness of the face, arm, or leg (most often on one side of the body).
- Sudden trouble seeing or loss of vision (often in only one eye).
- Loss of speech, or trouble speaking or understanding speech.
- Sudden, severe headache.
- Dizziness, unsteadiness, or sudden loss of consciousness.

A stroke occurs when blood flow to the brain is cut off, usually because of a blocked artery. Though a stroke can be fatal or disabling, prompt medical help may reduce some of its worst effects.

WHAT TO DO

- Call 911 or go to an emergency room **right away.**
- If you're waiting for medical help to arrive, check the **ABCs** (see box on page 14): Lift the chin to open the airway, then check for breathing and pulse. If the person is not breathing or has no pulse, begin **CPR** (see page 16).
- If the person is unconscious but breathing, support the head and roll him or her onto the side, into the **recovery position** (see box on page 25). **Caution:** Don't place the person in the recovery position if you suspect a **head, neck, or back injury** (see

page 38). Moving him or her could cause further injury.

- If the person is conscious, offer reassurance. Lay him or her down, with head and shoulders slightly raised by pillows. Loosen any tight clothing.
- If vomit or fluid is draining from the person's mouth, or if the person has trouble swallowing, turn him or her onto the side so the airway doesn't become blocked. **Caution:** Don't give anything to eat or drink.

Tick Bites

SIGNS AND SYMPTOMS

Lyme disease:

- A bull's-eye rash, often with a pale center, that may widen to several inches across. The rash begins to show 2 days to a month after the bite, and may last 2 to 4 weeks or longer.
- Flulike symptoms—such as headache, fatigue, fever, chills, and aching muscles and joints—starting within a month of the bite.

Rocky Mountain spotted fever:

- A pink rash that starts near the wrists and ankles 2 to 14 days after a tick bite, then spreads to the face, torso, and other areas of the body. The rash turns deep red, then looks like red pinpricks.
- Fever, chills, and severe headache.

The bite of the tiny deer tick may result in **Lyme disease** (see page 291), which can cause arthritis, heart problems, and vision and hearing problems, among other ailments. Bites of some other ticks can cause **Rocky Mountain spotted fever,** an infection that can be deadly if untreated.

WHAT TO DO

- If you can see the tick, remove it as soon as you can to prevent infection. Grasp it with tweezers close to the skin, then pull it out gently and steadily. If you don't have tweezers, use a glove, a piece of paper, or plastic wrap. (If you use your bare fingers, wash your hands right afterward.) Avoid squeezing or twisting the tick; this could spread bacteria into your skin or blood. Don't try to burn a tick off the skin. If you can't get all of the tick out, call a doctor for advice. Save the tick in a jar; rubbing alcohol will help preserve it.
- Wash the area of the bite with soap and water.
- Apply an antiseptic ointment or alcohol to prevent infection. An ice pack can help relieve pain, and calamine lotion will relieve itching.
- Watch for signs of Lyme disease or Rocky Mountain spotted fever.
- If you see symptoms, call a doctor for a prompt appointment. Bring the tick with you, if you saved it.

Tooth Knocked Out

WHAT TO DO

- Call a dentist **right away** or go to an emergency room. Teeth replanted within an hour or two can survive. Pick up the tooth by the crown (the part of the tooth that shows when it's in place), not the root. Use sterile gauze. The tooth must be kept as germ-free as possible.
- Wash the tooth quickly, either under running water or in saliva, and put it back in the socket at once. Bite down gently on the tooth or hold it in place with a sterile gauze pad for the trip to the dentist.
- If the tooth can't be put in the socket, hold it in the side of the mouth, or wrap it in sterile gauze (or paper towels) and put it in a closed container of cool milk for the trip to the dentist.
- If the socket is bleeding, cover it with a sterile gauze pad, then bite down to hold the gauze in place until you get to the dentist.

Problems & Solutions

In the normal course of life, the human body needs surprisingly little upkeep beyond some fairly regular feeding, rest, and exercise. But at some times, in some ways, things can go wrong. If that happens, you can do a lot to set your body right again. As a start, you can learn what's really going on and when it's time to call a doctor.

On the following 246 pages, in entries that cover a wide range of health problems, you'll find the facts you need. Each entry guides you through these logical steps: ➤ **Signs and Symptoms** ➤ **What You Can Do Now** ➤ **When to Call the Doctor** ➤ **How to Prevent It** ➤ **For More Help.**

You'll find a concise description of what your symptoms could mean, followed by clear suggestions for your best course of action. Each entry ends with a guide to useful hotlines, organizations, books, World Wide Web sites, and videos.

When you see the name of a condition in bold type—for example, **asthma**—you'll see the number of a page where you can read more about it. You'll also find charts that help you sort out, at a glance, the connections between symptoms that may seem similar, their possible causes, and what you can do.

In addition, the color illustrations on pages 161 to 176 give you a revealing new look at what can happen inside the body.

We trust that you will find helpful advice here on just about any problem your family is likely to encounter or worry about.

Head & Nervous System

Alzheimer's Disease

SIGNS AND SYMPTOMS

- Memory problems that get worse over time and disrupt normal life. A person with Alzheimer's often forgets what happened in the last half hour or asks the same question over and over.
- Confusion, faulty judgment and reasoning, loss of ability to complete simple tasks such as shopping or dialing new phone numbers.
- Growing tendency to lose things and to wander and get lost.
- Neglect of personal hygiene.
- Depression, suspicion, and anxiety—either as direct symptoms or as signs of the distress people feel over the baffling loss of basic skills.
- In later stages, failure to recognize places and people.
- Finally, near-total loss of memory, speech, and physical ability; the need for full-time care.

About 4 million Americans have Alzheimer's disease, a breakdown of the brain that leads to severe memory loss, confused thinking, and personality changes. It gets worse over time, and is always fatal. Still, people with Alzheimer's can live 10 years or more after symptoms first appear.

The cause of the disease is still unknown. It's most likely to appear in people over 65 and seems to run in families. A genetic link has also been found in some cases of early-onset Alzheimer's, a rare form that can strike people in their late 40s or in their 50s.

Alzheimer's has no cure, but new drugs that may slow its progress are being tested.

WHAT YOU CAN DO NOW

If you show signs of Alzheimer's, or a family member does:

- See a doctor. Memory loss and confusion don't always mean you have Alzheimer's (see box on **forgetfulness,** page 53, and **confusion** chart, page 207). If someone close to you shows signs of short-term memory loss, have his or her doctor check for other problems. These include depression, hypoglycemia, brain tumor, drug interactions or side effects, vitamin shortages, stroke, and other ailments in which memory problems may be reversible.
- If memory problems get worse over a few months, ask your doctor for the name of a specialist who can do further tests.

If you're taking care of someone who has Alzheimer's disease:

- Keep the home calm and neat. In the early stages, routines and aids such as checklists for daily tasks can help a person with Alzheimer's stay self-sufficient.
- Be patient. Forgetfulness, sudden mood changes, and rudeness come from the disease, not ill will.
- Help him or her remain active and main-

Dizziness

Dizziness can have many causes. Often it isn't serious. It can be a sign of illness, however, if it comes with other symptoms, is severe, recurs, or lasts a long time.

SYMPTOMS	WHAT IT MIGHT BE	WHAT YOU CAN DO
After blow to head: dizziness and brief loss of consciousness; headache, nausea, and vomiting.	Concussion (see head, neck, and back injuries, page 38).	Call 911 or go to emergency room **right away** after any blow to head that results in loss of consciousness.
Dizziness and fever over 104; no sweating; rapid pulse; confusion; hot, dry skin; loss of consciousness. Occurs in high heat.	Heat stroke (see page 40).	Call 911 or go to emergency room **right away.** If waiting for medical help to arrive, cool person with cold, wet cloths and fan.
Dizziness, palpitations, shortness of breath, sometimes chest pressure or pain.	Uneven heartbeat (see page 114). • Heart attack (see page 39).	Call 911 or go to emergency room **right away.**
Sudden dizziness and headache; weakness or numbness in face, arm, or leg; blurred vision or trouble speaking; confusion.	Stroke (see page 46).	Call 911 **right away.**
After head injury (often days or weeks later): dizziness and fatigue, weakness or numbness on one side of body.	Subdural hemorrhage and hematoma—bleeding and swelling in brain.	Call 911 or go to emergency room **right away.**
Dizziness; vomiting; sudden high fever; confusion; diarrhea; headache; red rash, often on palms of hands and soles of feet.	Toxic shock syndrome (see page 248). • Other bacterial infection in blood.	Call 911 or go to emergency room **right away.**
While working or exercising in hot weather without drinking enough fluids: dizziness, nausea, vomiting, and headache; cramps in arms, legs, or abdomen; cool, clammy skin; excessive sweating; rapid pulse.	Heat exhaustion (see page 40).	Call doctor for emergency advice. Watch for symptoms of heat stroke. Cool person with cold, wet cloths and fan. Give water or rehydration drink (see page 124), or dilute sport or fruit drink with equal amount of water.

(continued)

Dizziness *(continued)*		
SYMPTOMS	**WHAT IT MIGHT BE**	**WHAT YOU CAN DO**
Dizziness, frequent headaches, nausea and vomiting, double vision, seizures, confusion, memory loss.	Brain tumor.	Call doctor for prompt appointment.
Dizziness and headache, intense hunger, shaking, irritability, confusion, anxiety.	Hypoglycemia—low blood sugar, usually in people who take insulin.	People with diabetes should eat or drink something with sugar in it; for others, non-sugared foods. If symptoms persist, call doctor for advice and appointment. If person has seizure or loses consciousness, call 911 or go to emergency room **right away.**
Dizziness, weakness and fatigue, pale skin, shortness of breath.	Anemia (see page 278).	Call doctor for prompt appointment.
Earache, fever, chills, stuffy nose, blocked or full feeling in ear, muffled hearing, discharge from ear. In infants: tugging at ear, bad temper, restlessness, lack of appetite.	Middle ear infection (see page 73).	Call doctor for prompt appointment.
Sudden, severe dizziness, nausea, and vomiting; loss of balance or hearing.	Ménière's syndrome. • Labyrinthitis.	See ear and hearing problems chart, page 71.
Within 24 hours after head or neck injury: pain and stiffness in neck, dizziness, headache, nausea and vomiting, trouble walking (sometimes).	Whiplash, often caused by car collision.	Call doctor for prompt appointment if neck is injured. Apply ice packs and take pain relievers. Sleep with thin pillow under head and thin rolled-up towel under neck.
Dizziness, most often when moving head; nausea and vomiting.	Benign paroxysmal positional vertigo—dizziness related to inner ear.	Call doctor for advice and appointment.
Dizziness when sitting up or standing up quickly.	Hypotension—a brief drop in blood pressure.	Don't change positions quickly. Ask your doctor if drugs could be the problem.

tain family ties, friendships, and social contacts as long as possible.

- If the person with Alzheimer's tends to wander, have him or her wear a medical alert tag that says "Memory Impaired" and shows your phone number.
- Don't let a person with Alzheimer's drive. The disease impairs judgment and physical skills.
- Ask a doctor about ways to control symptoms such as insomnia, anxiety, and depression.
- Have someone take over for you now and then to ease some of your stress.
- Contact an Alzheimer's support group, which can help both you and the person with Alzheimer's.

HOW TO PREVENT IT

There is no known way to prevent Alzheimer's disease.

WHEN TO CALL THE DOCTOR

- If someone shows distinct symptoms of Alzheimer's. It's sometimes hard for people to see and accept their own symptoms, so it is often up to others to help.
- In the later stages, at the first sign of illness. Alzheimer's can weaken the immune system.
- If the person with Alzheimer's puts himself or herself or others in danger.
- If you take care of a person with Alzheimer's and feel you are getting to a breaking point.

FOR MORE HELP

Information line: National Institute on Aging Information Line on Alzheimer's Disease and Forgetfulness, 800-438-4380, M–F 8:30–5 EST. Staff answers questions, provides information, and refers to other organizations.

Information line: Alzheimer's Association, 919 N. Michigan Ave., #1000, Chicago, IL 60611-1676. 800-272-3900, 24-hour line. More than 200 chapters nationwide provide literature, referrals, and information on support groups. **Web site:** *http: //www.Alz.org.* Provides facts about current research as well as links to other Web sites and resources.

Book: *Alzheimer's: A Caregiver's Guide and Sourcebook*, by Howard Gruetzner. A complete resource for anyone coping with this disease. John Wiley & Sons, 1992, $14.95.

Book: *Alzheimer's & Dementia: Questions You Have... Answers You Need*, by Jennifer Hay. Easy-to-read book in a question-and-answer format. People's Medical Society, 1996, $12.95.

Book: *The 36-Hour Day: A Guide to Caring for Persons with Alzheimer's Disease, Related Dementing Illnesses and Memory Loss in Later Life,* by Nancy L. Mace and Peter V. Rabins, M.D. Revised edition of a classic. Warner Books, 1994, $6.50.

Web access: The Alzheimer's Page at Washington University in St. Louis. After logging on to the Internet, type: *http://www.biostat.wustl.edu/alzheimer.* This site offers e-mail discussion groups and loads of resources and facts. Sponsored by the National Institute on Aging.

Video: *Alzheimer's Disease at Time of Diagnosis.* Clear overview of causes and treatments, with 4 reports—Understanding the Diag-

A LITTLE FORGETFUL? DON'T FRET.

Everyone forgets things once in a while. Most middle-aged and older people find that their memory slows down a bit as they age. They may become more forgetful, and they may take a little longer to remember things than they used to. This does not mean they have Alzheimer's disease.

In people of any age, high fever, poor nutrition, head injuries, and reactions to medication can cause temporary forgetfulness. Older people may sometimes become confused or forgetful because of emotional problems as they deal with major life changes—retirement, the death of a loved one, or other upheavals. That's normal. But if memory problems persist and increase, call your doctor for advice.

nosis, What Happens Next?, Treatment and Management, and Issues and Answers. Time Life Medical, 1996, $19.95. Sold at many pharmacies; for one near you, call 800-588-9959.

Headaches

SIGNS AND SYMPTOMS

- Throbbing or steady dull pain in the head, sometimes on just one side. Often with other symptoms, such as nausea or dizziness (see **headaches** chart, next page).

Most headaches are mild and harmless, and go away with rest and a dose of aspirin. But others are more severe, and some can signal a serious problem, such as **stroke** (see pages 46 and 115) or **glaucoma** (see page 67). Some are chronic, meaning the symptoms come and go and may last a lifetime if not treated.

Ninety percent of headaches are tension headaches—a steady, dull pain in the scalp, temples, or back of the head. They are often the result of muscles getting tight because of stress or poor posture. Other common types include migraine, cluster, and sinus headaches.

Migraine pain can be severe, and may come with nausea and strange vision problems such as light flashes or partial blindness. Migraines begin when arteries that supply blood to the brain narrow and then widen; the swelling seems to affect nerves in the head. Stress and certain foods help bring them on. Migraines tend to run in families.

Cluster headaches can hurt even more than migraines, with pain that starts around one eye and spreads to that side of the head. They come and go over days or weeks—the "cluster"—before fading, often for months or years. Then they may return.

Sinus headaches are caused by sinus infections or congestion (see **sinusitis,** page 100).

Self-care or drug treatments can ease most headaches. In fact, several new prescription drugs can relieve and prevent chronic headaches better than ever before.

WHAT YOU CAN DO NOW

- Keep a headache diary. Note the time and date of each headache and its symptoms. Write down what you ate and drank, and what you did in the 6 to 8 hours before. Look for "triggers" for the headaches, and avoid them.
- Rest in a dark room, unless you have a cluster headache (see **headaches** chart, next page, for symptoms). Lying down often makes a cluster headache worse. Put an ice pack or a cold, wet cloth on your forehead, or a warm one if that feels better.
- Try over-the-counter painkillers such as acetaminophen (Tylenol), ibuprofen (Advil or Motrin), or aspirin. But don't take over-the-counter headache drugs daily for more than a few weeks; that will make your headaches worse. (Never give aspirin to a child under 12 who has chicken pox, flu, a cold, or any other illness you suspect of being caused by a virus; see box on **Reye's syndrome,** page 96.)
- Massage your forehead and temples for 10 minutes. Place 2 fingers at the middle of your forehead at the hairline. Using gentle pressure, work them slowly down the sides of the forehead to your temples.
- Stretch your neck by rolling your head, gently pressing forward at the base of your skull, and shrugging your shoulders. A self-massage of your neck can also ease the pain for a while. Starting where the neck muscles meet your skull, work your way down, across your shoulders, and up again to the base of the skull.
- Try a meditation class. Studies show the "relaxation response" can ease pain for people with chronic headaches (see **relax,** page 309).
- Imagine the pain away. Close your eyes and picture your headache as liquid filling a glass. Now visualize "pouring" the pain into a slightly smaller glass, without letting any of the liquid overflow. Keep pouring the liquid into smaller and smaller glasses; you may feel the pain decrease.

Headaches

Most people have an occasional pounding headache, but many Americans—some 50 million—have intense, chronic headaches. Symptoms vary from person to person; you may have all or only some of them. Headaches can also be a sign of serious illness.

SYMPTOMS	WHAT IT MIGHT BE	WHAT YOU CAN DO
Sudden, severe headache; paralysis, weakness, or numbness on one side of body; nausea, vomiting; delirium; often seizures or loss of consciousness; trouble speaking, moving, or seeing; dizziness and confusion; possibly fever.	Stroke (see page 46).	Call 911 **right away.**
Fever, headache, nausea and vomiting, stiff neck, aversion to light, red rash (sometimes), confusion.	Meningitis (see page 57).	Call doctor for emergency advice. If you can't get one, call 911 or go to emergency room.
Headache on waking that gets worse when you lie down, nausea and vomiting, double vision, dizziness, loss of memory, personality changes. Head pain comes on slowly but persists and grows worse over time (often months).	Brain tumor.	Call doctor for prompt appointment.
Intense eye pain, headache, nausea and vomiting, vision problems.	Glaucoma (see page 67).	Call doctor for prompt appointment.
Sudden, intense headache; dry mouth; sticky saliva; fatigue; thirst (sometimes).	Dehydration—particularly if headache follows nausea and vomiting (see page 133) or diarrhea (see page 122).	Call doctor for prompt appointment if symptoms are severe. Drink small amounts of liquids often.
Severe, throbbing pain, often on one side of head; vision problems; aversion to light and noise; dizziness; nausea, vomiting.	Migraine headache.	Use over-the-counter painkillers. Rest in dark room. Apply ice packs. See doctor about stronger medication or other help if pain persists or recurs.

(continued)

Headaches *(continued)*		
SYMPTOMS	**WHAT IT MIGHT BE**	**WHAT YOU CAN DO**
Extreme, nonthrobbing pain, usually around one eye; bloodshot or watery eye; red face; stuffed-up nose.	Cluster headache.	Apply ice packs and take hot showers. See doctor after first attack (symptoms could be caused by other, more serious problems). Doctor may prescribe medicine or pure oxygen (to be inhaled).
Lasting pain that can be dull or intense and often feels like a tight band around head; stiffness and tightness in neck, shoulders.	Tension headache.	Try over-the-counter painkillers. Get a deep muscle massage. Learn stress reduction, such as meditation. Apply ice packs and take hot showers. See doctor if pain persists.
Fever, pain behind forehead and eyes, with stuffed-up nose and sinus.	Sinus headache (see sinusitis, page 100).	Call doctor for advice and appointment. Infections can be treated with antibiotics. Use nasal decongestants, but for no more than 2 days.
Pain focused in front of and behind ear, sometimes spreading to face, neck, and shoulders; pain or clicking sound when opening mouth.	Temporomandibular disorder (see page 203).	Try over-the-counter painkillers. Try heat and massage. Call doctor for advice and appointment if symptoms persist.
Pounding headache and fatigue in coffee drinkers who skip their morning cup or quit abruptly.	Caffeine withdrawal.	Have cup of coffee for quick relief. Cut back slowly if you're trying to break caffeine habit.

- Ask your doctor if you should try biofeedback: You can use signals from your body—for instance, beeps from a device reading brain waves—to learn how to relieve headache pain.

WHEN TO CALL THE DOCTOR

Call 911 or have someone take you to an emergency room right away:

- If your headaches are sudden, severe, and come with symptoms such as dizziness or numbness. These could be signs of a serious problem such as stroke.

Call for an appointment right away:

- If your headaches are severe and come with other symptoms such as nausea, flashes of light, runny nose, or a stuffed-up nostril. These are signs of migraines or cluster headaches.

Call for an appointment:

- ➤ If your headaches are chronic—as often as once a week—or last longer than 24 hours.
- ➤ If your headaches often seem to be caused by allergies, sinus infection, or depression. Treatment for these ailments can ease the pain.

HOW TO PREVENT IT

- ➤ Avoid foods that contain the substance tyramine if they seem to cause your headaches. Such foods include ripe cheeses, nuts, peanut butter, pizza, and red wine.
- ➤ Reduce stress. Try exercise, taking a few breaks during a hectic day, or doing relaxation exercises.
- ➤ Practice correct posture. Sit up straight and don't keep your neck bent for long.
- ➤ Take rest breaks every hour if you're doing hard work such as moving furniture or digging in your garden.
- ➤ When reading or writing, make sure you have enough light, but not so much that it glares off the page; squinting can make muscles tighten. Take 10-minute rest breaks every hour.
- ➤ If your headaches seem to be caused by allergies, make sure your house is free of dust and mold. Don't go outside when pollen is high (see **allergies,** page 86, for other ways to prevent allergy attacks).
- ➤ Don't go hungry, sleep too little, or sleep too much on weekends. These can all produce headaches.
- ➤ Some drugs, such as birth control pills, provoke migraines. If your headaches seem to be caused by a drug, ask your doctor if you can switch.
- ➤ Don't smoke, and avoid smoky places such as bars. Smoke can cause migraines.
- ➤ Ask your doctor about new medications that can prevent headaches.

FOR MORE HELP

Hotline: National Headache Foundation, 428 West St. James Place, 2nd floor, Chicago, IL 60614-2750. 800-843-2256, M–F 9–5 CST. Also 24-hour recording. Staff answers questions about headache types, causes, and treatment. They'll send free brochures on headaches and a list of doctor members. For a $15 member's fee you get a quarterly newsletter, a list of foods to avoid, and handbooks on headaches.

Information line: American Council for Headache Education, 875 Kings Highway #200, Woodbury, NJ 08096. 800-255-2243, M–F 9–5 EST. For a $15 member's fee you get a quarterly newsletter, a package of pamphlets, and a list of doctors.

Book: *The Hormone Headache*, by Seymour Diamond, M.D. Describes the link between headaches and hormones and how to prevent and treat migraines and other headaches. Macmillan, 1995, $11.95.

Video: *Migraine & Other Headaches at Time of Diagnosis*. Clear overview of causes and treatments, with 4 reports—Understanding the Diagnosis, What Happens Next?, Treatment and Management, and Issues and Answers. Time Life Medical, 1996, $19.95. Sold in many pharmacies; for one near you, call 800-588-9959.

Meningitis and Encephalitis

SIGNS AND SYMPTOMS

The following symptoms need prompt treatment. Call your doctor. If not available, call 911 or go to an emergency room.

Meningitis in children:

- ■ Fever of 100 degrees or higher, with:
- ■ Headache or stiff neck. Lying down, the head can't be bent toward the chest (except in infants less than 1 month old) because of shooting pain in the neck and back.
- ■ Bad temper or listlessness.
- ■ Loss of appetite.
- ■ Turning away from bright lights.
- ■ Maybe nausea and vomiting.
- ■ In infants, bulging of the soft spot of the skull.

- Sometimes seizures.
- Rarely, a bumpy red or purple rash anywhere on the body.

Meningitis or encephalitis in adults:

- Fever, other flulike symptoms, and headache with:
- Eyes sensitive to light.
- Confusion, drowsiness, lethargy, or bad temper.
- Delirium, seizures, or coma.
- Sometimes, with encephalitis only, paralysis.
- Stiff neck, shoulders, or back. With meningitis only, shooting pain in the neck and back when head is bent forward.
- Rarely, with meningitis only, a bumpy red or purplish rash anywhere on the body.

Encephalitis in children:

- Same symptoms as in adults.
- In infants, bulging of the soft spot of the skull.

Meningitis and encephalitis are brain diseases with similar symptoms. Both need prompt medical treatment.

Meningitis is an inflammation of the fragile membranes that cover the spinal cord and brain. Bacteria, viruses, and fungi can cause it. Bacterial meningitis can follow an illness such as pneumonia or sinus or ear infections. A skull fracture or other head injury also raises the risk. Some forms of viral meningitis can spread through the air.

Bacterial meningitis can lead to death within hours if not treated, but early care most often results in complete recovery. Treatment includes a hospital stay and injected antibiotics.

Viral meningitis is usually a milder form of the illness that goes away on its own. It is treated with bed rest and plenty of liquids.

Encephalitis is an inflammation of the brain that is almost always caused by a virus. In the United States, it is most often caused by herpes simplex, the virus that brings cold sores. The illness can also be brought on by a chicken pox, mumps, or measles virus. Another form is spread by mosquitoes and ticks.

Severe encephalitis, which is rare, can lead to brain damage or death. People with a mild case most often recover in 2 to 3 weeks.

WHEN TO CALL THE DOCTOR

- If a child or an adult shows the symptoms listed, call your doctor for emergency advice. If not available, call 911 or go to an emergency room.

HOW TO PREVENT IT

- Get early treatment for any serious infection or high fever.
- Shots for meningitis are part of most childhood immunization series—be sure your child gets them.
- If you have had close contact with a person who has bacterial meningitis, or your child has, call your doctor for advice. You may be advised to take antibiotics (even if you show no symptoms) to prevent infection.
- Avoid ticks by wearing long pants and long-sleeved shirts in grassy or wooded areas (see **tick bites,** page 47).
- Prevent insect bites by using repellent.

FOR MORE HELP

Information line: Massachusetts Department of Public Health Epidemiology Program. 617-983-6800, M–F 9–5 EST.

Organization: National Institute of Neurological Disorders and Stroke, 31 Center

RED FLAG FOR CHILDREN

The bacterial form of meningitis, which strikes infants and young children more than adults, can lead to death within hours—or to permanent brain damage—if it isn't treated. Very young children are in special danger, because they can't describe their symptoms. Call 911 or go to an emergency room **right away** if a child has the symptoms listed. Early treatment usually results in full recovery.

Drive, MSC 2540, Bethesda, MD 20892-2540. 800-352-9424 and 301-496-5751, M–F 8:30–5 EST. Ask for the packet on meningitis and encephalitis.

Parkinson's Disease

SIGNS AND SYMPTOMS

Early symptoms:
- Weakness.
- Slight tremor of the head or hands.
- Depression (sometimes).
- Masklike face, almost no blinking.
- Muscle stiffness.
- Slowed movement.

Later symptoms:
- Loss of balance.
- Tremors in the hands and/or head when at rest.
- Confusion and memory loss (in severe cases).

Parkinson's disease most often shows up in people over 60. It occurs when nerve cells begin to die in the area of the brain that controls movement. Genes, brain injury, and environmental poisons may trigger the disease in some people, but in most cases its causes are unknown.

Parkinson's disease has no cure, but many people find that medication—most often levodopa, used with other drugs—controls their symptoms. Some drugs, such as selegiline, may even slow the progress of the disease.

WHAT YOU CAN DO NOW

- Some prescription drugs—most often those used to treat mental illness—can cause symptoms like those of Parkinson's. Check with your doctor. Changing the drug may stop your symptoms.

After diagnosis:
- Experts agree that it is good for people with Parkinson's to remain active and to exercise. But be careful not to tire yourself out, since stress and fatigue can make symptoms worse.
- Physical therapy, deep muscle massage, and yoga may help you move more easily. Talk to your doctor before starting any new program.
- Eat 7 times more carbohydrate (from vegetables, grains, and pastas) than protein (from meat and dairy products). Protein delays the body's production of levodopa, the chemical that people with Parkinson's lack.
- Constipation can be a problem. So eat plenty of vegetables and bran, and drink at least 6 glasses of water a day.
- Safeguard your home. Tape or tack down small rugs. Stick nonskid decals on the tub or shower floor. Put away shoes and small objects so you won't trip over them.
- Sit in chairs with armrests and firm seats to make getting up easier. Put a firm pillow on low chair seats.
- Use silky sheets and pajamas. They make it easier to move in bed. A cardboard box under the sheets at the foot of the bed will hold bedclothes off your feet.
- Join a support group. Many people with Parkinson's find that company eases the depression that can come with the disease.

WHEN TO CALL THE DOCTOR

- If you see symptoms of Parkinson's disease in yourself or someone close to you.
- If you have any new symptoms during treatment. They may be side effects of the medication you're taking or may mean the illness is getting worse.

HOW TO PREVENT IT

There is no known way to prevent Parkinson's disease.

FOR MORE HELP

Organization: American Parkinson's Disease Association, 1250 Hylan Blvd., Staten Island, NY 10305. 800-223-2732, M–F 9–5 EST. Can refer you to one of 500 support groups and 95 chapters nationwide. Also provides education, facts on diet and exercise, counseling, and names of doctors near you.

Organization: National Parkinson Foundation, 1501 NW Ninth Ave., Miami, FL 33136. 800-327-4545, M–F 8–5 EST. Provides free pamphlets about nutrition and general facts about Parkinson's.

Book: *Parkinson's Disease: The Complete Guide for Patients and Caregivers*, by Abraham N. Lieberman, M.D., and Frank L. Williams. An A–Z symptoms guide, complete with resources and advice on drug therapy, diet, and exercise. Fireside, 1993, $11.

Web access: The Parkinson's Web. After logging on to the Internet, type: *http://neurochief-e.mgh.harvard.edu/parkinsonsweb/main/pdmain.html.* Offers facts about Parkinson's disease, news, research reports, advice on coping skills, and a wide range of other resources.

Seizures and Epilepsy

SIGNS AND SYMPTOMS

- Many people with epilepsy get a warning sign, known as an aura, that lasts a few seconds. It's often marked by nausea, feelings of dread, unique smells and tastes, and warped vision. Auras vary widely, but each person tends to have the same aura before each seizure.

Petit mal, or absence, seizure:

- Person abruptly stops and stares blankly for several seconds, sometimes blinking or making chewing motions.

Grand mal, or tonic-clonic, seizure:

- Convulsions, jerking motions, and loss of consciousness, often with loss of bladder control and sometimes bowel control. Should stop after 1 to 2 minutes; followed by confusion and sleepiness.

Other epileptic seizures:

- Seeing or hearing things that aren't there.
- Incoherent talk or out-of-character actions and speech—sometimes taken for drug abuse.

Two and a half million Americans have epilepsy, an illness that results in seizures—brief events in which the brain's electrical system overloads and misfires.

A single seizure probably doesn't mean a person has epilepsy. It's not rare for a very young child with a high fever to have a seizure. This needs medical attention, but does not by itself mean the child has epilepsy (see **fever in children,** page 260). In adults and children, other triggers for nonepileptic seizures include diabetes, meningitis, and encephalitis. Pregnancy, poisoning, heat stroke, and alcohol or drug abuse can also bring them on.

Epilepsy can start at any age, even over 65, but it mostly begins when a person is a child or young adult. Children who have petit mal seizures often outgrow them. In a little more than half the cases of epilepsy, the cause is unknown. In the rest, causes include severe head injury, brain tumor, stroke, poisoning, infection, and brain damage. Experts believe genes can also play a role.

Up to 85 percent of people with epilepsy can control it with antiseizure drugs. Brain surgery may help those who can't control their seizures any other way.

WHAT YOU CAN DO NOW

If you have epilepsy, take steps to avoid seizures or to lessen their effects:

- Take your medication—missing doses can trigger a seizure. Consult a doctor before switching to a generic brand, since your body may absorb it differently than it does your regular brand.
- If you get a seizure warning sign, or aura, avoid a fall by lying down or moving away from any hazards.
- Be aware that stress, fatigue, and alcohol or drug abuse can bring on seizures.
- Keep a seizure diary, noting the kind of seizure, the time, and likely triggers. This can help you keep medication to a minimum and gain some control over the illness.
- Wear a medical alert tag to help others quickly understand the problem.
- Exercise and practice relaxation techniques to help reduce stress and tension.
- Ask your doctor if it is safe for you to drive.

If you are with someone who has a seizure:

- See **seizures,** page 43, for first aid.

WHEN TO CALL THE DOCTOR

Call 911 or go to an emergency room **right away:**

- If the seizure lasts more than 3 minutes, if a second seizure begins shortly after the first, or if the person does not seem to regain consciousness after the seizure.
- If the person is pregnant or diabetic.

Call your doctor for emergency advice, or if not available, call 911 or go to an emergency room:

- If your child has a high fever and has a seizure or what you suspect to be one.

Call for advice and an appointment:

- If someone you know, particularly a child, goes through times of blank staring, loss of consciousness, confused memory, fainting spells or falls, or odd blinking or chewing motions.
- If your doctor has prescribed antiseizure drugs and you have side effects such as drowsiness, hyperactivity, disorientation, or sleep problems.

HOW TO PREVENT IT

There is no known way to prevent most kinds of epilepsy. To guard against it, get good prenatal care, don't abuse alcohol or other drugs, and protect yourself and your children from head injuries by using seat belts and bicycle helmets.

FOR MORE HELP

Organization: Epilepsy Foundation of America, 4351 Garden City Dr., Landover, MD 20785. 800-332-1000 and 301-459-3700, in English and Spanish, M–F 9–5 EST. Staffs sends brochures, answers questions, and refers callers to other resources. Offers recreational and educational programs for children with epilepsy, as well as information on local chapters and support groups.

Organization: National Institute of Neurological Disorders and Stroke, 31 Center Drive, MSC 2540, Bethesda, MD 20892. 800-352-9424, M–F 8:30–5 EST. Ask for the epilepsy information packet.

Book: *Managing Seizure Disorders: A Handbook for Healthcare Professionals*, by Nancy Santilli. Complete sourcebook. Lippincott, 1996, $29.95.

Book: *Your Child and Epilepsy*, by Robert J. Gumnit, M.D. How you and your child can better understand and control epilepsy. Demos Vermande, 1995, $26.25.

Book: *A Guide to Understanding and Living With Epilepsy*, by Orrin Devinsky, M.D. Provides in-depth information about epilepsy and coping with the disease. F.A. Davis Company, 1994, $15.95.

Eyes

Cataracts

SIGNS AND SYMPTOMS

- Hazy or blurry vision.
- Discomfort or trouble seeing in bright lights.
- A feeling of film over the eyes or of looking through fog.
- Double vision or triple vision in only one eye.
- "Second sight"—a temporary change in near vision, so that you may find you don't need your reading glasses for a brief time.
- White or opaque area visible in the pupil of the eye (in advanced cataract).

A cataract is a fogging of the eye's clear lens (see color illustration, page 161). It can cloud vision like steam on a window. Cataracts often come on slowly, over years, and many people don't notice them until vision loss begins to interfere with the tasks of daily living, such as driving.

Most cataracts start as the lens breaks down with age. They can also come from some diseases, such as diabetes, as well as eye injuries, years of exposure to bright sunlight, and the prolonged use of drugs such as corticosteroids (prescribed for illnesses such as arthritis). Cigarette smoking may also increase the risk. Sometimes a baby is born with cataracts in one or both eyes if the mother had **German measles** (see page 263) during pregnancy.

Surgery is the only treatment for cataracts, though it's not needed unless the cataracts begin to cause problems with work or lifestyle. The entire lens of the eye, or the inside of the lens, is removed. It's most often replaced by a clear plastic lens. Less often, instead of a new lens, the doctor prescribes special eyeglasses or contact lenses after surgery. You can have the cataract operation in the doctor's office and go home the same day.

WHAT YOU CAN DO NOW

➤ If you think you have cataracts, call your doctor for advice on whether you should see an ophthalmologist (a medical doctor licensed to treat all eye conditions). He or she can tell you if you'll need surgery.

WHEN TO CALL THE DOCTOR

➤ If you have even a few of the symptoms, especially blurred vision or trouble with bright lights.

HOW TO PREVENT IT

➤ Be sure your sunglasses protect your eyes from the sun's ultraviolet A (UVA) and ultraviolet B (UVB) rays. Glasses that block out UVA and UVB light are labeled as "fulfilling the American National Standards Institute requirement." The label should

Eye and Vision Problems

This chart includes some of the most common eye and vision problems, as well as some of the most serious. If you have any concerns about your vision, call your doctor for advice right away.

SYMPTOMS	WHAT IT MIGHT BE	WHAT YOU CAN DO
Sudden vision changes, such as blindness, double vision, blurring, flashes of light, floating dark shapes, loss of peripheral (side) vision; acute, sustained pain.	Stroke (see page 115). • Transient ischemic attack—temporary blockage of artery, with symptoms like stroke. • Acute glaucoma (see page 67). • Optic neuritis—inflammation of optic nerve.	Call 911 or go to emergency room **right away** if you have sudden blindness, loss of part of visual field, or double vision.
Redness, watering, pain, or a feeling of having something in the eye.	Foreign body in eye (see eye injuries, page 34).	Call doctor for prompt appointment if something is in colored part of eye or if you can't get particle out of white of eye.
Blurred vision; slow loss of peripheral (side) vision; sudden, severe eye pain; halos around lights; teary, aching eyes; headache; nausea; vomiting.	Glaucoma (see page 67).	Call doctor for prompt appointment.
Blurred vision, sensitivity to light, ache or pain in eye, headache, redness (no discharge).	Iritis/uveitis—inflammation inside eye.	Call doctor for prompt appointment; prescription drugs may help.
Rapid or gradual vision loss; dim or distorted vision, especially when reading; dark, empty area in center of visual field; straight lines look wavy.	Macular degeneration—the macula, a tiny spot at center of retina, begins to break down or scar. Symptoms usually appear after age 55.	Call doctor for prompt appointment. Some forms can be slowed with laser treatment. **For more help:** Association for Macular Diseases, 210 E. 64th St., New York, NY 10021. 212-605-3719, M–F 10–1 EST.
Flashes of light, floating dark shapes, loss of peripheral (side) vision.	Retinal detachment—hole in retina. Risk increases with age, with severe myopia, and after cataract surgery.	Call doctor for prompt appointment. In early stages, vision can be restored with surgery.

(continued)

Eye and Vision Problems *(continued)*

SYMPTOMS	WHAT IT MIGHT BE	WHAT YOU CAN DO
Small, painful red bump at base of eyelash.	Stye.	See styes, page 69.
Red and itchy eyelids.	Blepharitis—inflammation and scaling of eyelids.	Wash eyelids with warm water containing a few drops of baby shampoo, or with over-the-counter eyelid wash. Call doctor for advice and appointment if ailment doesn't clear up with home treatment.
Hazy vision, blurriness around lights, frequent changes in eyeglass prescriptions, white area visible in pupil.	Cataracts.	See cataracts, page 62, and color illustration, page 161.
White of eye is bloodshot, sticky or watery discharge, itching.	Conjunctivitis.	See conjunctivitis, opposite page.
Blurred vision when looking at nearby objects, eyestrain, headaches.	Presbyopia, or farsightedness. Occurs with age as lens loses flexibility.	Call doctor for advice and appointment. Eyeglasses or contact lenses can correct it.
Blurred vision when looking at distant objects.	Myopia, or nearsightedness. May run in families.	Call doctor for advice and appointment. Eyeglasses or contact lenses can correct it.
Red spot on white of eye.	Subconjunctival hemorrhage—bleeding from small blood vessels in membrane over eyeball.	Harmless, though can look alarming. Usually no apparent cause; may follow injury, coughing, or sneezing. Should clear up in 2–3 days. Call doctor for advice if painful or if bleeding recurs.
Dry, hot, or scratchy eyes.	Lack of moisture due to aging, medications, or air pollution.	Moisten eyes with over-the-counter "artificial tears."
Spots or "threads" that float across field of vision.	Floaters—bits of tissue or cells floating in the jellylike liquid that fills the eye.	Usually harmless. Call doctor for advice the first time you see them.

also say they "eliminate 99 percent of UVA and UVB."

- If you are a woman and plan to become pregnant, protect your baby by getting vaccinated for German measles if you haven't had the disease already.
- Wear safety glasses to prevent eye injury during sports, or when using power tools or chemicals such as paint remover.
- Eat more green and yellow vegetables. These contain substances (antioxidants) that may help prevent cataracts.

FOR MORE HELP

Information line: National Eye Care Project Help Line, 800-222-3937, M–F 8–4 PST. Refers low-income senior citizens to ophthalmologists who provide medical care at no cost.

Organization: Prevent Blindness America, 500 E. Remington Rd., Schaumburg, IL 60173. 800-331-2020, M–F 8–5 CST. Provides material on eye diseases and has a national network of support groups.

Organization: National Eye Health Education Program, National Institutes of Health, Bldg. 31, Rm. 6A32, 31 Center Drive, MSC 2510, Bethesda, MD 20892-2510. 301-496-5248, M–F 8:30–4:30 EST. E-mail address: *2020@b31.nei.nih.gov.* Provides brochures, fact sheets, and advice about eye disease.

Book: *The Crystal Clear Guide to Sight for Life: A Complete Manual of Eye Care for Those Over Forty,* by Johnny L. Gayton, M.D., and Jan Roadarmel Ledford. Covers common eye problems, new treatments, and tips on choosing a doctor. Starburst Publishers, 1996, $15.95.

Web access: American College of Ophthalmology. After logging on to the Internet, type: *http://www.eyenet.org.* Click on *Eye Diseases and Conditions,* then click on *Cataracts.* Covers treatments and resources.

Web access: *Cataract in Adults: A Patient's Guide,* by the U.S. Department of Health & Human Services. After logging on to the Internet, type: *http://www.iacnet.com/health/14401248.htm.* Answers questions about cataracts and lists resources.

Video: *Cataracts at Time of Diagnosis.* Clear overview of causes and treatments, with 4 reports—Understanding the Diagnosis, What Happens Next?, Treatment and Management, and Issues and Answers. Time Life Medical, 1996, $19.95. Sold in many pharmacies; for one near you, call 800-588-9959.

Conjunctivitis

SIGNS AND SYMPTOMS

Redness of the whites of the eyes is common to all types of conjunctivitis. Other signs include:

In bacterial conjunctivitis:

- Discharge of pus from the eye or crusting on the eyelashes in the morning.

In viral conjunctivitis:

- Watery discharge, often from one eye only, occasionally with crusting.
- Sore throat and runny nose, with some viruses.

In allergic conjunctivitis:

- Itchy eyes.
- Burning and watery eyes.
- Swelling of the tissues around eye.
- Sneezing, runny nose.

In conjunctivitis caused by dirty air, fumes, or dust:

- Burning and watery eyes.
- A feeling of something in the eye.

Conjunctivitis is an inflammation of the membrane (conjunctiva) that covers the inside of the eyelid and the white of the eye. It is annoying but rarely serious. Causes include:

- Bacterial or viral infections (pinkeye).
- Allergies to such things as grass pollen, house dust, mold, or cosmetics.
- Smoke and fumes.
- In newborns (rarely): infection from the lining of the mother's birth canal. This is a serious problem that must be treated at once, as it can cause blindness.

THE EYE

An eyeball has 3 chambers filled with fluid. A thin fluid in the 2 front chambers, between the cornea and the lens, controls pressure inside the eye. A thicker fluid in the third and largest chamber keeps the eyeball firm.

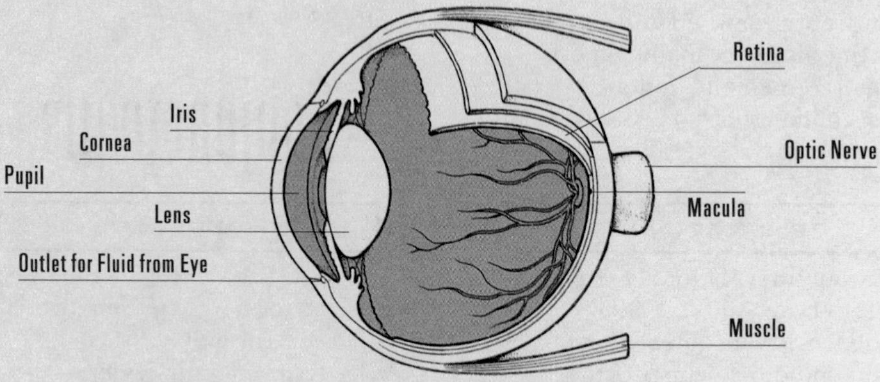

When caused by bacteria or a virus, conjunctivitis is easy to spread through direct contact or through towels, handkerchiefs, or washcloths. Your doctor can give you eyedrops or ointment to make the eye feel better and speed healing. Allergic conjunctivitis may be chronic—meaning it keeps coming back—or it may be a problem only in allergy season. You can't give it to others.

WHAT YOU CAN DO NOW

General:

- If bright light causes pain, wear dark glasses while out in the sun.
- Avoid things that irritate your eyes, such as tobacco smoke or the water in swimming pools.
- Don't wear eye makeup.
- Don't wear contact lenses.
- Use warm water to gently soak and wipe away any crusted or sticky discharge around the eyes.

Bacterial or viral conjunctivitis:

- To soothe infected eyes, apply a clean, warm, damp cloth. Wash used cloths in hot water with detergent so you don't spread the infection.
- If your child has it, keep him or her at home so it won't spread. The teacher and other parents will thank you.

Conjunctivitis caused by dirty air, fumes, or dust:

- To soothe sore eyes, use artificial teardrops, available over the counter.

Allergic conjunctivitis:

- Apply a cold, damp washcloth to the eyes to relieve itching.
- Try over-the-counter allergy eyedrops or pills to reduce redness and itching. Be aware that the pills can cause drowsiness.

WHEN TO CALL THE DOCTOR

Call for a prompt appointment:

- If your newborn's eyes redden and produce a discharge; this must be treated quickly to prevent eye damage.
- If conjunctivitis affects your vision or causes lots of pain or discharge; you may have a staph or strep infection. You may need treatment right away.

Call for advice:

- If you injure your eye; it could become infected and get ulcers on the cornea (the "window" at the front of the eye).
- If your conjunctivitis gets worse after a week of home care; you may need treatment for an infection.
- If you get conjunctivitis often.
- If you have symptoms of conjunctivitis that don't seem to be caused by an infec-

tion, a cold, or allergies. Several eye diseases can also cause redness and tears, including **glaucoma** (see this page).

➤ If you notice your vision is blurred, you're bothered by light, or your eyes are red; these may be signs of advanced glaucoma.

HOW TO PREVENT IT

➤ Don't share eye makeup or eyedrops.
➤ Replace eye makeup every 6 months, or after an infection.
➤ Don't share handkerchiefs, towels, or washcloths.
➤ If you wear contact lenses, wash your hands before touching them. Always soak them in fresh, sterile contact lens solution; never reuse solution.
➤ If you have conjunctivitis, don't touch your eye and then touch someone else; you can spread it to others.
➤ Wash your hands often if you have conjunctivitis, or if you live with someone who has it.
➤ If you have allergies, try to avoid the things that cause them, such as pollen, dust, mold, or pets.
➤ During allergy season, filter the air in your car and house by running the air conditioners, if you have them; keep the windows and doors in your home closed.
➤ Wear goggles on the job if you work around chemicals or fumes.

FOR MORE HELP

Information line: National Eye Care Project Help Line, 800-222-3937, M–F 8–4 PST. Refers low-income senior citizens to ophthalmologists who provide medical care at no cost.

Organization: National Eye Health Education Program, National Institutes of Health, 301-496-5248, M–F 8:30–4:30 EST. Provides facts about eye diseases.

Organization: American Academy of Ophthalmology, Box 7424, San Francisco, CA 94120-7424. 415-561-8500, M–F 9–5 PST. Provides fact sheets on eye diseases. Send a business-size, self-addressed, stamped envelope, and request a brochure on conjunctivitis.

Book: *Your Eyes... An Owner's Guide,* by James Collins, M.D., F.A.C.S. Provides information on eye care, eye problems, and new eye treatments. Prentice Hall, 1995, $10.95.

Glaucoma

SIGNS AND SYMPTOMS

Glaucoma often has no symptoms at first. By the time symptoms do appear, some vision may have been lost, so it's vital to spot and treat glaucoma early.

In chronic glaucoma:
- Blurred vision.
- Over time, loss of peripheral (side) vision.
- Teary, aching eyes.
- Headaches.

In acute glaucoma:
- Severe, sudden eye pain.
- Blurred vision.
- Halos around lights.
- Headaches.
- Nausea and vomiting.

In secondary glaucoma (after an injury or certain diseases):
- Blurred vision.
- Halos around lights.
- Headaches.

Think of the eye as a sink with a faucet and a drain. The "faucet" consists of many tiny blood vessels pouring fluid into the spaces in front of the lens. The "drain" lets out excess fluid, so the pressure inside remains constant. Glaucoma occurs when the drain becomes clogged; pressure builds up on the optic nerve and its small blood vessels. When not treated, glaucoma can cause vision loss and even blindness.

Glaucoma is one of the most common eye problems in people over 60. It runs in families. African Americans and people with severe myopia (nearsightedness) or diabetes are also at greater risk than others. Some drugs can cause glaucoma. These include certain antidepressants, as well as drugs for asthma or irritable bowel syndrome. People with past eye injuries may be prone to secondary glaucoma.

About 10 percent of glaucoma is acute—it gets worse quickly and requires prompt treatment. Chronic glaucoma accounts for the other 90 percent of cases. It's often called the "sneak thief" of sight because it comes on slowly to steal vision.

Glaucoma can usually be treated with eyedrops, pills, or shots that lower pressure in the eye. Doctors sometimes perform in-office laser surgery to widen clogged drains or to create new ones.

WHAT YOU CAN DO NOW

Glaucoma can be detected only with a test of eye pressure. Get regular eye checkups, above all if you're in a high-risk group.

WHEN TO CALL THE DOCTOR

- If you have symptoms of glaucoma. You'll need treatment right away.
- If you are being treated for glaucoma and another doctor prescribes drugs for some other ailment.
- If you are taking eyedrops or pills for glaucoma and you have side effects such as headaches; red eyes; stinging in the eyes; blurred vision; changes in heartbeat, pulse, or breathing; tingling fingers and toes; drowsiness; loss of appetite; bowel problems; kidney stones; or easy bleeding; or if you learn you have anemia.
- If you feel drowsy, tired, or short of breath after taking eyedrops for glaucoma. The drug may be making a heart or lung problem worse.

HOW TO PREVENT IT

- Get an eye exam with a glaucoma test every 3 to 5 years after age 39.
- Get an eye exam every 1 to 2 years if someone in your family has glaucoma or severe myopia, if you have African ancestors, if you have ever had a serious eye injury, or if you are taking antidepressants or any medications for asthma or irritable bowel syndrome.

FOR MORE HELP

Information line: National Eye Care Project Help Line, 800-222-3937, M–F 8–4 PST. Refers low-income senior citizens to ophthalmologists who provide medical care at no cost.

Information line: American Foundation for the Blind, 800-232-5463, M–F 10–12 and 2–4 EST. Covers visual impairment, including career advice for people who have trouble seeing.

Organization: National Eye Health Education Program, National Institutes of Health, Bldg. 31, Rm. 6A32, 31 Center Drive, MSC 2510, Bethesda, MD 20892-2510. 301-496-5248, M–F 8:30–4:30 EST. Provides brochures and fact sheets about eye disease. Reach them by e-mail at *2020@b31.nei.nih.gov*.

Organization: Glaucoma Research Foundation, 800-826-6693, 24-hour recording. 415-986-3162, M–F 8:30–4:30 PST. Sends free publications and coordinates a national telephone-based support network for glaucoma patients and their families. **Web site:** *http://www.glaucoma.org*. Covers glaucoma, current research, research centers, and links to local ophthalmologists.

Book: *The Crystal Clear Guide to Sight for Life: A Complete Manual of Eye Care for Those Over Forty,* by Johnny L. Gayton, M.D., and Jan Roadarmel Ledford. Covers common eye disorders, new treatments, and tips on choosing a doctor. Starburst Publishers, 1996, $15.95.

Web access: American Academy of Ophthalmology. After logging on to the Internet, type: *http://www.eyenet.org*. Click on *Eye Diseases and Conditions*, then *Glaucoma*. Answers common questions and provides information on treatment.

Styes

SIGNS AND SYMPTOMS

- A small, painful red bump on the upper or lower eyelid near the base of an eyelash.
- Burning, itching, or a feeling of having something in the eye.
- A teary eye.

A stye is a bacterial infection of a gland at the base of an eyelash. Styes are often painful, but they're rarely serious.

Styes usually swell, fill with pus, and break open within 3 to 7 days, easing the pain. They may also go away without bursting. They're easy to spread by touching your eyelid, by squeezing the stye, or by using contaminated makeup or towels.

WHAT YOU CAN DO NOW

- Don't rub the eye and don't squeeze or pick at the stye.
- Apply a soft, clean washcloth that has been soaked in warm water and wrung out. Hold for 10 to 15 minutes. Repeat 2 to 4 times a day until the stye goes away.
- Use a new washcloth each time so you don't spread the infection. Wash used cloths in hot water with detergent.
- If the stye comes to a head and bursts, gently wash the pus from the eyelid. Don't pick at the stye.

WHEN TO CALL THE DOCTOR

- If the stye does not respond to home care within a week. A doctor may prescribe antibiotic drops or ointment, or may lance and drain the stye.
- If you have some other infection. Your doctor may give you an antibiotic.
- If the stye swells but doesn't break open and drain.
- If styes keep coming back. Rarely, this can be a sign of cancer of the eyelid.
- If you have any signs of skin infection (redness and roughness) spreading on the eyelid.

HOW TO PREVENT IT

- Don't touch or rub your eyes. Styes can come back again if the bacteria spread.
- Wash your hands often with soap and water.
- Don't share towels or washcloths.
- Change towels and pillowcases often.
- Don't share eye makeup or eyedrops, and throw away used cosmetics after 6 months.
- If styes come back often, clean the outside of your eyelids every day: Dip a cotton swab into a cup of warm water and a few drops of baby shampoo. Wash the lashes of each closed eyelid with this mixture once or twice a day.

FOR MORE HELP

Organization: American Optometric Association, 243 N. Lindbergh Blvd., St. Louis, MO 63141. 314-991-4100, M–F 8–5 CST. Sends free pamphlets on eye and vision problems. For information on styes, send a self-addressed, stamped, business-size envelope to: Communications Center, Dept. FS14.

Organization: National Eye Health Education Program, National Institutes of Health, 301-496-5248, M–F 8:30–4:30 EST. Provides brochures and fact sheets about eye disease.

Ears

Airplane Ear

SIGNS AND SYMPTOMS

- Feeling of fullness in the ears.
- Pain in the ears.
- Ringing in the ears.
- Dizziness.

You may get "airplane ear" (barotrauma) when you take a plane trip, especially if you have a **cold** (see page 94), **sinusitis** (see page 100), or **allergies** (see page 86). But any rapid air-pressure change—from an elevator ride in a high-rise, say, or skin diving—can cause airplane ear.

The problem is in the middle ear. This is the part connected to the back of the nose by the eustachian tube (see illustration, page 75). A cold, sinusitis, or allergies can swell the tube, trapping air. You'll feel pressure in the ears, especially during descents.

WHAT YOU CAN DO NOW

- Yawning or swallowing opens the tube to the middle ear. Just before and during descent, chew gum or suck on candy so you'll swallow more often.
- When flying, don't sleep during descent. If swallowing and yawning don't work, try this: Take a deep breath; then close your mouth and hold your nose, and try to breathe out through the nose gently and slowly. This can force air through the tubes between your nose and ears. You may have to do this a few times.

If you're flying with an infant:

- Wake your baby before descent.
- Give your baby something to drink or a pacifier during landing. Babies can't "pop" their ears on purpose, but sucking on a bottle or pacifier may do the trick.

WHEN TO CALL THE DOCTOR

- If your ears don't clear, or if pain lasts for several hours after flying.
- If you're planning a plane trip and have just had ear surgery. Ask your doctor how soon you may fly safely.

HOW TO PREVENT IT

If you have a cold, a sinus infection, or an allergy attack—or a child traveling with you does—it's best to postpone a plane trip. If you can't:

- Some air travelers get relief from taking an over-the-counter decongestant pill or nasal spray about an hour before landing.
- People with allergies should also take their medication about an hour before landing.

FOR MORE HELP

Information line: American Speech-Language-Hearing Association, 800-638-8255, M–F 8:30–5 EST. Staff answers questions and gives written advice on airplane ear and other disorders.

Ear and Hearing Problems

Your ears serve two functions—hearing and balance. Some problems affect one or the other function, and some affect both. Try to find the cause of such a problem and treat it early; you can do a lot to prevent or treat most conditions that affect your ears.

SYMPTOMS	WHAT IT MIGHT BE	WHAT YOU CAN DO
Severe pain and swelling behind and in ear, fluid coming from ear, fever, temporary hearing loss.	Mastoiditis—inflamed mastoid bone behind ear.	Call doctor for prompt appointment. Antibiotics or surgical drainage may be required.
Pain, hearing loss, discharge or bleeding from ear.	Ruptured (perforated) eardrum—often caused by object pushed into ear. • Serious middle ear infection (see page 73). • Blow to ear or injury while diving or water-skiing.	Call doctor for prompt appointment. Treatment includes medications, patch over eardrum, or surgery. To relieve pain, cover ear with heating pad set on low and take painkillers.
Loss of balance, dizziness, ringing in ears, hearing loss, nausea or vomiting.	Labyrinthitis—infection often caused by a virus, in area of inner ear that controls balance.	Call doctor for advice and appointment. Treatment includes medications and bed rest.
Repeated sudden and severe dizziness, hearing loss, or ringing in ear; loss of balance; headache; nausea or vomiting.	Ménière's syndrome—from fluid buildup in inner ear.	Call doctor for advice and appointment. Treatment includes medications and sometimes surgery. Rest to reduce symptoms. Cut back on fluids and salt. Avoid alcohol, caffeine, tobacco. **For more help:** Ménière's Network, EAR Foundation, 800-545-HEAR, M–F 8–4:30 CST.
Hearing loss over time, dizziness, ringing in ear.	Otosclerosis—overgrowth of bone in middle ear. Often runs in families. More common in women; may get worse during pregnancy.	Call doctor for advice and appointment. Simplest treatment is hearing aid; surgery can help.
Trouble hearing, often at higher frequencies and with background noise; trouble understanding speech.	Presbycusis—hearing loss due to age. Usually begins between 40 and 50. Most common and severe in men.	Call doctor for advice and appointment. Hearing aid is usual treatment.

(continued)

Ear and Hearing Problems *(continued)*

SYMPTOMS	WHAT IT MIGHT BE	WHAT YOU CAN DO
Feeling of fullness, discomfort, or pain in ears during or after flying; temporary hearing loss; ringing in ears; dizziness.	Airplane ear.	See airplane ear, page 70.
Throbbing pain and/or tender lump in ear canal; discharge of pus or blood from ear.	Boil (see page 148).	Usually heals by itself. Antibiotic drops or heating pad may help.
Feeling of fullness or blockage in ear, temporary hearing loss, pain or discomfort, ringing in ear.	Earwax (see page 74). • Ear infection (see opposite page). • Early sign of throat cancer (rarely).	If symptoms persist, call doctor for advice.
Earache, fever and chills, stuffy nose, feeling of fullness or blockage in ear, muffled hearing, discharge from ear. In young children: tugging at ear, bad temper, restlessness, lack of appetite.	Middle ear infection.	See ear infections, opposite page.
Itchy or blocked ear, pain or tenderness, yellowish discharge, flaky skin around ear, temporary hearing loss.	Swimmer's ear—infection of outer ear canal.	See swimmer's ear, page 75.
Ringing or buzzing in ears—noise that can't be heard by others.	Tinnitus.	See tinnitus, page 76.
Earache with pain in jaw and/or face; headache; clicking noise or locked feeling when opening or closing mouth.	Temporomandibular disorder (TMD).	See temporomandibular disorder, page 203.

Ear Infections

SIGNS AND SYMPTOMS

In adults:

- Earache (either a sudden, sharp pain or a constant, dull pain).
- Muffled hearing.

Sometimes with:

- Fever of 100 degrees or above, perhaps with chills.
- Stuffy nose.
- Sore throat.
- Feeling of fullness in the ear.
- Pus or blood from the ear.
- Nausea or diarrhea.

In young children, especially those who aren't yet talking, watch for:

- Tugging at the ear.
- Bad temper.
- Restlessness.
- Lack of appetite.
- Fever of 100 degrees or above.
- Discharge from the nose or ear.

A middle ear infection (otitis media) is the most common cause of earaches. It's the number one reason children go to the doctor, but it also affects adults.

Ear infections are most often caused by **colds** (see page 94) or **flu** (see page 96). These ailments swell the tissues of the middle ear (see illustration, page 75), trapping fluids and making an ideal place for bacteria or viruses to thrive. **Allergies** (see page 86) or irritants such as smoke or fumes can have the same effect.

Infections that go on for weeks or happen again and again can cause permanent hearing loss. In young children, any hearing loss is cause for concern, as it may delay speech and language development; prompt treatment is vital.

An ear infection can lead to other problems, including mastoiditis (an inflamed mastoid bone behind the ear), perforated eardrum, **meningitis** (see page 57), and facial nerve paralysis.

WHAT YOU CAN DO NOW

- Hold a warm compress to the ear. Inhaling steam may also help. Or use a vaporizer if you have one.
- Gargle with warm salt water to soothe a sore throat and help open blocked ears.
- Drink plenty of water or other clear liquids.
- Use pillows to raise the head when lying down. This helps drain the middle ear.
- People with allergies may get relief from over-the-counter antihistamines. Some people use decongestant nasal sprays to open the ears. But after a couple of days, sprays can lead to "rebound" congestion that makes the problem worse.
- Over-the-counter drugs such as aspirin, ibuprofen, or acetaminophen may help with pain. (Never give aspirin to a child under 12 who has a cold, chicken pox, flu, or any other illness you suspect of being caused by a virus; see box on **Reye's syndrome,** page 96.)

WHEN TO CALL THE DOCTOR

- If your child has symptoms of an ear infection or trouble hearing.
- If an earache lasts more than 2 days.
- If your body temperature or your child's rises above 100 degrees.
- If you have frequent ear infections, or your child does.

HOW TO PREVENT IT

- Remove irritants and allergy-causing agents, such as dust, cleaning fluids, and tobacco smoke, from your home.
- If you have food allergies, or your child does, cut back on wheat products, corn products, or any other foods you know cause allergic reactions.
- Watch your baby's health closely if you're not breast-feeding. Bottle-fed babies are more likely to get ear infections. Hold your baby upright during bottle-feeding to keep milk from getting into the tube that connects the back of the nose and the ear.

FOR MORE HELP

Information line: American Speech-Language-Hearing Association, 800-638-8255, M–F 8:30–5 EST. Staff answers questions on hearing loss; ask for the pamphlet on otitis media.

Organization: National Institute on Deafness and Other Communication Disorders Information Clearinghouse, 800-241-1044, M–F 8:30–5 EST. Ask for the ear infections packet.

Organization: American Academy of Otolaryngology–Head & Neck Surgery, One Prince St., Alexandria, VA 22314-3357. 703-836-4444, M–F 8:30–5 EST. Ask for the brochure on earaches and otitis media.

Earwax

SIGNS AND SYMPTOMS

- Blocked or plugged feeling in ear.
- Trouble hearing.
- Ear pain or discomfort.
- Ringing in the ear.

Earwax coats and protects the outer ear canal that leads to the eardrum (see illustration, opposite page). Usually earwax is soft, drains easily, and doesn't cause trouble.

But sometimes the wax builds up and becomes hard and dry. Then it's one of the most common causes of hearing problems, especially when it mixes with dust, dirt, or water in the ear.

WHAT YOU CAN DO NOW

Infants and young children with built-up earwax should be taken to a doctor. Adults can try the following:

- Mix 1 tablespoon hydrogen peroxide with 1 tablespoon warm water. (Make sure it's warm—cold water in the ear can make you dizzy.)
  - Tilt your head, and put a few drops of the warmed liquid into your blocked ear. Leave it there for 3 minutes, keeping your head tilted.
  - Let the liquid run out onto a towel or tissue. The wax should be soft enough to be wiped away from the outer ear with a cotton ball. Repeat if needed.
  - If the wax is stubborn, soften it first with 3 or 4 drops of olive oil or glycerin. You may need to do this a few times.
- Over-the-counter liquid earwax softeners can help to loosen earwax. But don't use wax softeners if you suspect you have an **ear infection** (see page 73) or ruptured eardrum (see **ear and hearing problems** chart, page 71).
- Use a soft rubber bulb syringe to dislodge wax by gently rinsing the ear canal with warm water or a mixture of warm water and hydrogen peroxide. Don't do this if you have an earache, fever, discharge from your ear, or a punctured eardrum, or if you've just had ear surgery.
- Never attempt to remove earwax with a cotton-tipped stick or swab. You can damage your eardrum or cause an infection.

WHEN TO CALL THE DOCTOR

Call for a prompt appointment:

- If you have a sudden or total hearing loss in one or both ears.
- If pus, fluid, or blood drains from your ear. This can mean an ear infection or a punctured eardrum.

Call for advice and an appointment:

- If wax becomes so firmly lodged that home care doesn't work. Your doctor may need to clean the ear.
- If your infant or young child has wax blocking the ear. Don't try to remove the wax yourself.

HOW TO PREVENT IT

- Wear earplugs if you work around a lot of dust, which can trigger wax buildup.
- Don't let your child push objects into his or her ear canal.
- Each week, put 1 or 2 drops of mineral oil in each ear to keep wax soft.

THE EAR

The outer ear canal carries sound waves to the eardrum. From there, vibrations travel to the middle and inner ear. One part of the inner ear translates vibrations into signals that your brain "hears"; another part keeps you balanced. A second canal, the eustachian tube, connects the middle ear to the back of the nose and throat.

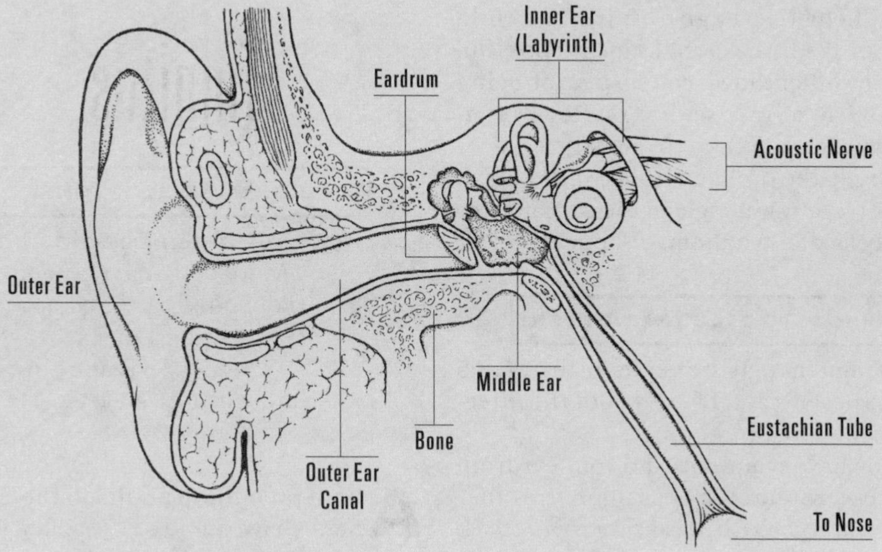

Ears

FOR MORE HELP

Information line: *Dial a Hearing Screening Test,* Swarthmore Medical Center, 300 S. Chester Rd., Swarthmore, PA 19081. 800-222-3277. Features a 2-minute hearing test, followed by names of doctors near you.

Swimmer's Ear

SIGNS AND SYMPTOMS

- Itching or blocked feeling in the ear.
- Ear pain and tenderness that is worse when you move your head or pull on your earlobe.
- Foul-smelling, watery, or yellow discharge from the ear.
- Patches of broken, flaky skin around the opening of the ear.
- Muffled hearing.

You don't have to be a swimmer to get "swimmer's ear" (otitis externa), an inflamed outer ear canal. It's often caused by moisture in the ear, perhaps from frequent showers or shampoos, or from swimming, particularly in polluted water.

The dampness can make the skin inside the ear canal crack or flake, letting bacteria or fungi invade. Some skin problems, such as **dermatitis** (see page 151) and **psoriasis** (see page 177), can also cause swimmer's ear. Another common cause is having too little earwax to protect the ear canal from moisture. Swimmer's ear is seldom serious.

WHAT YOU CAN DO NOW

Swimmer's ear often clears up on its own. If not, it responds quickly to treatment. Here's what you can do to speed recovery:

➤ Keep the infected ear dry. Wear earplugs or big, loose-fitting cotton balls coated with Vaseline when showering or washing your hair. Stay out of swimming pools.

- Use over-the-counter antiseptic eardrops. Or make your own, using equal parts rubbing alcohol and white vinegar. Warm the drops first. Leave them in your ear for a couple of minutes, then tilt your head to let them drain out.
- Hold a warm compress over the ear to relieve pain. Over-the-counter painkillers may help. (Never give aspirin to a child under 12 who has a cold, chicken pox, flu, or any other illness you suspect of being caused by a virus; see box on **Reye's syndrome,** page 96.)
- To keep the problem from coming back, don't let any water get in the ear canal for 3 weeks after symptoms disappear.

WHEN TO CALL THE DOCTOR

- If symptoms persist after more than 4 or 5 days of self-care. It's rare, but the infection can spread.
- If you have symptoms and your eardrum has ever ruptured or been injured in other ways, or if you've had ear surgery.
- If you have frequent bouts of swimmer's ear or already have an **ear infection** (see page 73).
- If you have diabetes or a weakened immune system.

HOW TO PREVENT IT

- Squirt lanolin eardrops (or baby oil) into your ears before you swim to protect them from the water. Tilt your head so the drops get to the bottom of the ear canal, then let the liquid drain out.
- Try to keep your ears dry. Wear earplugs while swimming (remove them right after), and pull a shower cap over your ears before showering.
- Dry the outer parts of your ears after swimming or showering, and use rubbing alcohol eardrops to help evaporate water inside.
- Use antiseptic eardrops if you get water in your ears and you tend to get swimmer's ear.
- Be careful when cleaning **earwax** (see page 74) from your ears. Don't use any object that could scratch the ear canal.

FOR MORE HELP

Organization: American Academy of Otolaryngology–Head and Neck Surgery, One Prince St., Alexandria, VA 22314. 703-836-4444, M–F 8:30–5 EST. Fax: 703-683-5100. Ask for the swimmer's ear brochure and names of doctors near you.

Tinnitus

SIGNS AND SYMPTOMS

- Ringing, whistling, buzzing, humming, or roaring that only you can hear. The sound can be constant or may come and go. It may vary in pitch or loudness; it is more distinct when other sounds are low.

About 50 million adults in the United States have tinnitus. Most often it is not a sign of anything serious, and it can go away on its own or when some problem behind it is treated. But when tinnitus is loud and constant, people can find it hard to concentrate, sleep, or work.

The older you are, the more likely you are to get tinnitus. It has many causes, including:

- Nerve damage from loud noises.
- Wax buildup (see **earwax,** page 74) in the ear canal.
- **Ear infection** (see page 73).
- A punctured eardrum.
- Side effects of many prescription and over-the-counter medications, such as aspirin, quinine, anti-inflammatories, antibiotics, diuretics, and antidepressants.
- Chronic stress (see **stress,** page 222).
- Too much alcohol or caffeine.

Tinnitus can also be a symptom of other health problems, such as:

- **High blood pressure** (see page 112).
- **Allergies** (see page 86).

If you have tinnitus along with dizziness, you might have fluid buildup in your inner ear or damage to the small bones in your middle ear (see Ménière's syndrome, otosclerosis, and labyrinthitis in the **ear and hearing problems** chart, page 71).

WHAT YOU CAN DO NOW

Tinnitus can't always be cured, but you can take steps to get relief:

- If you have trouble sleeping, cover the tinnitus with a recording of soothing sounds or music.
- Try a tinnitus masker, a small device worn like a hearing aid; it makes a pleasant sound to compete with the tinnitus.
- Stay away from caffeine, alcohol, tobacco, and aspirin—they can all make tinnitus worse.
- Exercise often. This may provide relief by bringing more blood to the head.
- If allergies cause your tinnitus, stay away from things that bring them on. Try a decongestant to relieve stuffiness (but don't use it for more than 2 days at a time, to avoid "rebound" congestion).
- Try to relax—practice deep breathing and meditation when tinnitus comes on; it may help (see **relax,** page 309).

WHEN TO CALL THE DOCTOR

Call for a prompt appointment:

- If you have sudden or total hearing loss.
- If you have tinnitus and feel dizzy.
- If you have tinnitus and pus or pain in your ear.

Call for advice and an appointment:

- If you think your tinnitus is caused by another health problem.
- If self-care doesn't work and tinnitus interferes with your concentration, daily activities, or sleep.
- If the sound bothers you.

HOW TO PREVENT IT

- Wear earplugs or earmuffs when exposed to loud noise. (Cotton balls don't block enough sound. Also, if you're not careful, they can lodge deep in the ear canal.)
- Keep the volume down when listening to music through earphones.
- Teach your children about the dangers of loud music.
- Cut down on salt. It can cause fluid to build up in your middle ear, and that raises your chances of having tinnitus.
- Get enough rest, avoid stress, and practice relaxation techniques.
- Don't let wax build up in your ears (see **earwax,** page 74).
- If you're taking any medications, ask your doctor if they could be causing your tinnitus. Are there alternatives?
- Keep a diary listing what you eat each day and when you're around dust, chemicals, or other irritants. Note when your tinnitus comes on. This may help you find the cause, so you know what to avoid.
- Allergy-proof your home—keep it free of dust, mold, pet hair, and other common causes of allergies. Change filters in your heater or air conditioner often.
- Wear a dust mask when you're cleaning house or working around chemicals, if you know this causes your tinnitus.

FOR MORE HELP

Information line: American Speech Language-Hearing Association, 800-638-8255, M–F 8:30–5 EST. Staff answers questions and sends out brochures on tinnitus and other ear disorders.

Organization: National Institute on Deafness and Other Communication Disorders Information Clearinghouse, 800-241-1044, M–F 8:30–5 EST. Ask for the tinnitus packet.

Organization: American Tinnitus Association, 1618 SW First Avenue, Suite 417, Portland, OR 97201. 503-248-9985, M–F 8:30–5 PST. Fax: 503-248-0024. E-mail: *tinnitus@ata.org*. Ask about publications, membership information, and support groups near you.

Mouth

Bad Breath

SIGNS AND SYMPTOMS

- Foul odor from the mouth.
- Bad taste in the mouth.
- Inflamed and bleeding gums.

Many people have bouts of bad breath (halitosis) not explained by the effects of strong-smelling food and drink. Most of the time, bad breath is no cause for alarm. But it can be a sign of a health problem, such as gum disease, tooth decay (see **toothache,** page 82), **sinusitis** (see page 100), **tonsillitis** (see page 103), **strep throat** (see page 271), or **diabetes** (see page 282).

Bad breath is mostly caused by bacteria mixed with food bits and saliva that form a smelly film on the teeth called plaque. Smoking is a major culprit, too. A dry mouth adds to the problem, causing "morning breath." Simply not drinking enough water can make it worse. So can some drugs, such as diuretics, tranquilizers, and antihistamines.

WHAT YOU CAN DO NOW

- Brush your teeth at least twice a day, and floss once daily.
- Gently clean the top of your tongue with the toothbrush. Be sure to reach in back.
- Postnasal drip—from a cold, allergies, or sinusitis—can cause bad breath. To flush away mucus and bacteria, try gargling with a saltwater mix: Dissolve one-half teaspoon of salt in 8 ounces of warm water. Use the same mix to flush out your nose: Squirt it in with a dropper or a bulb syringe, or put the mix in the palm of your hand and sniff it in, 1 nostril at a time. Wait a few minutes and then blow your nose gently.
- For a quick cover-up, eat fresh parsley or mint, an orange, an apple, or celery. Or use a mouthwash.

WHEN TO CALL THE DOCTOR OR DENTIST

- If your bad breath persists for no reason after you've flossed and cleaned your teeth, gums, and tongue extra well for a week.
- If you have a toothache with bad breath. You may have a cavity or an abscess.
- If your gums are inflamed and bleeding. This could be a sign of gum disease.
- If you also have a fever or cough and mucus. This can be a symptom of a lung abscess.

HOW TO PREVENT IT

- Brush at least twice a day and floss once.
- Brush your tongue every morning.
- Have your teeth cleaned every 6 months, and see a dentist once a year.
- Don't smoke.
- Go light on sugar, coffee, and alcohol;

Tooth and Mouth Problems

Even minor tooth and mouth problems can hurt. You can prevent many of them by brushing your teeth and flossing daily; seeing a dentist every year can help you take early action if a problem does come up.

SYMPTOMS	WHAT IT MIGHT BE	WHAT YOU CAN DO
White or red patch on gums; lump or discoloration anywhere in mouth; sore in mouth that bleeds and/or doesn't heal in 3–4 weeks; trouble swallowing; swelling in jaw or neck.	Oral cancer—tumors can occur anywhere in or around mouth or in upper throat.	Call doctor for prompt appointment. Most oral cancers can be treated if found early. **For more help:** Cancer Information and Counseling Hotline, 800-525-3777, M–F 8:30–5 MST.
Toothache and red, swollen, or bleeding gums; sometimes earache; often fever; facial swelling; bad taste in mouth.	Tooth abscess. See toothache, page 82.	Call dentist for prompt appointment.
Red, swollen gums that sometimes bleed; bad breath; loose teeth; pus discharge in mouth.	Periodontitis—advanced inflamed gums: end result of gingivitis (see below).	Call dentist for advice and appointment. Prompt treatment is needed to save teeth. **For more help:** American Academy of Periodontology, 737 N. Michigan Ave., Suite 800, Chicago, IL 60611-2690. Write for fact sheets and brochures on periodontitis.
Reddish, shiny, swollen gums that bleed easily; bad breath.	Gingivitis—also called gum disease. Most often caused by plaque buildup on teeth.	Call dentist for advice and appointment. Treatment includes removing plaque. Brush teeth after meals at least twice a day. Floss daily.
Red, swollen, painful gums; sore jaw; headache; bad taste in mouth; bad breath.	Impacted teeth—caused by lack of space in mouth.	Call dentist for advice and appointment. Treatment may include pulling a tooth.
Lump or sore in mouth or on tongue.	Noncancerous mouth or tongue tumors. Cause is unknown.	Call doctor for advice and appointment if lump or sore doesn't clear up in 3 weeks.

(continued)

Tooth and Mouth Problems *(continued)*

SYMPTOMS	WHAT IT MIGHT BE	WHAT YOU CAN DO
Creamy yellow patches in mouth that leave raw, red spots when rubbed.	Thrush—a fungal infection (see page 155); common in people with HIV and infants. Caused by some antibiotics and steroid inhalers.	Call doctor for advice and appointment.
Painful, swollen glands under tongue, behind ear, or in neck; bad taste in mouth; dry mouth; fever.	Salivary gland disorders. Causes include mumps (see page 268) and bacterial infection.	Call doctor for advice and appointment. Treatment may include antibiotics. Avoid spicy foods and citrus fruits.
Jaw, mouth, and facial pain; headache; clicking noise when opening or closing mouth.	Temporomandibular disorder (see page 203).	Call doctor or dentist for advice and appointment.
Pain and/or tightness in face and jaw muscles; toothache; worn teeth.	Tooth grinding (see page 85).	Call dentist for advice and appointment.
Gray film on gums; red, painful, bleeding gums; bad breath; bad taste in mouth.	Trench mouth—bacterial infection of gums; appears suddenly, often returns.	Call dentist for advice and appointment. Left untreated, can cause permanent gum damage, loss of teeth.

spicy foods such as garlic, hot peppers, and salami; and strong-smelling foods such as anchovies and tuna.

➤ Drink at least 8 glasses of water every day.

FOR MORE HELP

Information line: Richter Center for the Treatment of Breath Disorders, 800-210-2110, M–F 8–8 EST. Treats people with chronic bad breath and provides facts about the condition.

Web access: American Dental Association. After logging on to the Internet, type: *http://www.ada.org.* Select *Consumer Information,* then click on *Cleaning Your Teeth and Gums* or *Your Diet and Dental Health.* You'll find advice on proper brushing and flossing and a list of dentists by state.

Canker Sores

SIGNS AND SYMPTOMS

- Painful sores on the gums and tongue and inside lips. They can be white, gray, or yellowish, with a red rim.
- A tingling feeling just before a sore appears.
- Pain that may increase when eating or talking.
- Fever and swollen glands (sometimes).

A tear or break in the flesh inside the mouth can lead to canker sores. They're a common ailment; teenagers and women are the most likely to get them. Most often, they heal themselves in 7 to 10 days. The causes aren't clear, but some triggers include:

- Injury to the mouth's lining from chipped or jagged teeth, dental work, or dentures.
- Damage from rough toothbrushing.
- Burns from hot foods or liquids.
- Soreness from sour foods (such as lemons) or acidic foods (tomatoes or oranges).
- Food allergies.
- Vitamin and mineral shortages.

WHAT YOU CAN DO NOW

Home treatments can ease the pain of canker sores. Try these:

- Rinse your mouth about 4 times a day with 8 ounces of warm water mixed with one-half teaspoon of salt. Don't swallow.
- Rub an ice cube or Popsicle on the sore.
- Apply a paste of baking soda and water.
- Avoid spicy, sour, or acidic foods, which may make the sore worse.
- Put a wet tea bag on the sore area.
- Use an over-the-counter salve or an antiseptic mouthwash made for canker sores.

WHEN TO CALL THE DOCTOR OR DENTIST

- If you get sores and a fever of 100 degrees or higher, or swollen glands.
- If the sores last longer than 3 weeks; this may mean a serious problem, such as oral cancer.
- If you have severe pain. Your doctor may prescribe painkillers or antibiotics.
- If you suspect that tooth or denture problems are causing your canker sores. Talk to your dentist; the sores are not likely to heal until the cause is fixed.

HOW TO PREVENT IT

- Clean your teeth gently with a soft brush, and floss daily. Buy toothpaste that's free of the detergent sodium lauryl sulfate, which may dry out the lining of the mouth, leaving the insides of the cheeks and the gums easy to irritate.
- Don't eat foods that seem to trigger the sores.
- Take a multivitamin/mineral supplement.

FOR MORE HELP

Organization: The American Academy of Otolaryngology–Head and Neck Surgery, One Prince Street, Alexandria, VA 22314-3357. 703-836-4444, M–F 8:30–5 EST. Ask for the brochure on canker sores and fever blisters.

Web access: Healthtouch. After logging on to the Internet, type: *http://www.healthtouch.com/level1/leaflets/101228/101300.htm.* Click on *Canker Sores.* Offers advice and suggests treatments.

Cold Sores

SIGNS AND SYMPTOMS

- Painful blisters on or around the lips or mouth.
- Tingling, prickling, or itching on the lips or mouth (often just before cold sores appear).
- Fever and swollen neck glands with the first outbreak only.

Cold sores are caused by the herpes simplex virus. After a first outbreak, often during childhood, the virus may lie dormant for years, but it can become active at any time. Triggers include fever (the sores are sometimes called fever blisters), infection, stress, sun or windy weather, and certain foods such as chocolate, nuts, or seeds.

Like **canker sores** (see opposite page), they are common and aren't a major health concern unless your immune system is weakened by some other illness, such as **AIDS** (see page 224).

But they are catching, so take care not to spread the virus by contact. Don't touch a cold sore and then touch your eyes: You could cause a serious eye infection. Also, herpes cold sores on the mouth can be spread to the genitals (see **sexually transmitted diseases** chart, page 225). When you have a cold sore or are with someone who does, don't kiss or have oral sex.

WHAT YOU CAN DO NOW

Cold sores most often clear up on their own in 7 to 10 days. You can't cure them, but to relieve pain:

- Apply an ice cube to the sore spot for a few minutes at a time.
- Don't eat sour, spicy, or acidic foods. They may make the sores worse.
- Use a lip salve—plain petroleum jelly works well—to ease dryness and prevent cracked lips.
- If you get cold sores often, ask a doctor to prescribe medicine you can use when you feel the first signs of an outbreak.

WHEN TO CALL THE DOCTOR

Call for a prompt appointment:

- If you have a cold sore and feel any eye pain, or if your vision is affected. You may have a herpes infection in your eye.

Call for advice:

- If you get sores and a fever of 100 degrees or higher and/or chills.
- If your cold sores last longer than 2 weeks or come back often.

HOW TO PREVENT IT

- Get a new toothbrush after you've had cold sores.
- Wear a hat and use sunblock on your lips if sun appears to trigger cold sores.
- If stress seems to bring on cold sores, find ways to relax: Exercise and practice yoga or meditation (see **relax,** page 309).

These sores are catching. To keep from spreading them:

- Wash your hands often, and don't share tableware, towels, or razors.
- Don't share lip products or kiss anyone during an outbreak.
- Don't touch the infected area.
- Don't touch a cold sore and then touch your eye. This can cause a serious eye problem.

FOR MORE HELP

Organization: The American Academy of Otolaryngology–Head and Neck Surgery, One Prince Street, Alexandria, VA 22314-3357. 703-836-4444, M–F 8:30–5 EST. Ask for the brochure on fever blisters and canker sores.

Web access: Healthtouch. After logging on to the Internet, type: *http://www.healthtouch.com/level1/leaflets/101228/101300.htm.* Click on *Fever Blisters.* Offers advice and suggests treatment.

Toothache

SIGNS AND SYMPTOMS

Tooth decay:

- Sharp pain in a tooth, often when you bite or chew.
- Ache or soreness in teeth, gums, or jaw.
- Bad breath or bad taste in your mouth—a sign of severe decay or an abscess (infection).

Tooth abscess:

- Severe pain in the tooth or jaw.
- A loose tooth.
- Red, swollen, or bleeding gums.
- Fever.
- Earache.
- Swollen glands in the neck.

Cavities are the most common reason for toothache. They are caused by dental plaque, a sticky substance made up of food bits, saliva, and bacteria. Plaque makes acids that eat away the enamel on teeth. A toothache can also be caused by a bit of food stuck between the gum and a tooth, or something as serious as:

- Impacted teeth (teeth that don't grow out fully or that come in at a bad angle) pressing on other teeth or trapping food.
- **Tooth grinding** (see page 85), which can crack teeth.
- Gum disease.
- Pressure from infected or stuffed-up sinuses (see **sinusitis,** page 100).
- Jaws that don't line up right (see **temporomandibular disorder,** page 203).

SENSITIVE TEETH

If heat or cold makes a tooth hurt, you could have an ailment known as dentinal hypersensitivity. This occurs when enamel, the outer covering of the tooth, thins, cracks, or wears away. It's brought on by age, receding gums, dental surgery, or repeated brushing with hard-bristled toothbrushes or "whitening" toothpastes with abrasives.

You can help relieve it and prevent further damage by using a toothpaste made for sensitive teeth and a brush with soft bristles. If pain persists, see your dentist.

WHAT YOU CAN DO NOW

You'll need to see the dentist, above all if you have signs of an abscess. Until then, these home treatments can relieve some pain:

- Use dental floss to remove trapped food bits. Rinse with warm salt water (see **tips on tooth and gum care,** page 84).
- Suck on an ice cube to numb your gum, or put a cold pack on your jaw.
- If cold doesn't work, try heat. Put a hot compress on your jaw, and rinse your mouth with warm salt water.
- Put a wet tea bag (black tea) on a sore gum for 30 minutes to ease soreness, or to stop bleeding.
- Put oil of cloves on an aching tooth with a cotton swab every 20 minutes for pain.
- Make a temporary filling for a broken or lost filling from an over-the-counter product sold in many drugstores.
- Take an over-the-counter pain reliever. Don't take aspirin if you think you might be about to have dental work—it can increase bleeding. (Never give aspirin to a child under 12 who has chicken pox, flu, a cold, or any other illness you suspect of being caused by a virus; see box on **Reye's syndrome,** page 96.)
- Don't put aspirin directly on the gums—it can burn the tissues.

WHEN TO CALL THE DENTIST

Call for a prompt appointment:

- If you have any symptoms of an abscess. You may need emergency care.

Call for advice:

- If your toothache lasts longer than a day or two; if you have throbbing pain in a tooth that doesn't go away; or if heat, cold, or pressure makes the tooth hurt. You may have a cavity.
- If you have swollen, red, and painful gums. You may have gum disease or an impacted tooth.

HOW TO PREVENT IT

- Brush at least twice a day using a toothpaste with fluoride and a soft-bristled toothbrush. Floss every day. Replace your toothbrush every few months.
- Don't eat sweet and sticky foods, which damage tooth enamel.
- Get a cleaning every 6 months, and see a dentist every year.

FOR MORE HELP

Organization: American Dental Association, Department of Public Education and Information, 211 E. Chicago Ave., Chicago, IL 60611. 312-440-2593, 8:30–5 CST. Write for pamphlets on caring for teeth and gums. **Web site:** *http://www.ada.org*. Select *Consumer Education*.

Organization: American Academy of Periodontology, 737 N. Michigan Ave., Suite 800, Chicago, IL 60611-2690. Write to request brochures on dental care. Include a business-size, self-addressed, stamped envelope.

Book: *Tooth Fitness: Your Guide to Healthy Teeth,* by Thomas McGuire, D.D.S. A reader-friendly guide to tooth care. St. Martin's Press, 1994, $16.95.

TIPS ON TOOTH AND GUM CARE

Safeguard your smile by cleaning your teeth and gums at least twice a day. Before you buy a toothbrush, toothpaste, or floss, look for the American Dental Association's seal of approval.

- Get a good toothbrush. Soft, "end-rounded" bristles are best. Make sure the brush fits your mouth—you should be able to reach every tooth easily. Be sure your child's toothbrush isn't too big or too hard.
- Replace your toothbrush every 3 to 4 months, or sooner if the bristles get bent or splayed out. Worn brushes don't clean well and can hurt your gums. Many brushes have color markers that change when it's time to buy a new one.
- Keep your brush clean, and don't let others use it.
- An electric toothbrush can be a help if you use it right. And it may get a child to brush more often. Ask your dentist for advice.
- Devices that use a jet of water to remove food particles from teeth are helpful for people who wear braces, bridges, or partial dentures. But they are meant to improve—not replace—regular flossing and brushing.
- Use a toothpaste or gel with fluoride, which helps protect teeth from decay.
- Some products that claim to whiten teeth may not be safe. They can harm the enamel. Ask your dentist before you use these or other tooth products with special claims.
- Start dental care with your baby's first teeth. Don't let your child fall asleep with a bottle of milk or juice—sweet liquids cling to baby teeth and invite decay that can cause tooth loss.
- Take your child to the dentist before his or her first birthday—sooner, if you think there is a problem.

Cleaning tips

- Don't rush. Take enough time to reach all the surfaces of all of your teeth.
- Hold the brush at a 45-degree angle to your gums so the tips of the bristles point into the gumline. Move it gently back and forth in very short strokes, brushing about half a tooth at a time.
- Be sure to brush the inner surfaces of your teeth. Get the inside of your front teeth as well.
- Don't forget to brush your tongue, but be gentle.

How to floss

Floss once a day to clean places your toothbrush can't reach.

- Floss comes in many types: Choose one that feels comfortable and that doesn't cut your gums.
- To floss: Break off about 18 inches of dental floss and wind it around the middle finger of each hand. Pinch it between your thumbs and forefingers, leaving about an inch of floss. Use a gentle sawing motion to slip it between your teeth. Do not jerk or snap the floss into the gums.
- When the floss reaches the gumline, curve it into a C shape against one tooth. Slide it gently up under the gum. Don't press hard; you don't want to cut the gum.
- Hold the floss against the tooth. Scrape the side of the tooth gently, moving the floss away from the gum. Repeat the flossing on the back side of your last tooth.
- Your gums may bleed a bit the first 5 or 6 days after you begin flossing. But if they bleed after that, call your dentist. You may be hurting your gums.
- You can buy other products besides floss for cleaning between teeth—picks, sticks, and small brushes.

Tooth Grinding

SIGNS AND SYMPTOMS

- Tension, tightness, or pain in the face and jaw muscles.
- Toothache.
- Mild to severe headache or migraine.
- Looseness or aching in the teeth, often upon waking.
- Worn or broken teeth.

Tooth grinding (bruxism) is a common problem, mostly among women. It's thought to be caused by many factors, such as an abnormal bite, crooked or missing teeth, high levels of stress, or a **sleep disorder** (see page 292).

Until you have symptoms, you may not know you're grinding or clenching your teeth, above all if you do it in your sleep. But you may be wearing down your teeth and cracking them.

WHAT YOU CAN DO NOW

➤ During the day, practice letting your jaw relax while keeping your teeth slightly apart.

➤ Don't chew gum, tobacco, pencils, or any other nonfood object.

➤ Hold a warm washcloth to the side of your face. This may help to relax your jaw.

➤ If you suspect that stress is the problem, try to reduce it with exercise and relaxation techniques such as meditation, deep breathing, or yoga (see **stress,** page 222, and **relax**, page 309).

WHEN TO CALL THE DOCTOR

➤ If you still have symptoms after a month of home treatment, or if you think a bad bite or a missing tooth is causing the problem. You may need to have your dentist fit you with a mouth guard or bite plate.

➤ If you have tooth pain or a jaw ache for more than a day or two. These symptoms could be the result of tooth decay (see **toothache,** page 82) or a sign of **temporomandibular disorder** (see page 203).

➤ If you think stress is still causing problems. You may want to seek counseling or ask your dentist to prescribe a jaw muscle relaxant.

HOW TO PREVENT IT

➤ Learn how to ease your stress and stay as relaxed as you can, especially around bedtime. Take a warm bath or shower before bed, listen to soothing music, and practice meditation, deep breathing, or yoga.

➤ Cut down on food and drinks with caffeine, such as coffee, tea, colas, and chocolate.

➤ Practice good posture. Slouching or hunching can trigger teeth clenching.

FOR MORE HELP

Organization: American Dental Association, Department of Public Education and Information, 211 E. Chicago Ave., Chicago, IL 60611. 312-440-2593, 8:30–5 CST. Write for the pamphlet "Do You Grind Your Teeth?"

Nose, Throat, Lungs, & Chest

Allergies

SIGNS AND SYMPTOMS

Hay fever (allergic rhinitis):
- Frequent sneezing.
- Itchy or runny eyes.
- Runny or stuffy nose.
- Itching in back of throat or on roof of mouth.

Allergic asthma:
- Sneezing, wheezing, and coughing.
- In some cases, trouble breathing.

Food allergies:
- Outbreaks of itchy, red, or bumpy skin.
- Upset stomach.

Drug allergies:
- Outbreaks of itchy, red, or bumpy skin, sometimes with flulike symptoms such as headache, low fever, and joint pain.

When your immune system overreacts to things that are mostly harmless, you have allergies. In fighting what it spots as an invader, the immune system produces a substance called histamine that can provoke the sneezing, itching, and other symptoms of allergies.

Hay fever is one of the most common allergies—nearly 1 in 5 Americans has it. Pollen, bits of animal skin called dander, household dust, and molds can set it off.

Food allergies—which are rare—occur more often in children than adults; children tend to outgrow them by the age of 3. The foods that most often cause allergies include nuts, eggs, and milk. Seafood and peanuts tend to produce the strongest reactions, even shock or death in rare cases; the treatment is a shot of epinephrine. People seldom outgrow seafood and peanut allergies. Reactions to drugs such as penicillin or to insect stings can be just as deadly (see **bee and wasp stings,** page 27, and **shock from allergy,** page 24).

Many allergies can be handled at home. If yours are severe, though, your doctor might prescribe antihistamines, steroid nasal sprays, or shots to relieve your symptoms. Some people with allergies find relief in alternative treatments such as homeopathy, acupuncture, or herbs.

WHAT YOU CAN DO NOW

- If you're allergic to pollen, stay indoors with the air conditioning on (if you have it) on days with high pollen counts.
- Don't smoke, and avoid smoky places, dust, and insect sprays. Stay inside on days with high pollution levels.
- If you have hay fever, try over-the-counter antihistamines and keep track of which ones work best. Don't mix antihistamines with prescription drugs or other over-the-counter drugs without checking with your doctor or pharmacist. (**Note:** Phenylpropanolamine—found in some decongestants—has in rare cases been linked to

Breathing Problems and Coughs

The causes of most breathing problems and coughs—flus, colds, and allergies—clear up with time. If your problem doesn't go away, it could signal an illness that needs treatment.

SYMPTOMS	WHAT IT MIGHT BE	WHAT YOU CAN DO
Wheezing; tight chest or throat; itching and hives; swollen eyes, lips, and tongue; panic; stomach cramps or vomiting; bluish skin (sometimes).	Shock from allergy (see page 24).	Call 911 **right away.**
Shortness of breath; crushing chest pain, pressure, or squeezed feeling (perhaps spreading to jaw, neck, back, or arms); sweating; nausea.	Heart attack (see page 39).	Call 911 **right away.**
Shortness of breath, sharp chest pain, dry cough; symptoms of shock—cold hands and feet, rapid pulse, confusion, moist skin.	Collapsed lung.	Call 911 or go to emergency room **right away.**
Wheezing and shortness of breath; lasting wet (mucus-making) or dry cough.	Chronic bronchitis or emphysema (see page 92). • Croup (see page 258).	If skin turns blue or purple, call 911 or go to emergency room **right away.** If not, call doctor for prompt appointment.
Sudden shortness of breath and sharp chest pain, cough (sometimes with bloody phlegm), anxiety, loss of consciousness (sometimes).	Blood clot that travels through body to block artery in lungs.	Call 911 or go to emergency room **right away.**
Wheezing; quick, shallow breathing; coughing (sometimes with thick mucus); tightness in chest; gasping for breath.	Asthma (see page 89).	If skin turns blue or person becomes confused, call 911 or go to emergency room **right away.** If not, call doctor for prompt appointment.

(continued)

Breathing Problems and Coughs *(continued)*		
SYMPTOMS	**WHAT IT MIGHT BE**	**WHAT YOU CAN DO**
"Smoker's cough" (sometimes with bloody mucus), wheezing and shortness of breath, chest pain, fatigue, weight loss, lack of appetite.	Lung cancer (see page 97). • Pneumonia (see page 98). • Tuberculosis (see page 105).	Call doctor for prompt appointment.
Cough; fever; runny nose; sore throat; muscle aches; red, itchy bumps all over body.	Measles (see page 267).	If bumps start to bleed or seizures occur (very rare), call 911 or go to emergency room **right away.** If they don't, treat at home with rest and fluids. Call doctor for advice if symptoms last longer than a week.
In children ages 6–12: first symptoms like a cold; after 2 weeks, cough becomes almost constant and is followed by whooping sound, vomiting, choking.	Whooping cough (see page 273).	If child turns blue or stops breathing, call 911 and start **CPR** (see page 19). Call doctor for advice if symptoms linger or get worse.
Sharp, sudden chest pain that gets worse with deep breathing; fever and chills; headache; weakness; dry cough.	Pleurisy—inflamed lining of lungs.	Call doctor for prompt appointment.
Cough, hoarseness, and lost voice (sometimes); sore throat; fever (sometimes).	Laryngitis—inflamed voice box. May be caused by bacterial or viral infection, or by strained vocal cords.	Call doctor for advice. Avoid talking, drink lots of fluids, and take nonprescription throat lozenges.
Coughing and sneezing, congestion, runny nose, sore throat, headache, aching muscles, fever and fatigue (sometimes).	Flu (see page 96). • Cold (see page 94).	Rest, drink lots of fluids, and take over-the-counter painkillers. Don't give aspirin to child under 12 (see box on **Reye's syndrome,** page 96).

stroke. Use decongestants with pseudoephedrine instead.)

- If you're allergic to insect stings or have severe reactions to some foods, ask your doctor for an emergency kit with an antihistamine and an epinephrine shot. Always carry the kit with you.
- If you often have itchy or teary eyes, try over-the-counter eyedrops, or ask your doctor to prescribe antihistamine eyedrops.

WHEN TO CALL THE DOCTOR

Call 911 **right away:**

➤ If you get a rapid heartbeat and skin welts along with flushing, itching, dizziness, and trouble breathing. You could be having a potentially fatal reaction called **shock from allergy** (see page 24).

Call 911 or go to an emergency room **right away:**

➤ If it becomes very difficult or painful to breathe. You may be having an attack of **asthma** (see this page).

➤ If you have severe stomach cramps, vomiting, bloating, or diarrhea. This could signal a reaction to a food.

Call for advice:

➤ If you have recurring allergies. Your doctor may refer you to an allergy specialist, who can test you to find out what causes your attacks.

HOW TO PREVENT IT

➤ Learn what you're allergic to, and avoid it. (If you're allergic to a common drug such as penicillin, wear a medical alert tag.)

➤ If you're allergic to cats or dogs, stay away from them—or at least see that your pets are bathed often and keep them out of your bedroom.

➤ If you're allergic to molds, keep your house clean and dry. Key spots are bathrooms (chiefly shower stalls), refrigerator drip trays, basements, and closets.

➤ If you sneeze and cough year-round, you may be among the millions of people allergic to dust mites (tiny bugs that live in house dust). Try to keep your house—your bedroom most of all—dust-free. Encase mattresses in nonallergenic covers. Wash your bedding weekly in hot water. Leave your floors bare or use washable area rugs instead of carpets. Avoid upholstered furniture and other dust-catchers. Also, vacuum often (use a nonporous bag), or better yet, have someone else do it.

➤ If you have a severe food allergy, read package labels. When dining out, ask what's in dishes before you order.

FOR MORE HELP

Information line: National Jewish Center for Immunology and Respiratory Medicine, 1400 Jackson St., Denver, CO 80206. 800-222-5864, M–F 8–5 MST. Nurses answer questions, make referrals, and send brochures. 800-552-5864, Lung Facts, offers recorded facts on breathing problems.

Book: *The Best Guide to Allergy,* by Nathan Schultz, M.D., Allan V. Giannini, M.D., Terrance T. Change, M.D., and Diane Wong. Humana Press, 1995, $14.50.

Book: *Empty Your Bucket: Practical Steps to Overcome Allergy and Allergic Asthma,* by Stephen Astor, M.D. Two A's Industries, 1994, $14.95.

Web access: American Academy of Allergy, Asthma & Immunology. After logging on to the Internet, type: *http://execpc.com/~edi/aaaai.html.* Scroll to *Public Education Materials,* then click on any of the *Tips to Remember* brochures.

Asthma

SIGNS AND SYMPTOMS

Mild or moderate attack:

- Coughing.
- Feeling of tightness in the chest.
- Noisy breathing (wheezing).
- Trouble catching your breath.

Severe attack:

- Rapid, shallow breathing.
- Trouble talking because of rapid breathing.
- Racing pulse.
- Panic.

Asthma clogs the airways in your lungs. If you have it, you can breathe normally most of the time, but not during an asthma attack. Then the tiny airways in your lungs called bronchial tubes swell and fill with mucus, making you cough, wheeze, and gasp for breath (see color illustrations, page 168). Attacks can come on fast. They can last from a few minutes to a day or longer.

No one knows why some people have asthma and others don't; we do know, though, that most asthma comes from allergies, mainly to things you inhale. Dust, pollen, pet dander (bits of skin), germs, molds, smoke, and chemical fumes can spark an attack. So can exercise, cold air, certain foods—seafood or peanuts, for instance—emotional peaks and dips, a common cold, and pregnancy. About a third of women with asthma find that it gets worse when they're pregnant. Recent research also points to impaired lung muscles as a cause. For a few people, aspirin and some other painkillers can start an attack.

Asthma is a chronic disease. That means you may have it the rest of your life, with symptoms that can come and go. It often starts during childhood, and it's more common and more serious among African American children than others. Many youngsters seem to outgrow it, but it can return when they're adults.

Without prompt medical help, severe asthma can be fatal. Once you know how to manage it, though, chances are you can control it by taking medications and by staying away from things that trigger an attack.

WHAT YOU CAN DO NOW

- Remain calm and quiet. Staying relaxed will help you breathe better.
- Don't lie down. You can breathe better when you sit upright and lean forward slightly, resting your elbows on a table.
- Keep all your medicines in one place. They may include a bronchodilator—a spray drug to open your airways—in an inhaler that controls the dose. Rinse your mouth with water each time you use it to prevent thrush, a yeast infection (see **fungal infections,** page 155).
- Use your medication exactly as your doctor has told you to. Write down each dose and the time you took it; overdoses can be dangerous.
- Ask a friend, coworker, teacher, or family member to stay with you.

WHEN TO CALL THE DOCTOR

Call 911 or go to an emergency room **right away** if you note these signs of a lack of oxygen:

- Trouble talking because you feel you're suffocating.
- Nostrils flaring with the extra effort needed to pull in air.
- Skin between the ribs looking sucked-in as you inhale.
- Lips and nails tinged blue.

Call for a prompt appointment:

- The first time you have long-lasting trouble with breathing, with or without coughing and wheezing.
- If the medicine your doctor prescribes fails to work as quickly as it's supposed to.
- If you cough up green, yellow, or bloody mucus.
- If you feel strange new symptoms. These may be side effects of your drugs or may mean your asthma is getting worse.

HOW TO PREVENT IT

Anyone with asthma should be under a doctor's care. Ask if you should learn to use a peak flow meter. It measures how much air your lungs can push out in a single breath; when you use it every day, it can give early warning of a coming attack. Ask if you should use an inhaler, or pills, to reduce swelling in your bronchial tubes. Also:

- Track your attacks by keeping a diary: How frequent? How severe? What happened just before? Notice whether certain foods, drugs, or actions seem to bring on an attack. You can't avoid everything that might bring on an attack. Still, keep an eye on:
  - Pollen and dirty air. Keep windows closed and use air conditioning if you have it.
  - Dust. Vacuum often, wearing a dust mask. Or, if you can, ask someone else to do it.
  - Humidity. Dust mites and molds (common allergy triggers) love damp air, so use a dehumidifier to control them. Clean the tank often.
  - Dust-catchers in the bedroom, such as large shelves of books. Move them out.

- Bedding. Use foam-rubber pillows. Avoid wool blankets and down comforters; use washable cotton blankets instead. Wash blankets every week. Wash sheets and pillowcases more often if you can. Use a dryer; pollen sticks to anything hung outside.
- Pets. If being around cats or dogs causes attacks, don't keep pets with hair or fur. If you can't bear to part with Kitty or Fido, try to bathe your pet every week and keep it out of the bedroom.

➤ Don't smoke, and stay out of smoky rooms (see **smoking and illness,** page 220).

➤ Exercise regularly, but don't overdo it. Swimming is good—unless chlorine in pools bothers you—since humidity helps ease breathing. If a certain exercise triggers your asthma, try others.

➤ Lower your risk of colds and flu by washing your hands often and getting a flu shot every year.

➤ Learn relaxation methods such as yoga, meditation, or deep breathing; easing stress can reduce the number and strength of attacks (see **relax,** page 309).

FOR MORE HELP

Information line: National Jewish Center for Immunology and Respiratory Medicine, 1400 Jackson St., Denver, CO 80206. 800-222-5864, M–F 8–5 MST. Nurses answer questions, make referrals, and send brochures. 800-552-5864, Lung Facts, offers recorded information on breathing problems.

Information line: Asthma and Allergy Foundation of America, 800-727-8462, 24-hour recording. 202-466-7643, M–F 9–5 EST. Fax: 202-466-8940. Lists local support groups and books, pamphlets, and videos for sale.

Organization: Allergy and Asthma Network/Mothers of Asthmatics, 3554 Chain Bridge Rd., Suite 200, Fairfax, VA 22030-2709. 800-878-4403, M–F 9–5 EST. Provides phone information and brochures on asthma. **Web site:** *http://www.podi.com/health/aanma/index.html.*

Book: *The Asthma Self-Help Book,* by Paul J. Hannaway, M.D. A thorough, easy-to-read book about living with asthma. Prima Publishing, 1994, $13.95.

Web access: American Lung Association. After logging on to the Internet, type: *http://www.lungusa.org/homepage.html.* Click on *Learn About Lung Health,* then on *Asthma* or *Asthma in Children.*

Video: *Asthma in Children at Time of Diagnosis.* Clear overview of causes and treatments, with 4 reports—Understanding the Diagnosis, What Happens Next?, Treatment and Management, and Issues and Answers. Time Life Medical, 1996, $19.95. Sold in many pharmacies; for one near you, call 800-588-9959.

Bronchitis, Acute

SIGNS AND SYMPTOMS

- Hacking dry or wet cough that brings up green, gray, or yellowish mucus.
- Wheezing and shortness of breath.
- Pain in the upper chest, made worse by fits of coughing.
- Fever of 100 degrees or higher.

Acute bronchitis is a swelling in the branches of the windpipe (the bronchial tubes) that carry air to and from the lungs. When these air tubes become irritated and swollen, they produce extra mucus that clogs the airways and causes fits of coughing.

Most people have had an attack of acute bronchitis, which comes on fast and doesn't last long. It can come when a virus that causes a cold or throat infection spreads to the airways. The illness can also be brought on by agents such as tobacco smoke, chemical fumes, or dust. If your heart and lungs are healthy, bronchitis most often clears up in a few days and vanishes when the infection that brought it on does.

If bouts of bronchitis keep coming back, you may have **chronic bronchitis** (see page 92).

WHAT YOU CAN DO NOW

➤ Take acetaminophen or ibuprofen to fight

fever and pain. (Never give aspirin to a child under 12 who has a cold, chicken pox, flu, or any other illness you suspect of being caused by a virus; see box on **Reye's syndrome,** page 96.)

- If you have a lasting dry cough, try an over-the-counter cough medicine. (If you have a cough that is bringing up mucus, don't take medicine labeled as a cough suppressant; doing so could cause mucus to build up in your lungs.)
- Stay home in a warm room, and rest.
- Inhale steam from a vaporizer or a pot of hot water, or take hot showers (see **humidifiers and vaporizers** box, opposite page). This will loosen mucus in your lungs.
- Drink a lot of liquids—at least 8 to 10 big glasses a day.
- Get a massage for sore back and chest muscles.

WHEN TO CALL THE DOCTOR

- If symptoms don't ease in 3 or 4 days, or if your bronchitis keeps coming back.
- If the person with bronchitis is an infant or elderly.
- If your mucus increases or becomes darker or thicker. You may have a bacterial infection that requires antibiotics.
- If you have a lung disease or heart disease and you suffer a bronchitis attack.
- If you cough up blood or become more short of breath.
- If you have a fever of 102 degrees or higher.

HOW TO PREVENT IT

- Don't smoke (see **smoking and illness,** page 220). Avoid smoky places and other places with lots of fumes.
- Treat colds and flus promptly.
- On days with poor air quality, avoid exercise, outdoor work, or long outings.

FOR MORE HELP

Information line: National Jewish Center for Immunology and Respiratory Medicine, 1400 Jackson St., Denver, CO 80206. 800-222-5864, M–F 8–5 MST. Nurses answer questions, make referrals, and send out brochures. 800-552-5864, Lung Facts, offers recorded advice on breathing problems. **Web site:** After logging on to the Internet, type: *http://www.njc.org/MFhtml/URI_MF.html.*

Information line: American Lung Association, 800-LUNG-USA (586-4872), M–F 9–5 your time. Connects you to a local ALA chapter, which provides advice on bronchitis and other lung diseases and can refer you to support groups and programs for quitting smoking.

Chronic Bronchitis and Emphysema

SIGNS AND SYMPTOMS

Chronic bronchitis:

- Usually begins with a "smoker's cough"—a morning cough that brings up mucus.
- As the disease goes on, coughing more often and shortness of breath.
- In the final stages, coughing and wheezing almost nonstop.

Emphysema:

In the early stages, you may have no symptoms. Later symptoms include:

- A frequent dry cough.
- Shortness of breath: at first, only with exertion; later, with any activity.
- In the late stages, chest that is swollen and barrel-shaped from air trapped in lungs.
- Weight loss.
- Lung infections that keep coming back.

Chronic bronchitis and emphysema often come on at the same time. ("Chronic" means you may have it the rest of your life, with symptoms that come and go.) Together, they're known as chronic obstructive pulmonary disease, or COPD. They damage the lungs and the bronchial tubes—the branches of the windpipe that carry air to and from the lungs—making it hard to breathe.

Chronic bronchitis: When you cough up mucus for 3 months or more, 2 years in a row, you have chronic bronchitis. It is usually linked to smoking, although dirty air, fumes, dust, and allergies can also play a role. If you don't treat it and you still smoke or breathe fumes, you leave yourself open to other diseases, such as **pneumonia** (see page 98) or emphysema.

Chronic bronchitis affects 7.5 million Americans. Early treatment—and quitting smoking—can ease symptoms and slow the disease. A small number of cases are fatal.

Emphysema: When the lungs are damaged by tobacco smoke (and often by the coughing of chronic bronchitis), the millions of tiny air sacs inside them can't pass along enough oxygen to the bloodstream. You use more and more energy gasping for breath; you tire quickly and lose weight. Even a short walk may leave you breathless. Because emphysema makes the heart work harder, it can lead to heart disease. It also leaves you open to lung diseases such as pneumonia.

The disease, which can't be cured, most often strikes people over 50, although a small group of those with a defect in their genes may get symptoms in their 20s and 30s. A blood test can tell who has this problem; these people should never smoke.

Emphysema kills more Americans—90,000 a year—than any other chronic lung disease. There are 2 important things to know about it: 1) If you don't smoke, you have very little chance of getting it. 2) If you do smoke, you should quit even if you think you're in good health. Because emphysema often has no symptoms in the early stages, it can sneak up on you. By the time most people find out they have it, they have lost 50 to 70 percent of their lung capacity.

Treatment is limited. A therapist may design a program to help you exercise more. Your doctor may prescribe a bronchodilator—a drug to open your airways—and, in later stages, pure oxygen, which helps some people breathe better.

HINTS ON HUMIDIFIERS AND VAPORIZERS

Humidifiers put cool moisture into the air. Vaporizers make steam. Many people with chronic dry noses and throats, sinus problems, or lung ailments use one or the other to boost the moisture in the air so they can breathe more easily. People who live in dry climates, such as parts of the American Southwest, also find them helpful.

Ask a doctor before using either device, and take extra care when using one in a child's room. Humid air promotes the growth of both molds and household dust mites, so it can cause problems for people with allergies or asthma. You can also get a problem called "humidifier lung"—an allergic reaction to mold and other organisms that can grow in the device—so clean your humidifier daily using bleach. Scalding water from a vaporizer can inflict burns, and water and electricity together always pose a danger of shock.

For more help: You can order a paper on cleaning humidifiers from the Lung Line, sponsored by the National Jewish Center for Immunology and Respiratory Medicine, by calling 800-222-5864, M–F 8–5 MST.

WHAT YOU CAN DO NOW

- Don't smoke (see **smoking and illness,** page 220), and stay away from smoky places. Smoking is the main cause of emphysema and chronic bronchitis. Studies show that giving up tobacco—even after symptoms appear—can greatly slow lung damage.
- Get a flu shot every year and a vaccination against pneumonia.
- Stay inside if the air is very polluted.
- Exercise gently but daily in good-quality air.
- Take good care of yourself, and if you get a lung infection, have it treated promptly.

WHEN TO CALL THE DOCTOR

- If you have a mild cough that doesn't go away for months.
- If you often become breathless after mild exertion, such as climbing a flight of stairs.

HOW TO PREVENT IT

- Don't smoke.
- Treat bronchitis promptly to guard against emphysema.

FOR MORE HELP

Information line: National Jewish Center for Immunology and Respiratory Medicine, 1400 Jackson St., Denver, CO 80206. 800-222-5864, M–F 8–5 MST. Nurses answer questions, make referrals, and send brochures. 800-552-5864, Lung Facts, offers recorded facts on breathing problems.

Information line: American Lung Association, 800-LUNG-USA (586-4872), M–F 9–5 your time. Connects you to a local ALA chapter, which has advice on COPD and other lung diseases and can refer you to support groups and programs for quitting smoking.

Brochure: Agency for Health Care Policy and Research. 800-358-9295 M–F 9–5 EST. Ask for "You Can Quit Smoking."

Book: *Shortness of Breath: A Guide to Better Living and Breathing,* by Andrew L. Ries, M.D. Tells people with bronchitis, emphysema, and other breathing problems how to manage their illness. Mosby Co., 1995, $9.95.

Web access: American Lung Association. After logging on to the Internet, type: *http://www.lungusa.org/homepage.html.* Click on *Learn About Lung Health,* then on *Lung Diseases.* Scroll to *Chronic Bronchitis* or *Emphysema.*

Colds

SIGNS AND SYMPTOMS

- Runny nose.
- Sore throat and hoarseness.
- Watery eyes.
- Coughing.
- Low fever, below 100 degrees.

If you have a scratchy throat, runny nose, and cough, you've most likely caught a viral infection of the head and throat known as the common cold. Colds are caused by more than 200 viruses that get into the body chiefly through the nose and tear ducts.

You can't catch a cold from getting your feet wet or sitting in a drafty room—you get it from a virus. But a few simple safety measures can help protect you from this contagious ailment.

WHAT YOU CAN DO NOW

Nobody has found a cure yet for the common cold, but there are things you can do to feel less sick. They start with staying home from work or school for the first 3 or 4 days—not only to rest and recover, but also to prevent your cold from spreading to other people. Then:

- Drink lots of fluids to avoid dehydration.
- Take a painkiller for aches and fever. (Never give aspirin to a child under 12 who has a cold, chicken pox, flu, or any other illness you suspect of being caused by a virus; see box on **Reye's syndrome,** page 96.)
- If you have a sore throat, try gargling with salt water a few times a day. (Mix 1 teaspoon salt in 8 ounces warm water. Don't swallow.)
- To clear up a stuffy nose, try over-the-counter saline drops or sprays. You can also make your own (mix ½ teaspoon salt in 8 ounces lukewarm water). Use a dropper or a bulb syringe to squirt it into your nose 2 to 4 times a day. Or you can put the solution in the palm of your hand and sniff it in, 1 nostril at a time. Wait a few minutes and then blow your nose gently.

- Don't smoke, and avoid smoky places.
- Taking one 500-milligram tablet of vitamin C four times a day may shorten your cold and make it milder, some researchers say. But taking too much vitamin C can cause diarrhea.
- Use a cool-mist humidifier or a vaporizer or take hot, steamy showers to keep your nasal passages from drying out (see box on **humidifiers and vaporizers**, page 93).

WHEN TO CALL THE DOCTOR

Call for a prompt appointment:

- If you have a fever of 100 degrees or higher and facial swelling and/or severe pain in the ears; you may have an **ear infection** (see page 73).
- If you have severe throat pain and your tonsils or throat have a white or yellow coating; you may have **tonsillitis** (see page 103) or **strep throat** (see pages 101 and 271).
- If you have a severe cough with thick, colored mucus; a cough that lasts more than 10 days; or bluish lips or nails. You may have **pneumonia** (see page 98).

Call for advice:

- If you have a headache with pain around the face, a sore upper jaw, or yellow or green mucus coming from your nose or throat; these are signs of a sinus infection (see **sinusitis,** page 100).
- If a fever lasts longer than 4 days or goes higher than 102 degrees.
- If your cold hasn't improved after 10 days or has gotten worse.

HOW TO PREVENT IT

Cold viruses can be spread through handshakes and can lurk on doorknobs, telephones, and counters. Wash your hands often, above all during cold season in the fall and winter. Also:

- Keep your hands away from your eyes, nose, and mouth.
- Move away from people who are coughing and sneezing.
- Drink lots of fluids.
- Since stress, allergies, and menstrual periods may make you more open to disease, try to rest more and take good care of yourself when you're feeling under the weather.

WHAT TO LOOK FOR IN COLD AND COUGH MEDICINES

Cold medicines are a $1.9 billion-a-year industry. Many combine far more ingredients than you need, and some may even make you feel worse.

Doctors suggest you buy generic drugs with only 1 ingredient—such as aspirin, a cough suppressant, or an oral decongestant—rather than brand-name "mega" formulas, which try to tackle many symptoms at once. Here are some drugs that don't really do much to relieve cold symptoms:

- **Antihistamines.** Although they help to clear up runny noses and sneezing, they can also dry out the nasal passages too much. Also, in older men, they may cause urination problems.
- **Expectorants.** There is no proof that these loosen mucus.
- **Nasal decongestant sprays.** Although they help shrink swollen nasal passages, they often have a "rebound effect," meaning that the nasal tissues may swell back up, sometimes even worse, after a few days of use.

Cough suppressants (antitussives) also have pros and cons. Some coughs are "productive"—that is, they bring up mucus from the lungs—so it's better not to suppress them. Dry, hacking coughs, though, are best treated with an antitussive syrup or lozenge. The medicine may make you sleepy, so don't drive if you take it. Also, don't take decongestants with certain antidepressants (see chart on **drug combinations to avoid,** page 323).

FOR MORE HELP

Book: *77 Ways to Beat Colds and Flu: A People's Medical Society Book*, by Charles B. Inlander and Cynthia K. Moran. Bantam, 1996, $4.99.

Flu

SIGNS AND SYMPTOMS

- Fever over 103 degrees.
- Chills and muscle aches.
- Fatigue and weakness.
- Headache and eye pain.
- Sore throat.
- Dry cough.

Flu (influenza) is a contagious disease caused by a virus that gets in through the nose or mouth and often invades the lungs. Flu shows up mainly in winter and early spring. The virus changes from year to year, making the rounds of schools, offices, and other public places. Sometimes it mutates—makes a big change in its form—leading to more severe outbreaks.

Children are more likely than others to get the flu, and it's most often mild. Older adults and people with lung disease or other chronic illness have a high risk as well, but for them the disease is often more severe.

Flus and colds are much alike, but flus are more severe, with higher fevers and aches and pains. A bad case of the flu may send a healthy person to bed for 3 to 5 days, but he or she will most likely be well within 1 to 2 weeks.

WHAT YOU CAN DO NOW

The more rest you get, the sooner you'll get well. And staying home keeps you from spreading it at school or work: Flu is catching for 3 or 4 days after symptoms appear. To get well quickly:

- Drink as many fluids—water, juice, hot tea—as you can. Have some frozen juice bars for a change.
- Have chicken soup and bouillon; the heat may relieve the stuffed-up feeling.
- Take a painkiller for aches and fever. (Never give aspirin to a child under 12 who has a cold, flu, chicken pox, or any other illness you suspect of being caused by a virus; see box on **Reye's syndrome,** this page.)
- Avoid over-the-counter medicines aimed at treating more than 1 symptom (see box on **cold medicines,** page 95).
- Ask your doctor about rimantadine, a virus-fighting drug that can reduce the length and strength of Type A flu—the type behind most epidemics—even after the first symptoms appear. By taking it, you may also help family members avoid catching your flu.

REYE'S SYNDROME

This rare disease causes vomiting and sometimes leads to delirium, coma, or even death. Reye's syndrome reached its peak in the late 1970s and early 1980s, with hundreds of cases reported each year, but there are now fewer than 20 cases a year. No age group is immune, although the disease almost always strikes young people, from infants to teens. While its exact causes are unknown, it is connected with aspirin taken during viral infections such as chicken pox and flu.

For this reason, doctors warn that you should never give aspirin to a child under 12 who has chicken pox or any other illness you suspect of being caused by a virus, such as a cold or the flu. Instead, use acetaminophen.

If your child or teenager has a viral infection, begins to vomit, and becomes drowsy or delirious, or confused, disoriented, or eager to fight, he or she may have Reye's syndrome. Call your doctor promptly.

WHEN TO CALL THE DOCTOR

Flus are a special danger for people with chronic illness such as cancer; diabetes; respiratory, heart, or kidney disease; cystic fibrosis; or recurring anemia. If you have one of these—or if you are HIV positive—call your doctor at the first sign of flu symptoms.

Call for a prompt appointment:

- If you have a fever or chest pain that keeps coming back, or if you cough up thick, colored, or bloody mucus; you may be getting **pneumonia** (see page 98) or **bronchitis** (see page 91).

- If you have an earache, facial swelling, drainage from your ear, or severe pain in your face or forehead. These may signal some other illness, such as **sinusitis** (see page 100) or an **ear infection** (see page 73).

Call for advice:

- If you have a fever higher than 102 degrees or that lasts more than 3 to 4 days.

HOW TO PREVENT IT

The flu virus changes every year, so you can't become immune. Also, a flu vaccine might not work if it's designed for a virus different from the one that comes to your area. But if you are over 65 or have a chronic illness, a flu shot every fall is a good idea.

- If you are pregnant, ask your doctor before getting a flu shot.
- If you are allergic to eggs, or think you are, ask your doctor about whether to get a flu shot.

The flu virus is spread in the spray from coughs and sneezes, so keeping away from people who have the flu may lessen your chances of getting it. Also:

- Wash your hands often to reduce your risk of catching a cold or the flu.
- Don't smoke, and stay away from smoky places.
- Keep your immune system healthy by eating well, getting enough sleep, keeping stress levels low, and drinking lots of water.

FOR MORE HELP

Information line: Centers for Disease Control and Prevention's Voice Information System, 404-332-4555, 24-hour automated line. Choose from several topics about the flu and flu shots; you can get information by voice, fax, or mail.

Organization: American Academy of Otolaryngology–Head and Neck Surgery, One Prince Street, Alexandria, VA 22314-3357. 703-836-4444, M–F 8:30–5 EST. Call for their brochure on flu, or look it up on the Internet at: *http://www.netdoor.com/com/entinfo/flu.html.*

Book: *77 Ways to Beat Colds and Flu: A People's Medical Society Book,* by Charles B. Inlander and Cynthia K. Moran. Bantam, 1996, $4.99.

Lung Cancer

SIGNS AND SYMPTOMS

In its early stages, lung cancer has no symptoms. By the time a tumor has grown large enough to cause symptoms, it's often in an advanced stage. Then, symptoms include:

- An increase in a chronic, hacking "smoker's cough," sometimes with blood-streaked mucus. These are often the first signs.
- Recurring bronchitis—inflamed air passages in the lungs.
- Shortness of breath; wheezing; dull, lasting chest pain or sharp chest pain off and on.
- Shoulder, arm, or hand pain and weakness.
- Weight loss or loss of appetite.
- Lasting low fever (below 100 degrees).

Before the widespread use of cigarettes, lung cancer was a rare disease. Today it causes 25 percent of all cancer deaths in the United States. Although lung cancer remains more common among men than women, it now kills more women than breast cancer does.

Smoking is by far the main cause of lung cancer. But genes, other lung disease, and exposure to other cancer-causing substances are also factors.

When a normal cell in the lungs becomes cancerous, it begins to reproduce uncontrollably. It forms a tumor, or mass of tissue, that slowly invades and destroys healthy lung tissue. If not treated, the cancer cells may spread through the blood and the lymph system to other parts of the body, where they can form new tumors. Only 13 percent of all lung cancer patients live for 5 years or longer, but chances increase greatly when it's found and treated early.

WHAT YOU CAN DO NOW

Lung cancer is not something you can treat yourself. But once it is found, your doctor will work with you to decide which treatment—surgery, chemotherapy, radiation, or a combination—is best for you.

You can do much during treatment to improve your chances of recovering and leading an active life:

- Don't smoke, and stay away from smoky places.
- Ask your nurse or doctor to show you exercises that strengthen your chest muscles.
- Join a support group for people with cancer and their families. Studies show emotional support helps people live longer.

WHEN TO CALL THE DOCTOR

- If you have the symptoms listed here.
- After you are diagnosed if you get any new symptoms or get worse.

HOW TO PREVENT IT

- Don't smoke. Even long-term smokers improve their chances of avoiding lung cancer by quitting (see **smoking and illness,** page 220).
- Quitting smoking will not only reduce your risk of getting lung cancer, it will reduce the risk for those close to you; the spouses of smokers have at least a 30 percent higher risk of getting lung cancer from secondhand smoke than do the spouses of nonsmokers.
- Eat plenty of fresh fruits and vegetables. They contain substances (antioxidants) that help the body resist cancer.
- Reduce stress through relaxation, visualization, meditation, or yoga.

FOR MORE HELP

Information line: Cancer Information Service, National Cancer Institute, 800-422-6237, M–F 9–4:30 your time. Provides information, literature, lists of doctors, and news of clinical trials, free of charge.

Information line: American Cancer Society's Cancer Response System, 800-227-2345, M–F 9–5 your time. Provides pamphlets and can refer you to cancer support groups in your area.

Book: *The Stop Smoking Workbook,* by Lori Stevic-Rust and Anita Maximin. A do-it-yourself guide to kicking the habit. New Harbinger Publications, 1996, $17.95.

Web access: American Lung Association. After logging on to the Internet, type: *http://www.lungusa.org/homepage.html.* Click on *Learn About Lung Health,* then *Lung Diseases.* If you're a smoker, click on *Smoking and Tobacco Control.*

Pneumonia

SIGNS AND SYMPTOMS

Common:

- Shaking, chills, and fever as high as 105 degrees.
- Chest pain.
- Mucus that is greenish, greenish-yellow, rust-colored, or streaked with blood.
- Shortness of breath.

Sometimes:

- Sweating, rapid pulse, and rapid breathing.
- Bluish lips and nails.
- Delirium.
- Diarrhea, headache, or pain in the muscles.
- Nausea, vomiting, or abdominal pain.

Pneumonia is a severe infection: Parts of the lungs fill with pus or other liquid that clogs air sacs and prevents oxygen from reaching the bloodstream. Symptoms can range from those of "walking pneumonia"—fatigue and congestion that can linger without sending you to bed—to more severe cases that require prompt hospitalization. Call your doctor right away if you think you have any form of the illness.

The most common causes include:

- **Bacteria.** If untreated, bacterial pneumonia can sometimes be fatal, most of all for people with emphysema and other chronic illnesses. It can spread from the lungs to the rest of the body.
- **Viruses.** There are no drugs for viral pneumonia, but most people get better with bed rest and care.
- **Fungi.** Certain fungi that cause a mild form of pneumonia in healthy people can cause severe disease in people with AIDS or other immune system problems. One of the most common causes of pneumonia in people with AIDS is *Pneumocystis carinii*, which may be a fungus. It is most often treated with antibiotics, sometimes with steroids such as cortisone.

The people most likely to get severe pneumonia are those under age 2 and over 75, and people with chronic health problems such as heart trouble, cancer, emphysema, HIV, or asthma. The risk is high for people who are bedridden or who have just had surgery, because lying flat on the back makes it harder to cough up mucus.

WHAT YOU CAN DO NOW

- Drink lots of fluids.
- Don't take cough suppressants if you have a wet cough: Coughing up mucus will help you recover.
- Try using a cool-mist humidifier in your bedroom. Clean it daily with bleach, and fill it only with distilled water (see box on **humidifiers and vaporizers,** page 93).
- Put hot compresses on your chest. Wet a small towel in hot water, wring it out, and put it in a plastic bag. Wrap it in a cloth before you put it on your skin.
- Don't smoke, and avoid smoky places.
- To prevent a relapse, which can be worse than the first bout, be sure to take all the medicine your doctor prescribes.
- Get plenty of rest and don't rush recovery.

WHEN TO CALL THE DOCTOR

Pneumonia often comes on the heels of some other chest illness, such as a cold. Call for a prompt appointment if you have been sick and these symptoms appear:

- Change in color of mucus, or mucus streaked with blood.
- Lasting fever over 100 degrees, with chills or sweats.
- Shortness of breath and/or pain when breathing.

If the recently ill person is at high risk (very young, over 65, or someone with a chronic illness), be on guard for the first signs of pneumonia and call a doctor.

HOW TO PREVENT IT

If you are in a high-risk group, talk to your doctor about getting shots for bacterial pneumonia as well as a yearly flu shot. Also:

- Don't smoke, and avoid smoke-filled rooms and heavy drinking: These all weaken your ability to fight off disease.
- Avoid close contact with people who have a cold, the flu, or any other chest disease.
- Eat healthy foods: fruits, vegetables, and grains. Plant-based foods are high in vitamins and fiber (see **eat well,** page 302).
- Exercise daily. You'll increase your energy and strength, and build your body's resistance to colds and flu.
- If you're bedridden, sit up for 1 or 2 hours after eating, so you don't inhale bits of food; they can lead to pneumonia. If you have just had surgery, ask about breathing exercises to help prevent pneumonia.

FOR MORE HELP

Information line: National Jewish Center for Immunology and Respiratory Medicine, 1400 Jackson St., Denver, CO 80206. 800-222-5864, M–F 8–5 MST. Nurses answer questions, make referrals, and send information. 800-552-5864, Lung Facts, offers recorded information on breathing problems. **Web site:** *www.njc.org/MFhtml/PNE_MF.html.*

Organization: American Lung Association, 800-LUNG-USA (586-4872), M–F 9–5 your time. Connects you to an ALA chapter that can send a pamphlet on pneumonia.

WHERE YOUR SINUSES ARE

The paranasal sinuses—air spaces in bones around the nose—have 2 main features: They are sound chambers for the voice and they make the skull lighter. Their walls are lined with mucus membranes, which can swell and trap infections.

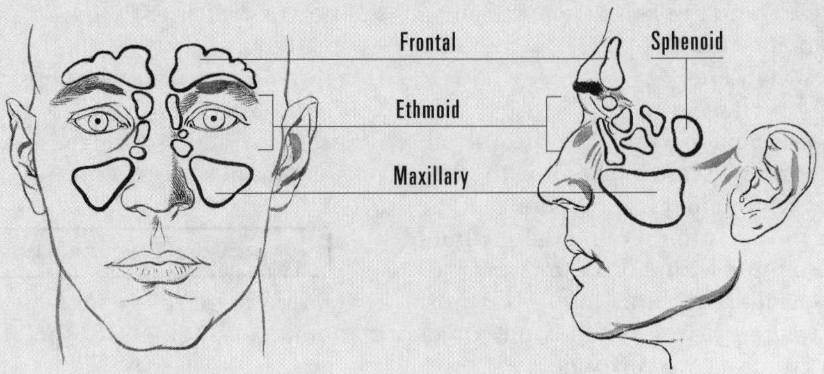

Sinusitis

SIGNS AND SYMPTOMS

Acute sinusitis:

- Stuffy nose and trouble breathing, and a cold for longer than a week.
- Green or yellow nasal discharge, sometimes tinged with blood. It may drip into the back of your throat, making you cough.
- Pain or pressure in or around the eyes and forehead. The pain may travel to the back of your head and be worse in the morning or when you're leaning forward.
- Foul smell in your nose, bad breath.

Sometimes:

- Fever.
- Pain in the upper jaw or teeth.

Chronic sinusitis:

- Nasal discharge and sinus congestion that come back or last for months.

Sinusitis is an inflammation of the sinuses, the air-filled pockets in the bones around the nose and eyes.

When allergies, infections, or smoke, dust, and dirt in the air irritate the inside of your nose, the membranes there swell and clog the tiny openings to your sinuses. Bacteria grow in the mucus trapped in the sinuses, causing pressure and pain—sometimes severe—in the forehead and cheeks, or behind and around the eyes.

People who smoke, have allergies, or are often exposed to germs—such as schoolteachers and health care workers—are among the most likely to get sinus infections.

Symptoms of **acute sinusitis** caused by bacteria most often last only a few days if treated with antibiotics. Sinusitis caused by a virus most often goes away by itself. The symptoms of **chronic sinusitis** can be milder than those of the acute form: Chronic sinusitis seldom causes severe headaches. But it can cause congestion and nasal discharge for months or years. Chronic sinusitis occurs when a sinus opening is blocked for a long time, sometimes as a result of small growths in the nose called nasal polyps, or of a deviated septum (in which the wall between the nostrils is crooked and reduces the flow of air).

WHAT YOU CAN DO NOW

- Make the air in your home more moist (see **humidifiers and vaporizers,** page 93).
- Inhale steam for relief, take a hot shower, or place a warm, damp cloth over your nose.

- Drink plenty of liquids—at least 8 to 10 glasses a day.
- Try decongestant pills or nasal sprays. They may help you breathe, but they should not be used for more than 2 days without asking a doctor, because their "rebound effect" can make symptoms worse.
- Flush your nose with salt water to wash away mucus and bacteria. You can buy saline solution or make your own: Mix ½ teaspoon salt in 8 ounces lukewarm water. Use a dropper or a bulb syringe to squirt it into your nose 2 to 4 times a day. You can also put the solution in the palm of your hand and sniff it in, 1 nostril at a time. Wait a few minutes and then blow your nose gently.
- Soothe a throat sore from postnasal drip with a saltwater gargle: Mix 1 teaspoon salt in 8 ounces warm water. Don't swallow.
- Take a painkiller for headache. (Never give aspirin to a child under 12 who has a cold, chicken pox, flu, or any other illness you suspect of being caused by a virus; see box on **Reye's syndrome,** page 96.)

WHEN TO CALL THE DOCTOR

Call for a prompt appointment:

- If your face swells or your vision blurs; you may have a dangerous infection.

Call for advice:

- If symptoms last more than 7 days without getting better. If a bacterial sinus infection goes untreated, it can last for years, causing chronic pain. The postnasal drip of infected mucus can lead to bronchitis, chronic cough, or asthma.

HOW TO PREVENT IT

Since sinus problems often follow ailments such as allergies, colds, or the flu, you should treat those problems to prevent sinusitis.

- If you have **allergies** (see page 86), learn their triggers so you can avoid an attack.
- Sleep with your head higher than your body to help your sinuses drain.
- Don't smoke, and stay away from smoky places and dirty air, fumes, and dust.
- Don't blow your nose hard.

FOR MORE HELP

Organization: National Jewish Center for Immunology and Respiratory Medicine, 1400 Jackson St., Denver, CO 80206. 800-222-5864, M–F 8–5 MST. Nurses answer questions, make referrals, and send brochures. 800-552-5864, Lung Facts, offers recorded information on breathing problems. **Web site:** *http://www.njc.org/MFhtml/SIN_MF.html.*

Pamphlet: "Sinus Pain, Pressure, and Drainage," by the American Academy of Otolaryngology. Send a business-size, self-addressed, stamped envelope to AAO, One Prince St., Alexandria, VA 22314. Or fax your request to 703-683-5100.

Sore Throat

SIGNS AND SYMPTOMS

- Pain when talking or swallowing.
- Throat that looks red all over or in streaks when you say "Aahhh."
- Swollen, tender glands in the neck.

Sometimes:

- Fever.
- Headache.
- Earache.
- Hoarseness or "lost voice."

Strep throat:

- Sore throat that comes on quickly, with fever, swollen neck glands, headache, or bright red tonsils, sometimes with white pus spots.

Mononucleosis:

- Same symptoms as strep throat, plus fatigue and loss of appetite.

Most sore throats result from a virus—from flu, a cold, or a sinus infection. Dirty air, allergies, tobacco smoke, and the dry air of winter heating can also bring them on. Even shouting can cause soreness.

A few sore throats come from bacteria—usually streptococcus (or strep). **Strep throat** is most common in children (see page 271). Because strep can invade other parts of the body and cause serious trouble such as **rheumatic fever** (see page 269) or a kidney infection—and because it's impossible to tell without a test—you should see your doctor promptly if you suspect you have it. A doctor can take a throat culture or give you a new rapid strep test. If you have strep, antibiotics should knock it out.

Children often get painful sore throats with **measles** (see page 267) and **chicken pox** (see page 255). A sore throat can also signal problems such as epiglottitis (a serious infection of the larynx) or mononucleosis.

WHAT YOU CAN DO NOW

- Drink lots of liquids. Warm ones such as soup or herbal tea are soothing.
- Gargle with warm salt water every few hours. (Mix 1 teaspoon salt in 8 ounces warm water. Don't swallow.)
- Don't smoke, and avoid smoky places.
- Take a nonaspirin painkiller to ease pain and inflammation. (Never give aspirin to a child under 12 who has a cold, chicken pox, flu, or any other illness you suspect of being caused by a virus; see box on **Reye's syndrome,** page 96.)
- Suck on throat lozenges or cough drops to keep your throat moist.
- Use a vaporizer or humidifier to moisten bedroom air (see box on **humidifiers and vaporizers,** page 93).
- For laryngitis, rest your voice by not talking or whispering. Don't clear your throat.

WHEN TO CALL THE DOCTOR

Call 911 or go to an emergency room **right away:**

- If you can't swallow liquids or you have trouble breathing.

Call for a prompt appointment:

- If you have a fever over 101 degrees.
- If the glands in your neck are swollen.
- If your tonsils are bright red or have spots of white pus on them.
- If your sore throat lasts longer than the 5-to-7-day span of a cold.

HOW TO PREVENT IT

- Don't smoke. Stay away from smoky places and dirty air, fumes, and dust.
- Stay away from people who have strep throat or a sore throat.

FOR MORE HELP

Pamphlet: "Sore Throats: Causes and Cures," from the American Academy of Otolaryngology. For the pamphlet and a list of qualified doctors in your state, send a business-size, self-addressed, stamped envelope to AAO, One Prince St., Alexandria, VA 22314. Or fax your request to 703-683-5100.

Web access: American Academy of Family Physicians' brochure on sore throat. After logging on to the Internet, type: *http://www.iacnet.com:80/health/16151054.htm.*

Swallowing Difficulty

SIGNS AND SYMPTOMS

- Pain while swallowing.
- Trouble getting food to go down.
- Feeling of a lump in the throat.

Pain and trouble swallowing can signal a disease of the throat or the esophagus, the tube that connects the throat to the stomach (see color illustrations, pages 172 and 174).

Or the problem could be something (such as a fish bone) stuck in the throat. This could become an emergency if it stops a person from breathing (see **choking,** page 20).

If you have problems swallowing, with a sore throat and maybe a fever and hoarseness, you might have **tonsillitis** (see page 103); an infected larynx, or "voice box" (laryngitis); or an inflamed pharynx or throat (pharyngitis).

Often, acid pushed up from the stomach can burn the esophagus and produce a feeling like **heartburn** (see page 127). This is called esophagitis; it can also cause chest pain and, rarely, vomiting. Symptoms like these also occur when part of the stomach squeezes up into the chest cavity—a hiatal **hernia** (see page 129)—or when the esophagus is narrowed by a buildup of scar tissue caused by stomach acid.

Other causes of swallowing trouble are cancers of the mouth and esophagus; myasthenia gravis; Lou Gehrig's disease (ALS); **Parkinson's disease** (see page 59); and multiple sclerosis.

WHAT YOU CAN DO NOW

- Don't smoke, and avoid smoky places.
- For burning pain in the throat or a feeling of heartburn, take antacids.
- For the feeling of a lump in the throat, drink lots of water with meals and practice relaxation techniques to reduce stress (see **relax,** page 309).

WHEN TO CALL THE DOCTOR

Call 911 or go to an emergency room **right away:**

- If something is caught in your throat.

Call for a prompt appointment:

- If you have swallowing troubles that last for more than a few days, or if you also are losing weight and vomiting.

Call for advice:

- If you suspect you have tonsillitis, laryngitis, or pharyngitis.
- If you can swallow food or drink yet still feel as if you have a lump in your throat, even after trying relaxation techniques.

HOW TO PREVENT IT

- Don't smoke. Smoking can cause oral cancer and problems of the esophagus (see **smoking and illness,** page 220).
- Take antacids for stomach acid or acid blockers to reduce the amount of acid your stomach makes.
- Avoid spicy foods and alcohol, which can worsen heartburn.
- If you are overweight, losing weight may help with swallowing and ease heartburn from a hiatal hernia.

FOR MORE HELP

Organization: National Digestive Diseases Information Clearinghouse, 2 Information Way, Bethesda, MD 20892-3570. Ask for the fact sheet on gastroesophageal reflux disease, which includes facts about heartburn and hiatal hernia.

Book: *Gastrointestinal Health,* by Steven Peikin, M.D. HarperCollins, 1992, $12.

Tonsillitis

SIGNS AND SYMPTOMS

Mild cases:

- Sore or raw throat.
- Hoarse or "throaty" voice that gets worse.

More severe cases:

- Tonsils that are red or have white or yellow spots.
- Tonsils so swollen that they fill the back of the throat.
- Tender or swollen lymph glands in the neck.
- Fever of 100 degrees or higher, headache, or vomiting.
- Ear or stomach pain.

In children:

- Not eating because it hurts to swallow.

In adults:

- Foul-smelling white debris and a burning in the back of the throat.

Thirty years ago, "having your tonsils out" was almost a rite of passage for youngsters. Doctors would remove children's tonsils—pink masses of lymph tissue on both sides of the back of the throat—to prevent tonsillitis, a viral or bacterial infection. Now doctors know that children often outgrow these infections. (Adults can get tonsillitis, too, although it's more common in children.)

Besides, as it turns out, tonsils may help the nose and throat fight off infections such as colds, especially in young children. Most doctors now feel they don't need to be taken

ABOUT ADENOIDS

Tonsillitis should not be confused with enlarged adenoids, which often come along with a tonsil infection. The adenoids are grapelike clusters of tissue in the upper part of the throat where you can't see them, behind the nose. They begin to grow when a child is about 3; at about 5, they usually begin to shrink, and by the teens they are gone.

A child who snores or breathes through the mouth rather than the nose, and who develops a twangy, nasal voice, may have enlarged adenoids. These can cause sleep apnea, in which the child may stop breathing for several seconds at a time while asleep (see **sleep disorders,** page 292). Call a doctor if any symptoms of enlarged adenoids last for more than a week.

out unless children have repeated tonsil infections that make them miss weeks of school.

WHAT YOU CAN DO NOW

If your child's tonsils are simply red (with no swelling or white or yellow coating) and he or she does not have a fever or any problems swallowing, you can often get good results with home treatment (see **sore throat,** page 101).

- Keep your child warm and rested, with a cool-mist humidifier in the bedroom (see **humidifiers and vaporizers,** page 93).
- Give lots of liquids, along with ice cream or frozen yogurt, to soothe the throat.
- Use a saltwater gargle to help dull the pain and cleanse the tonsils. (Mix 1 teaspoon salt in 8 ounces warm water. Gargle every few hours. Don't swallow.)
- Give acetaminophen for fever and pain. (Never give aspirin to a child under 12 who has a cold, chicken pox, flu, or any other illness you suspect of being caused by a virus; see box on **Reye's syndrome,** page 96.)
- Sponge the face with cool water to reduce fever.

WHEN TO CALL THE DOCTOR

In children:

- If the tonsils have a white or yellow coating or spots on them. (Use a flashlight to help you look.)
- If the tonsils are so swollen that they touch; this may mean a bad infection such as **strep throat** (see page 271).
- If a sore throat is severe and lasts more than 2 days.
- If your child has a fever above 100 degrees or goes 24 hours without eating.
- If your child has greenish, yellowish, or rusty-colored mucus or has nausea, skin rashes, chest pain, seizures, inflamed or painful joints, or a fever that returns after being absent for a day or two. These may signal a system-wide staph or other infection.

In adults:

- If you have trouble swallowing or opening your mouth, and severe jaw or throat pain.

HOW TO PREVENT IT

Tell children to avoid infections by:

- Moving away from people who are coughing and sneezing.
- Not sharing cups or silverware.
- Washing their hands often.
- Keeping their hands away from their mouths.

FOR MORE HELP

Pamphlet: American Academy of Pediatrics, Box 927, Elk Grove Village, IL 60009-0927. Send a business-size, self-addressed, stamped envelope, and request a copy of "Tonsils and Adenoids."

Web access: University of Washington/Seattle, Department of Otolaryngology. After logging on to the Internet, type: *http://weber.u.washington.edu/~otoweb/tonsil.html.* Covers tonsillitis and its treatment.

Tuberculosis

SIGNS AND SYMPTOMS

Tuberculosis (TB) infection:
Note: You may have TB even if you have no symptoms at all.
- Mild cough (sometimes).

Active TB disease:
- Coughing, sometimes with bloody mucus.
- Slight fever.
- Weight loss and fatigue.
- Night sweats.
- Chest pain.

Tuberculosis, or TB, is a chronic infection that most often affects the lungs. But it can also spread throughout the body, chiefly to the brain, kidneys, and bones.

Tuberculosis was once so common that it killed 1 in 5 adults in Europe and the United States. With the use of antibiotics, the disease all but vanished until the mid-1980s, when it began to spread among people deprived of medical care or whose immune systems had been weakened by AIDS. Also, new types of TB appeared that outsmarted common antibiotics.

You are at high risk for TB if:
- You are HIV positive.
- You have spent a long time with someone who has the disease, or you work in a homeless shelter, a hospital, a nursing home, a prison, or other public place.
- You are an IV drug user.
- You have spent a long time in crowded living quarters in a country where TB is known to be a problem.

Tuberculosis comes in 2 stages, inactive and active. In the first, TB bacteria enter the lungs and multiply but the body's immune system often stops the infection within 2 to 10 weeks.

Only about 10 percent of the people with TB go on to get the active disease, half of those within 1 to 2 years. People who get active TB can spread it to others through long-time close contact. It is rarely spread by casual contact or on buses and airplanes.

Most TB can be treated with antibiotics. But a rarer, drug-resistant TB kills about half of those it infects.

WHAT YOU CAN DO NOW

- If you have the disease, get medical care and follow your doctor's advice closely.

WHEN TO CALL THE DOCTOR

- If you have symptoms of the disease.
- If you suspect you have been exposed to TB for a long time.
- If you are being treated for TB and you get new symptoms.

HOW TO PREVENT IT

Most people are not at risk of getting TB, so they need no special safeguards. On the other hand, if you are in a high-risk group, talk with your doctor about screenings, prevention, or a preventive vaccine (the vaccine is not 100 percent effective).

Also, if TB has shown up in your children's school, they should be tested.

FOR MORE HELP

Information line: National Jewish Center for Immunology and Respiratory Medicine, 1400 Jackson St., Denver, CO 80206. 800-222-5864, M–F 8–5 MST. Nurses answer questions, make referrals, and send brochures. 800-552-5864, Lung Facts, offers recorded facts on breathing problems.

Information line: Centers for Disease Control and Prevention, 404-639-1819, M–F 8–4 EST. Voice-mail system allows you to hear about TB, request brochures by mail or fax, and talk with staff members.

Web access: New York City Bureau of Tuberculosis Control and Columbia University. After logging on to the Internet, type: *http://www.cpmc.columbia.edu/tbcpp.* Covers tuberculosis and lists other sources of facts.

Heart & Circulation

Artery Disease

SIGNS AND SYMPTOMS

Artery disease (atherosclerosis) can damage your health before you have any symptoms. That's why it's vital to prevent artery disease, or to find and treat the problem early. Watch for symptoms of the following:

Heart disease:

- Dull chest pain (angina) or simply a feeling of tightness or heavy pressure. It's most often in the center of the chest but can spread into the arms and jaw. With rest, angina goes away in 30 seconds to 5 minutes.

Heart attack:

Call 911 **right away:**

- If the pain lasts, gets worse, comes more often, or comes during rest; this could mean you're having a heart attack.

Stroke:

Call 911 **right away:**

- If you lose your balance, speech, or vision; or have trouble moving; or have a sudden tingling, numbness, or loss of movement in a limb.

Peripheral vascular disease:

- Muscle fatigue, weakness, or pain in the buttocks or legs, most often in the calves when you walk.
- Cold feet.
- Discolored skin, sores that won't heal, and sudden sharp pains in the legs or feet when you rest.

The walls of a healthy artery are smooth and elastic, so blood flows freely. But sometimes a substance known as plaque builds up inside an artery; the process is called atherosclerosis. The walls of the vessel thicken and grow rough and stiff, narrowing the artery. (See color illustrations, page 169.)

Plaque deposits build up when a person has high levels of cholesterol in the blood. The problem runs in some families. Lack of exercise, a high-fat diet, smoking, and untreated **high blood pressure** (see page 112) or **diabetes** (see page 282) also increase your chances of having it.

The risk rises with age; heavy people are more at risk than those who are lean. Men are in more danger than women, up to a point: The risk for women goes up sharply once they reach menopause. Women over 35 who smoke and take birth control pills may also increase their risk.

Most of us are likely to have some narrowed arteries by the time we're in our 50s or 60s. But even before symptoms appear, atherosclerosis can make a person feel tired or generally unwell.

When the disease is more advanced, it can cause many health problems, including:

Heart disease: This is the leading cause of death in the United States. It occurs when the arteries that supply blood to the heart

Chest Pain

Never ignore chest pain, especially in an adult. It's hard to tell one kind of chest pain from another, so if it is severe or lasts more than a few minutes, call 911.

SYMPTOMS	WHAT IT MIGHT BE	WHAT YOU CAN DO
Crushing pain, pressure, or squeezing in center of chest that may spread to jaw, neck, back, or arms (often left arm); sweating, nausea, or shortness of breath.	Heart attack (see page 39).	Call 911 **right away.**
Pain or chest tightness with breathing. In adults: sudden, sharp chest pain with shortness of breath that gets worse. In young people: possibly vague or minor pain that spreads to neck or back with some trouble breathing.	Collapsed lung. Sometimes occurs in young people for no apparent reason, or in adults who have asthma or chronic bronchitis. May follow a recent chest injury.	Call 911 **right away.**
Severe, stubborn, ripping chest pain that may spread to abdomen and upper back; dizziness and fainting.	Aortic aneurysm—weak spot with rip or tear in main artery from heart. Most often caused by artery disease (see opposite page) or high blood pressure (see page 112).	Call 911 **right away.** Surgery may be needed to repair aorta.
Sharp chest pain, worse when breathing in; shortness of breath; possibly fever.	Pleurisy—inflamed sac around lungs; often a complication of pneumonia (see page 98) or tuberculosis (see page 105).	Call 911 or go to emergency room **right away.**
Dull pain, pressure, or squeezing in center of chest that may feel like stomach upset or heartburn; may spread to jaw, neck, back, or arms (usually left arm); brought on or made worse by stress or activity, easing with rest in 30 seconds to 5 minutes.	Angina. • Coronary artery disease (see artery disease, opposite page, and heart attack, page 39).	Call doctor for prompt appointment, but if symptoms persist 10 minutes or longer, call 911 **right away.**

(continued)

Chest Pain *(continued)*

SYMPTOMS	WHAT IT MIGHT BE	WHAT YOU CAN DO
Chest pain, trouble breathing, easy fatigue, uneven heartbeat (palpitations), fainting (sometimes).	Problem with heart rhythm. • Mitral valve prolapse—heart valve allows blood to leak backward. Affects many more women than men; may run in families.	Call doctor for prompt appointment. For mitral valve prolapse, beta-blockers may ease palpitations and chest pain. Antibiotics should be taken before dental work or surgery to prevent infection of heart's lining. **For more help:** American Heart Association, 800-242-8721, M–F 8–5 your time.
Pain or tightening in chest; rapid heartbeat; shortness of breath; numbness or tingling in hands; fear.	Anxiety. • Panic attack. • Hyperventilation—rapid breathing that lowers level of carbon dioxide in blood (see anxiety and phobias, page 210).	If you can't function as usual, call doctor for advice.
Burning or pressure in chest or upper abdomen, worse on bending over or lying down, especially when stomach is full; belching. Symptoms can resemble heart attack.	Heartburn. • Esophageal reflux—stomach acid backs up into esophagus when muscle that prevents this becomes weak. • Ulcer. • Gastritis.	See heartburn, page 127, or ulcers and gastritis, page 136.
Severe burning or aching pain on one side of chest that may spread to back, not affected by breathing; followed a few days later by blisters and itchy rash.	Shingles.	See shingles, page 178.
Sharp pain that gets worse with movement or deep breathing, or when area is pressed; may follow severe coughing or sneezing, or chest injury.	Pulled muscle. • Inflamed cartilage. • Injured rib.	Rest, apply an ice pack (a bag of frozen peas wrapped in a dishcloth works well) several times a day, 10–15 minutes at a time. Take a painkiller—aspirin, ibuprofen, or acetaminophen.

muscle become narrowed. If these coronary arteries can't supply enough blood to the heart during exertion or strong emotions, your heart complains and you feel chest pain (angina). A heart attack happens when a blood clot forms in a coronary artery and blocks blood flow to a part of the heart. This most often happens where plaque has built up and damaged the artery's walls.

Stroke: Some types of **strokes** (see page 115) occur when clots form in vessels in the brain or leading to it. As in coronary artery disease, this often happens where the vessel is narrowed by plaque. Another type of stroke happens when a weakened vessel bursts and leaks blood into the brain.

Peripheral vascular disease: This occurs when arteries that go to the arms and legs become narrowed. While not always life-threatening, if untreated it can lead to gangrene and the loss of a limb, most often a leg.

If your doctor suspects you have narrowed arteries, he or she may suggest diet and lifestyle changes, and maybe drugs to reduce high cholesterol or control high blood pressure. A technique called balloon angioplasty can sometimes open blocked arteries, or surgery can bypass them.

WHAT YOU CAN DO NOW

There is no quick fix. But changes in lifestyle can make a big difference. They'll help you prevent artery disease and cut your risk of heart disease, stroke, and other problems. If your arteries have already begun to narrow, these same changes can slow the progress of the disease and even reverse it.

➤ Exercise. Like any muscle, your heart gets stronger with regular work. And a strong heart pumps blood with less effort than a weaker one. Exercise also helps open up clogged arteries, lowers blood pressure, makes clots less likely to form in narrowed arteries, helps keep off extra weight, and helps reduce stress (see **get some exercise,** page 298).

The idea of exercising may be a little scary if you haven't been active over the years, or if you've been told you have narrowed arteries, but exercise is extra important then. To make it safer and easier:

- Check with your doctor first if you're at risk for narrowed arteries.
- Start by being just a bit more active each day. Any exercise is better than none. Take the stairs instead of the elevator. Walk your dog for 15 minutes each evening. Your dog and your arteries will thank you.
- When you're used to being more active, add more things that make you breathe harder, sweat a bit, and get your heart pumping. Brisk walking, jogging, biking, cross-country skiing, and swimming are all great for your heart. But find something you like—you'll be more likely to stick with it. Take a couple of months to work up to getting exercise 2 or 3 times a week for 20 to 30 minutes at a time.

➤ Eat right. A low-fat, low-cholesterol diet can help prevent and even reverse narrowing of arteries (see **eat well,** page 302).

You need some fat and cholesterol to stay healthy. They provide energy and help maintain cell walls. But when you eat extra fat and cholesterol, you store some of it as body fat, and some of that ends up clogging your arteries.

Build your meals around fruits, vegetables, and grains. They have little fat and no cholesterol and are loaded with vitamins, minerals, and fiber. Fiber is important. It lowers cholesterol and blood pressure and helps keep your arteries open. Foods rich in fiber include apples, oranges, potatoes, squash, peas, carrots, soybeans and other beans, oats, and barley.

Simple things you can do to cut fat and cholesterol:

- Read food labels to know what you're eating. The important things to look for are: calories, calories from fat, total fat, saturated fat, and cholesterol. The American Heart Association says to keep your fat intake under 30 percent of your total calories each day. Some experts think it should be 20 percent or under.
- If you eat red meat, make it a once-in-a-while treat. Eat no more than 6 ounces

of meat, poultry, or fish a day. Keep servings to 3 ounces—a cut of meat about the size of a deck of cards, half a skinless chicken breast or leg, or three-quarters of a cup of flaked fish.
  - Don't fry foods. Bake, broil, steam, or sauté in a nonstick pan.
  - If you eat dairy foods, choose the low-fat or nonfat versions.
  - Go easy on eggs—they have lots of cholesterol. Eat no more than 3 or 4 of them in a week.

➤ Don't smoke. With the first puff, your risks for narrowed arteries and heart attack go way up. A man who smokes a pack a day has twice the risk of a nonsmoker. For a woman, it's even more dangerous—a pack a day increases her risk 5 to 10 times.

  The good news: As soon as you stop smoking, your body begins to recover. Within a year, your risk for heart disease drops to half that of a smoker. Fifteen years after stopping, your risk is the same as that of a person who never smoked (see **smoking and illness,** page 220).

➤ If you have **high blood pressure** (see page 112), do what you can to lower it. Your blood pressure is too high if it's above 140/90. Lose weight if you're overweight, exercise regularly, eat right, and reduce daily stress.

➤ Have your cholesterol level checked. If it's too high, do what you can to bring it down. Best is a total cholesterol reading under 200 milligrams per deciliter of blood. Borderline is 200–239. Too high is 240 and over. But total cholesterol tells only part of the story. What's in it also counts. Experts now say it's good to have a high level of high-density lipoproteins (HDLs) and a low level of low-density lipoproteins (LDLs). Your HDLs should make up at least 25 percent of your total cholesterol. Eating right and exercising will help. If lifestyle changes don't work, your doctor can prescribe medication.

➤ If you're overweight, take steps to lose the extra pounds (see **maintain a healthy weight,** page 301).

➤ Be careful with alcohol. Moderate drinking may help cut the risk of narrowed arteries. But too much can make your heart pump faster and raise blood pressure. It can also damage the heart muscle. What's "moderate"? No more than 2 drinks a day for men, 1 for women. (A drink is 1.5 ounces of hard liquor, a 12-ounce can of beer, or a 5-ounce glass of wine.)

WHEN TO CALL THE DOCTOR

Call 911 **right away:**

➤ If you feel crushing pain in your chest. You may also have nausea, vomiting, sweating, shortness of breath, weakness, or intense feelings of anxiety. You may be having a heart attack.

➤ If you've had chest pain before, but this time it doesn't go away in 5 to 10 minutes.

➤ If you've had chest pain before, but it's getting worse or you have it while resting.

➤ If you have any symptoms of a stroke, such as loss of speech or balance, or numbness.

Call for a prompt appointment:

➤ If you have symptoms of peripheral vascular disease, such as pain in the legs or feet.

HOW TO PREVENT IT

Follow the guidelines in What You Can Do Now, above. See **eight ways to feel your best,** page 298, for more details.

➤ Vitamin E (found in foods such as vegetable oils, wheat germ oil, and almonds) may help prevent heart attack (see **the nutrition top ten,** page 304).

➤ Take a baby aspirin (81 mg) every day, or an adult-strength aspirin (325 mg) every other day. This over-the-counter medicine helps keep blood from clotting and cuts your risk of a heart attack. Check with your doctor before starting this routine.

➤ Don't stress out. Too much stress is hard on the heart. Do what you can to relax: Try deep breathing, meditation, or simply a "time-out" now and then (see **relax,** page 309).

➤ Enjoy your friends (see **stay involved,** page 307). Friendships can do wonders for your heart. Volunteer, take classes, or join a support group to talk with others who know what you're going through.

FOR MORE HELP

Information line: American Heart Association, 800-242-8721, M–F 8–5 your time. Staff answers questions and sends out brochures. **Web site:** *http://www.amhrt.org/heartg/athero.html.*

Organization: National Heart, Lung, and Blood Institute Information Center, Box 30105, Bethesda, MD 20824-0105. 800-575-WELL, 24-hour recording. 301-251-1222, M–F 8:30–5 EST. Fax: 301-251-1223. Staff answers questions on narrowed arteries and sends brochures.

Organization: Coronary Club, Cleveland Clinic Foundation, 9500 Euclid Ave., Cleveland, OH 44195. 800-478-4255, M–F 9–3 EST. Provides information on heart health and healing, and offers support to patients with heart problems.

Book: *Dr. Dean Ornish's Program for Reversing Heart Disease,* by Dean Ornish, M.D. A step-by-step guide to reversing heart disease without drugs or surgery. Ivy Books, 1996, $6.99.

Book: *American Heart Association Guide to Heart Attack: Treatment, Recovery, and Prevention.* Times Books, 1996, $23.

Web access: The Franklin Institute. After logging on to the Internet, type: *http://www.fi.edu/biostat/heart.html.* This user-friendly tour of the heart and blood system provides links to other heart-related sites.

Video: *Coronary Artery Disease at Time of Diagnosis.* Clear overview of causes and treatments, with 4 reports—Understanding the Diagnosis, What Happens Next?, Treatment and Management, and Issues and Answers. Time Life Medical, 1996, $19.95. Sold in many pharmacies; for one near you, call 800-588-9959.

Congestive Heart Failure

SIGNS AND SYMPTOMS

- Weakness and fatigue.
- Shortness of breath, even during light activity or while lying down. This might cause wheezing that is mistaken for asthma.
- Need to sleep on more pillows than normal or to sleep sitting up.
- Swelling in the feet, ankles, and legs.
- Dull ache or pain in the chest.
- Stubborn cough with foamy, blood-specked mucus.
- Stomach feels full.
- Weight gain from fluid buildup.
- Frequent need to urinate, most often at night.
- Swelling of neck veins.
- Nausea, vomiting, loss of appetite.
- Irregular or rapid heartbeat.

Despite its scary name, congestive heart failure is not always a life-threatening disease when the causes are found and treated. It occurs when the heart muscle is damaged, usually by **high blood pressure** (see page 112), a **heart attack** (see page 39), **palpitations** (see page 114), **artery disease** (see page 106), valve problems, or an illness called cardiomyopathy, which may be caused by a virus, alcohol abuse, or inherited heart defects. As a result, the heart can't keep the blood flowing well, causing swelling, most often in the legs and ankles. Sometimes fluid collects in the lungs and makes it hard to breathe. Congestive heart failure also makes it harder for the kidneys to get rid of excess sodium and water, which can make the swelling worse.

Congestive heart failure is the most common reason that people over 65 go to the hospital. With treatment, though, a person who has it can most often go on to lead an active life.

WHAT YOU CAN DO NOW

After diagnosis:

- ➤ Get plenty of rest at first. Later, as your symptoms ease, staying on the move will help you get better.
- ➤ To make breathing easier when lying down, raise your head by putting a wedge under your mattress, or use extra pillows.
- ➤ Put your legs up when sitting.
- ➤ Eat less salt; it makes you retain fluid and swell.
- ➤ Don't eat or drink anything with caffeine; if you're having heart palpitations, caffeine can make them worse.
- ➤ Use elastic support stockings to control swelling in your legs. Ask your pharmacist about them.

WHEN TO CALL THE DOCTOR

Call 911 **right away:**

- ➤ If you have severe chest pain or trouble breathing.

Call for a prompt appointment:

- ➤ If you often become breathless and tired after mild activity.

Call for advice:

- ➤ If you're being treated for congestive heart failure and your symptoms get worse.
- ➤ If you gain weight rapidly.

HOW TO PREVENT IT

- ➤ Eat sensibly and exercise daily to prevent the causes, such as high blood pressure.
- ➤ If you know you have high blood pressure or heart disease, follow your doctor's advice about treating the problem.
- ➤ Drink moderately, if at all.

FOR MORE HELP

Information line: American Heart Association, 800-242-8721, M–F 8–5 your time. Staff answers questions and sends out literature.

Organization: National Heart, Lung, and Blood Institute Information Center, Box 30105, Bethesda, MD 20824-0105. 800-575-WELL, 24-hour recording. 301-251-1222, M–F 8:30–5 EST. Fax: 301-251-1223. Staff answers questions and sends out brochures.

Book: *Living Well, Staying Well,* by the American Heart Association and the American Cancer Society. A guide to heart wellness with practical, step-by-step advice. Times Books, 1996, $25.

Book: *The Stanford Life Plan for a Healthy Heart,* by Helen Cassidy Page, John Speer Schroeder, M.D., and Tara Coghlin Dickson, M.S., R.D. Covers heart disease and includes more than 200 recipes. Chronicle Books, 1996, $29.95.

Web access: Heart Information Network. After logging on to the Internet, type: *http://www.heartinfo.com.* Scroll to the topic you want. Covers latest heart news, answers questions about heart disease, and lists other patient resources.

High Blood Pressure

SIGNS AND SYMPTOMS

High blood pressure, or hypertension, is often called the "silent killer." In most cases, there are no clear warning signs, even as the illness harms your health.

Blood pressure refers to the force of blood pushing against artery walls as it courses through the body. It's normal for your blood pressure to rise and fall through the day with changes in your activities and moods. But when it remains high most of the time, it can force your heart to work too hard, which can threaten your health. High blood pressure is the most common of all cardiovascular diseases. It is the leading cause of **heart attack** (see page 39) and **stroke** (see pages 46 and 115).

Blood pressure is measured with a device that records 2 numbers. It's too high if the first number (the peak pressure when your heart beats) is 140 or higher most of the time, or if the second number (the pressure when your heart relaxes between beats) is above 90 most of the time. Best is around 110/70.

While the causes of most cases of high blood pressure aren't known, the risk factors are—they include things you can't control and things you can. If high blood pressure runs in your family, your risk is doubled. The risk goes up with age. African Americans have a high risk. If you weigh too much, don't get enough exercise, or have a lot of stress, you're also at risk. Sometimes high blood pressure is a sign of other problems, such as **diabetes** (see page 282) or kidney disease.

High blood pressure can be treated with lifestyle changes and, often, with drugs.

WHAT YOU CAN DO NOW

- If you're in a high-risk group, have your blood pressure checked as often as your doctor advises. Your doctor can check your blood pressure; your community may offer free or low-cost screenings; or you can buy a blood pressure cuff and check it yourself, though this takes some practice.
- Don't smoke, and avoid smoky places (see **smoking and illness,** page 220).
- Exercise often—try brisk walking, swimming, or biking. If you haven't been active, check with your doctor before starting an exercise program.
- Eat no more than 2,000 milligrams of salt a day. (One teaspoon of salt equals about 2,100 mg.) Fresh vegetables and fruits are low in salt; fast food and processed foods contain a lot of it.
- Find a healthy outlet for **stress** (see page 222). Try meditation or yoga to **relax** (see page 309).

WHEN TO CALL THE DOCTOR

Call for emergency advice (if you can't get it, call 911 or go to an emergency room):

- If you have or suspect you have high blood pressure and you have any of these: recurring headaches, chest pain or tightness, frequent nosebleeds, numbness and tingling, confusion, or blurred vision.

Call for advice:

- If you check your blood pressure over a number of days and it stays much higher than before.
- If you're pregnant and get high blood pressure. This can harm both you and your unborn child (see **pregnancy,** page 244.)
- If you have high blood pressure and lifestyle changes don't help.
- If you're taking drugs to control your high blood pressure and you start to feel dizzy or sleepy, or you become constipated or impotent. You may need a different drug. But never stop taking your blood pressure medication without telling your doctor; stopping suddenly can cause problems.

HOW TO PREVENT IT

Follow the suggestions above in What You Can Do Now. Also:

- Lose any extra pounds.
- If you drink alcohol, drink moderately—no more than 2 drinks a day for men, 1 for women. (A drink is 1.5 ounces of hard liquor, a 12-ounce can of beer, or a 5-ounce glass of wine.)
- If you use birth control pills, give some thought to other methods. The Pill can cause high blood pressure in some women (see **birth control health risks,** page 228).
- Make sure you get enough potassium (orange juice and potatoes have lots), magnesium (leafy greens and whole grains), and calcium (leafy greens and dairy products). These minerals help control blood pressure (see **the nutrition top ten,** page 304).
- Cut fats in your diet—eat less fatty meat, butter, and whole dairy products, and more vegetables, fruits, and grains (see **eat well,** page 302).

FOR MORE HELP

Information line: American Heart Association, 800-242-8721, M–F 8–5 your time. Staff answers questions and sends literature, including pamphlets on groups at risk, such as African Americans and women. **Web site:** *http://www.amhrt.org/heartg/hbpcause.html.*

Organization: National Heart, Lung, and Blood Institute Information Center, Box 30105, Bethesda, MD 20824-0105. 800-575-WELL, 24-hour recording. 301-251-1222, M–F 8:30–5 EST. Fax: 301-251-1223.

Staff answers questions on high blood pressure and sends fact sheets.

Pamphlets: Citizens for Public Action on Blood Pressure and Cholesterol, Box 30374, Bethesda, MD 20824. Provides information on high blood pressure.

Book: *Eating Well, Living Well With Hypertension,* by Connie W. Bales, Ph.D., R.D., and the Duke University Medical Center. Viking, 1996, $12.95.

Book: *Good News About High Blood Pressure: Everything You Need to Know to Take Control of Hypertension—And Your Life,* by Thomas Pickering, M.D. New research and treatments. Simon & Schuster, 1996, $22.50.

Book: *From Stress to Strength: How to Lighten Your Load and Save Your Life,* by Robert S. Eliot, M.D. Outlines a program for coping with stress. Bantam, 1994, $11.95.

Video: *High Blood Pressure at Time of Diagnosis.* Clear overview of causes and treatments, with 4 reports—Understanding the Diagnosis, What Happens Next?, Treatment and Management, and Issues and Answers. Time Life Medical, 1996, $19.95. Sold in many pharmacies; for one near you, call 800-588-9959.

Palpitations

SIGNS AND SYMPTOMS

Rapid heart rate:

- A nagging awareness of your heartbeat.
- A fluttering, thumping, pounding, or racing beat.
- Shortness of breath, chest pain, light-headedness, or fainting.

Slow heart rate:

- Fatigue, shortness of breath, light-headedness, or fainting.
- Nausea.

Palpitations are caused by changes in the electrical impulses that control the heart muscle. Nearly everyone has an uneven heartbeat now and then, and it's most often harmless. But a frequent or lasting change in the heart's rhythm can mean a health problem.

The older you are, the greater your chances of having palpitations. Anxiety, stress, thyroid problems, and some drugs, including nicotine, caffeine, and alcohol, can also set them off. But the most important causes are **high blood pressure** (see page 112) and **artery disease** (see page 106). These health problems can damage the heart muscle, causing a "short circuit" in its electrical system.

Mild palpitations can often be controlled with drugs or surgery. Sometimes devices such as pacemakers are put into the chest to control more severe palpitations.

WHAT YOU CAN DO NOW

Call your doctor for a prompt appointment if you have palpitations often—even once a day—if they make you feel dizzy, or if they're bad enough that you become very aware of your heartbeat.

WHEN TO CALL THE DOCTOR

Call for a prompt appointment:

- If you have fainting spells.
- If you notice a strange heartbeat and feel light-headed or dizzy.
- If you have uneven heartbeats that are intense, painful, or more than fleeting.
- If you are taking drugs your doctor has given you for palpitations and you notice a new, uneven heartbeat pattern; or you are nauseated, vomit, faint, or have diarrhea or a rash.

HOW TO PREVENT IT

- Cut out caffeine (in coffee, tea, chocolate, and caffeinated soft drinks).
- Don't smoke, and stay away from alcohol, decongestants, diet pills, and stimulant drugs such as cocaine or amphetamines.

Do what you can to keep your heart in good shape:

- Get plenty of exercise, such as brisk walking, jogging, swimming, or bicycling, to help control your resting heart rate (see **get some exercise,** page 298).

- ➤ Find a healthy outlet for **stress** (see page 222). Try meditation, yoga, or deep breathing (see **relax,** page 309).
- ➤ Eat balanced, low-fat meals (see **eat well,** page 302). Your doctor may also suggest mineral supplements; calcium, magnesium, and potassium help control the heartbeat (see **the nutrition top ten,** page 304).

FOR MORE HELP

Information line: American Heart Association, 800-242-8721, M–F 8–5 your time. Staff answers questions and sends out literature.

Organization: National Heart, Lung, and Blood Institute Information Center, Box 30105, Bethesda, MD 20824-0105. 800-575-WELL, 24-hour recording. 301-251-1222, M–F 8:30–5 EST. Fax: 301-251-1223. Staff answers questions and sends fact sheets.

Stroke

SIGNS AND SYMPTOMS

If you have any of the following, or if someone with you does, call 911 **right away.**

- Abrupt weakness or numbness of the face, arm, or leg, often on one side of the body.
- Sudden trouble seeing or loss of vision—especially in just one eye.
- Trouble talking or making sense of someone else's speech.
- Sudden and severe headache.
- Dizziness or sudden loss of consciousness.

A person has a stroke when blood flow to part of the brain is blocked. A stroke needs treatment right away, since parts of the brain can begin to die within minutes, damaging speech, vision, and movement. Strokes disable more people in the United States than any other cause.

There are three main kinds of strokes:

Cerebral thrombosis, the most common, occurs when a blood clot forms and blocks blood flow in an artery in the brain or leading to it. These clots most often form in arteries narrowed by a fatty substance called plaque.

Cerebral embolism occurs when a clot forms in some other part of the body, then is carried to the brain.

These 2 types of stroke often follow a transient ischemic attack (TIA), in which a clot briefly blocks an artery in the brain or leading to it, cutting off oxygen. The symptoms are similar to those of cerebral thrombosis or cerebral embolism, but they come on quickly and most of the time last only a few minutes. TIAs cause no lasting damage, but they are an important warning sign that you're at risk of a stroke.

Cerebral hemorrhage occurs when a weakened artery in the brain bursts and bleeds into the tissues near it. Sometimes a vessel on the surface of the brain breaks and bleeds into the area between the brain and the skull. The blood presses on the brain and can cause damage.

The single most important risk factor for stroke is **high blood pressure** (see page 112). Smokers, people over 65, men, African Americans, and people with a family history of stroke all have higher than normal chances of having a stroke. Women using birth control pills (see **birth control health risks,** page 228) have a greater risk of stroke if they also smoke. They have an even higher risk if they are over 35 or have high blood pressure.

Many people who have had strokes recover fully following physical or occupational therapy combined with other treatments, such as medications to improve circulation and prevent clots, and lifestyle changes to prevent another stroke.

WHAT YOU CAN DO NOW

Get help—call 911 **right away**—if you are with someone who has symptoms of a stroke. While waiting for help to arrive, follow these steps (for more details, see page 46):

- ➤ Check the person's **ABCs** (see box on page 14).

- Begin **CPR** (see page 16) if the person is not breathing or you can't find a pulse.
- If the person is not conscious but is breathing, support the head and roll him or her into the **recovery position** (see box on page 25).
- If vomit or fluid is draining from the person's mouth, or he or she is having trouble swallowing, turn the person onto his or her side so the airway isn't blocked. Don't give anything to eat or drink.
- If the person is conscious, offer comfort.

WHEN TO CALL THE DOCTOR

Call 911 **right away.** Don't try to drive the person to an emergency room yourself—wait for help to come, and follow the steps above. The sooner a person gets help, the better his or her chances for recovery. A drug widely used against heart attack—t-PA—can limit the damage from a stroke, if it is given within 3 hours.

HOW TO PREVENT IT

- If you have **high blood pressure** (see page 112), do what you can to control it.
- Find a healthy outlet for **stress** (see page 222), such as meditation, yoga, or deep breathing (see **relax,** page 309).
- Get plenty of **exercise** (see page 298), and eat plenty of low-fat, high-fiber foods—fresh fruits and vegetables and whole grains (see **eat well,** page 302).
- Don't smoke, and avoid smoky places (see **smoking and illness,** page 220).
- If you have **artery disease** (see page 106), your doctor may suggest aspirin or prescription drugs to reduce the chance of clots. Your doctor may also discuss surgery to widen narrowed vessels in your neck.
- If you have **diabetes** (see page 282), take steps to control it. This disease can damage blood vessels and increase the risk of stroke.

FOR MORE HELP

Information line: Stroke Connection of the American Heart Association, 800-553-6321, M–F 8:30–5 CST. Provides information about strokes and support groups near you.

Information line: National Stroke Association, 800-787-6537, M–Th 8–4:30, F 8–4 MST. Provides facts about strokes and a list of support groups.

Information line: National Institute of Neurological Disorders and Stroke, 800-352-9424, M–F 8:30–5 EST. Provides free brochures on strokes.

Book: *American Heart Association Family Guide to Stroke Treatment, Recovery, and Prevention,* by Louis R. Caplan, M.D., L. Dyken, M.D., and J. Donald Easton, M.D. Times Books, 1996, $14.

Web access: American Heart Association's on-line Heart and Stroke Guide. After logging on to the Internet, type: *http://www.amhrt.org/heartg/battack.html*. Defines stroke and lists other resources.

Video: *Stroke at Time of Diagnosis.* Clear overview of causes and treatments, with 4 reports—Understanding the Diagnosis, What Happens Next?, Treatment and Management, and Issues and Answers. Time Life Medical, 1996, $19.95. Sold in many pharmacies; for one near you, call 800-588-9959.

Varicose Veins

SIGNS AND SYMPTOMS

- Swollen, twisted clusters of blue or purple veins.
- Swollen legs.
- Legs ache or feel heavy.
- Itching around affected veins.
- Brown discoloring of skin.
- Sores.

In healthy veins, valves allow blood to flow only one way. Varicose veins form when these valves fail, allowing blood to back up and pool inside the vein, making it swell. These veins can hurt, and they may look bad, but they're rarely harmful.

Varicose veins can occur anywhere on the body, but they show up mostly on the legs, sometimes within patches of thin red capillaries or green veins known as spiders. Hemorrhoids are varicose veins around the anus.

Varicose veins run in families. Women, often those of German or Irish descent, are twice as likely as men to develop them. Anything that puts pressure on the legs, such as standing for a long time, pregnancy, and being overweight, can cause them.

Most varicose veins are near the surface of the skin. Deeper ones can't be seen, but poor circulation can swell, darken, and harden the skin above them. In severe cases, sores may form, often around the ankles. Varicose veins can be removed with surgery or treated with medications.

WHAT YOU CAN DO NOW

- Wear elastic support stockings. They keep blood from pooling in the legs. You can find them at most drugstores.
- If your varicose veins are bothering you, stay off your feet as much as you can. Take breaks often. When you can, sit or lie with your feet above chest level. Sleep with your legs raised to relieve swelling.
- If you have to stand still for a long time, flex your calf muscles and toes. This helps pump blood toward the heart and prevents pooling.

WHEN TO CALL THE DOCTOR

Call for a prompt appointment:

- If you cut a varicose vein—it may bleed heavily. First, lie down, raise the injured leg, and apply gentle, firm pressure with a clean cloth. Get help as soon as you can after the bleeding has slowed.

Call for advice:

- If varicose veins make walking or standing painful.
- If you develop sores.

HOW TO PREVENT IT

The steps in What You Can Do Now will help prevent varicose veins. Also:

- If you are overweight, take steps to lose the extra pounds.
- Exercise often. Activities that work the leg muscles, such as walking or jogging, help pump blood toward the heart.
- Don't wear garters, girdles, or other tight clothing.
- Don't cross your legs.
- Avoid long periods of sitting or standing.
- Sit or lie down with your legs about hip level or higher at least twice a day for 30 minutes at a time.

FOR MORE HELP

Organization: National Heart, Lung, and Blood Institute Information Center, Box 30105, Bethesda, MD 20824-0105. 800-575-WELL, 24-hour recording. 301-251-1222, M–F 8:30–5 EST. Fax: 301-251-1223. Ask about varicose veins.

Book: *Varicose Veins: A Guide to Prevention and Treatment,* by Howard C. Baron, M.D., and Barbara Ross. Facts on File, 1995, $24.95.

Stomach, Abdomen, & Digestive System

Colon Cancer

SIGNS AND SYMPTOMS

Cancers of the colon and rectum often show no symptoms in the early stages. First warning signs may be:

- Changes in bowel habits (such as constipation or diarrhea, not being able to empty the bowel all the way, or bleeding from the rectum) that last for more than 10 days.
- Stools with areas of dark blood, or that are long and slim.
- Black, sticky stools; they may mean internal bleeding.
- Stomach pain, which may include cramps, and/or pain from gas and bloating.
- Fatigue, weakness, weight loss, or lack of appetite for no known reason.

Colon cancer is one of the most common cancers in the United States. The disease—a malignant tumor in the large intestine (see color illustration, page 174)—is most common among people over 40. Anyone with a family history of this cancer or who has had colon polyps (benign tumors) or **inflammatory bowel disease** (see page 131) may be at high risk. So are people who have been exposed to asbestos.

The food you eat seems to affect the risk as well. People who eat a lot of animal fat and don't eat enough fiber (found in fruits, vegetables, and unrefined grains) seem to be more likely to get this type of cancer than those with a low-fat, high-fiber diet.

Recent research also suggests aspirin may slow the growth of colon tumors and help prevent polyps in the colon from turning into cancers.

People whose cancer is caught early have a good chance of a full recovery. Everyone should get a digital rectal exam once a year beginning at about 40.

People over 50 should have an annual stool test to screen for traces of blood and an internal rectal exam (sigmoidoscopy) every 3 to 5 years. Anyone with a history of benign colon polyps, inflammatory bowel disease, or a family history of colon cancer may also need regular exams in which a tube is used to view the entire colon (colonoscopy).

WHAT YOU CAN DO NOW

➤ If you have colon cancer, surgery, radiation, or chemotherapy may cure or help control it.

WHEN TO CALL THE DOCTOR

Call for a prompt appointment:

➤ If you get symptoms of anemia (pale skin, fatigue, rapid heartbeat).

Call for advice:

➤ If you notice a change in your bowel movement habits.

➤ If you bleed from the rectum, pass tarry stools, or notice blood in or on your stool.

Abdominal Pain

Abdominal pain is most often a sign of a mild ailment such as indigestion or stomach flu. But severe pain can be an emergency, and long-lasting pain may signal a serious illness.

SYMPTOMS	WHAT IT MIGHT BE	WHAT YOU CAN DO
Sharp, ongoing pain in abdomen that moves to back and chest; fever; nausea; vomiting; swollen abdomen; sweaty skin.	Pancreatitis—inflamed pancreas.	Call 911 or go to emergency room **right away.** Acute pancreatitis can cause shock, which can be fatal if not treated quickly.
Sharp abdominal pain, perhaps with other acute symptoms.	Intestinal blockage. ● Appendicitis (see page 26). ● Pelvic inflammatory disease (see page 242). ● Heart attack (see page 39). ● Perforated stomach ulcer (see page 137). ● Shock from allergy (see page 24). ● Diabetic emergency (see diabetes, page 282). ● Poisoning (see page 42).	Call 911 or go to emergency room **right away.**
Pain in upper right side of abdomen; may spread to upper back, chest, or right shoulder; nausea; vomiting; gas.	Gallstones (see page 125).	In a first attack, call doctor for emergency advice. If you can't get one, call 911 or go to emergency room. Do not eat or drink anything.
Severe pain in side that moves toward groin or abdomen; need to urinate often, or painful or stopped-up urination; murky, smelly, or bloody urine; nausea and vomiting; sweating.	Kidney stones (see page 138). ● Kidney infection.	Call doctor for prompt appointment. Then drink lots of water to help stone pass, and take a nonaspirin pain reliever if you need to (see pain relief, page 317).
Cramping or pain in abdomen, nausea, diarrhea, vomiting, fever, fatigue, weakness, gas.	Stomach flu (see nausea and vomiting, page 133). ● Food poisoning (see page 36).	If, with vomiting and pain, you have blurred or double vision, muscle weakness, or trouble speaking or swallowing, call 911 or go to emergency room **right away;** these may be signs of botulism, a sometimes fatal bacterial food poisoning.

(continued)

Abdominal Pain *(continued)*

SYMPTOMS	WHAT IT MIGHT BE	WHAT YOU CAN DO
Pain or cramps in abdomen, diarrhea, bloody stool, fever, fatigue, weight loss.	Crohn's disease. • Ulcerative colitis. • Bacterial dysentery, particularly if you have been overseas.	See inflammatory bowel disease, page 131. If you think you have bacterial dysentery, call doctor for prompt appointment.
Pain that is worse when sore spot on abdomen is touched; severe abdominal cramping, often more painful on the left; nausea; fever; chills; diarrhea, constipation, or thin stools.	Diverticulitis.	See diverticulitis, page 124.
Ache or pain in abdomen or groin when lifting or bending over, swelling or bulge under skin in abdomen or groin.	Hernia.	See hernia, page 129.
Ache or pain in abdomen with diarrhea or constipation, or bouts of both; extreme gas or bloating; nausea, most often after eating; fatigue.	Irritable bowel syndrome.	See irritable bowel syndrome, page 132. (For self-care, also see diarrhea, page 122, and constipation, opposite page.)
Pain in upper abdomen, nausea, vomiting, diarrhea, loss of appetite, burping or gas, heartburn.	Stomach ulcer. • Gastritis.	See ulcers and gastritis, page 136.
Pain and cramps after drinking milk or eating other dairy foods, gas and bloating, diarrhea, nausea, rumbling sounds from abdomen.	Lactose intolerance—trouble digesting cow's milk, cheese, butter, ice cream, and other dairy foods.	Eat fewer dairy foods or none. Try soy milk and acidophilus yogurt, which may agree with you better than milk.

(Don't just assume you have hemorrhoids.)

- If you have lasting abdominal pain, or are weak or losing weight. These signs can have other causes but should be checked right away to rule out cancer.

HOW TO PREVENT IT

- Eat lots of whole grains, fresh fruits, and vegetables—at least 5 servings of fruits and vegetables each day (broccoli, cauliflower, and cabbage are good choices).

- Cut back on red meat and animal fats. Beans, nuts, and soybean products such as tofu are also good sources of protein (see **eat well,** page 302).
- Eat more fiber. Try adding bran or wheat germ to breakfast food. Begin with 1 tablespoon and work up to 3 or 4.
- Get a fecal occult blood test every year after age 50.
- Get plenty of exercise. Studies show that brisk walking, jogging, swimming, and other activities reduce the risk of colon cancer, perhaps by speeding "transit" time of waste matter through the colon.

FOR MORE HELP

Hotline: Cancer Information and Counseling Hotline, AMC Cancer Research Center, 800-525-3777, M–F 8:30–5 MST. Trained staff counsels, answers questions, and sends pamphlets, brochures, and fact sheets.

Information line: The Wellness Community, 310-314-2555, M–F 9–5 PST. Free psychological and emotional support for cancer patients and their families.

Book: *What to Do If Cancer Strikes.* To order, send $2 for postage and handling to: Cancer Research Institute, Box 5199, FDR Station, New York, NY 10150-5199, or call 800-992-2623.

Book: *Your Gut Feelings,* by Henry D. Janowitz, M.D. Covers intestinal problems, including colon cancer. Oxford University Press, 1994, $11.95.

Web access: Cansearch: A Guide to Cancer Resources. After logging on to the Internet, type: *http://www.access.digex.net/~mkragen/cansearch.html.* A step-by-step guide to on-line cancer resources.

Video: *Colon & Rectal Cancer at Time of Diagnosis.* Clear overview of causes and treatments with 4 reports—Understanding the Diagnosis, What Happens Next?, Treatment and Management, and Issues and Answers. Time Life Medical, 1996, $19.95. Sold in many pharmacies; for one near you, call 800-588-9959.

Constipation

SIGNS AND SYMPTOMS

- Dry, over-firm stools that are hard or painful to pass.
- Feeling of fullness after having a bowel movement or of not being able to finish it.
- No bowel movement after 3 days (for adults) or 4 days (for children). How "regular" you are depends on your age, diet, and daily activity. Three bowel movements a week is normal for some, 3 a day for others.
- Swelling, bloating, or pain in the abdomen.

Constipation is a common ailment—and one of the most frustrating. Our fast modern lifestyle is often at fault: eating fast foods that are low in fiber, drinking too little water, getting too little exercise, and failing to respond right away to the urge to move the bowels. Emotional problems play a role. So do some drugs and food supplements.

Stubborn, chronic constipation may signal a more serious illness, such as **irritable bowel syndrome** (see page 132), **colon cancer** (see page 118), or **diabetes** (see page 282).

WHAT YOU CAN DO NOW

Most cases respond to home treatment, such as diet changes and exercise. If constipation isn't caused by disease, simply eating more fiber (found in fruits, vegetables, and whole grains) and drinking lots of water (at least 8 glasses a day) should soften your stools and make you "regular" once more. Also:

- Don't use over-the-counter laxatives unless your doctor suggests them. You might become hooked. If you must take one, try a bulk-forming psyllium laxative, which is more gentle than other kinds. But don't use a laxative if you have stomach pain, nausea, or vomiting, or if you are pregnant.
- Don't take mineral oil as a laxative unless your doctor advises it.

A FOLK REMEDY TO TRY

An age-old way to get the bowels moving is to mix the juice of a whole lemon into a glass of warm water and drink it in the morning. Or try a glass of water with a teaspoon of apple cider vinegar and a teaspoon of honey mixed in.

➤ If infants under 6 months are mildly constipated, be sure they are getting enough water. Prune juice can help: Start with a half teaspoon. Increase to 4 tablespoons bit by bit. Make sure the infant does not get diarrhea. Toddlers, older children, and adults can have strained or whole prunes. (Remove pits for toddlers.)

➤ Don't use an enema unless your doctor advises you to.

WHEN TO CALL THE DOCTOR

Being constipated every now and then shouldn't send you to the doctor's office, but 2 weeks or more of the problem should. Call for a prompt appointment:

➤ If you also have fever and lower abdominal pain, and the stools you do have are thin. You may have **diverticulitis** (see page 124).

Call for advice and an appointment:

➤ If your stools are bloody. This may be from an anal fissure or a **hemorrhoid** (see page 128), but it could also be a sign of **colon cancer** (see page 118).

➤ If you get constipation after taking a new prescription drug or food supplements. Changing the dosage may help.

➤ If you are elderly or disabled and haven't had a bowel movement for a week or more; the problem may be an impacted stool.

➤ If you are losing weight.

➤ If exercise and eating more fiber haven't helped after 2 weeks.

HOW TO PREVENT IT

➤ Exercise. A brisk 30-minute walk every day will help regulate your bowel movements.

➤ Drink plenty of water—at least 8 glasses every day.

➤ Get lots of fiber by eating at least 5 servings a day of fresh fruits, vegetables, and other good sources of fiber, including bran and other whole-grain cereals, and raw or cooked dried fruits such as raisins and prunes, beans, and nuts.

➤ Allow enough time for bowel movements. A pattern—the same time every day, after breakfast or dinner—is best.

FOR MORE HELP

Hotline: Nutrition Hotline of the American Dietetic Association, 800-366-1655, M–F 9–4 CST. A registered dietitian answers questions about constipation and can give you names of dietitians near you.

Organization: International Foundation for Bowel Dysfunction, Box 17864, Milwaukee, WI 53217. 414-241-9479, M–F 9–5 CST. Offers support and printed materials on bowel disorders.

Web access: National Institute of Diabetes and Digestive and Kidney Diseases of the National Institutes of Health. After logging on to the Internet, type: *http://www.niddk.nih.gov/Constipation/Constipation.html.* Explores the causes and treatment of constipation.

Diarrhea

SIGNS AND SYMPTOMS

- Loose, watery stools.
- Frequent bowel movements.
- Abdominal pain or cramping.

Diarrhea occurs when stools move faster than usual through the intestines (see color illustration, page 174), before the body can take out the water they contain. Its causes can include viruses, a reaction to food, **food poisoning** (see page 36), **stress** (see page 222), too much alcohol, and some drugs, especially antibiotics. Diarrhea can also result from drinking untreated water that contains giardia, a common parasite that attacks the intestines, or from other parasites and amoebas.

In some cases, diarrhea may indicate a more serious disease (see **colon cancer,** page 118, **diverticulitis,** next page, **inflammatory bowel disease,** page 131, or **irritable bowel syndrome,** page 132).

WHAT YOU CAN DO NOW

- Don't eat solid food at first, to let your digestive tract rest.
- Don't take over-the-counter antidiarrhea products for the first few hours; let your system get rid of whatever is causing the problem. If you do use such products, don't take them for more than a day or two without asking your doctor.
- Sip clear, warm liquids (water, tea, or broth), sports drinks, or flat sodas (ginger ale, cola, or other sodas that have been left open to lose their fizz). Drink only small amounts for the first few hours, then as much as your stomach can handle.
- If your stomach takes the fluids, try eating bland, bulk-adding foods such as bananas, white rice, or toast.
- While you are recovering, don't drink alcohol or milk, or eat dairy foods or fiber-rich foods such as salads and fruit.
- If your diarrhea is severe, watch out for dehydration. The signs include dry mouth, sticky saliva, and dark yellow urine in smaller amounts than usual. You can buy rehydration drinks such as Pedialyte (for infants) and sports drinks to help replace lost fluids and minerals—or you can make your own (see box on page 124).

WHEN TO CALL THE DOCTOR

Call for emergency advice (if you can't get any, call 911 or go to an emergency room):

- If the diarrhea comes with severe cramping, light-headedness, chills, vomiting, or fever over 101 degrees.
- If you notice signs of severe dehydration—dry mouth, sticky saliva, dizziness or weakness, and dark yellow urine. Dehydration can be dangerous for older people and for young children.

Call for a prompt appointment:

- If stools are bloody or tarry, or contain mucus or worms. (Some medicines and iron may make the stools look black, which isn't anything to worry about.)

Call for advice and an appointment:

- If you have diarrhea often, or if you get it while you are taking a medication.
- If diarrhea lasts for more than 2 days (1 day for a child under 3, or 8 hours for an infant under 6 months).
- If you have been traveling and may have been drinking untreated water.
- If diarrhea and constipation come and go in turn for more than a few weeks. You may have **irritable bowel syndrome** (see page 132) or—though less likely—**colon cancer** (see page 118).

HOW TO PREVENT IT

- Avoid foods you know your body can't handle well.
- When traveling in foreign countries, drink

DIARRHEA IN CHILDREN

Infants and young children need special care when they have diarrhea. If it's severe, an infant can become very dehydrated in less than a day.

- Breast-fed infants should continue regular feedings. If you use formula, ask your doctor about diluting it with water to half strength for 24 to 48 hours. If the diarrhea doesn't improve, try soy-based formula until your child is better.
- Don't give soda, fruit juice, or sports drinks to infants or young children. To help prevent dehydration, give a few sips of a rehydration drink such as Pedialyte every few minutes.
- Don't give antidiarrhea medicine to infants or young children.
- For older babies, try feeding rice cereal, bananas, toast, and other foods that add bulk to the stool. But don't give babies solid food if they are vomiting.
- Call your doctor if you see signs of dehydration—sticky saliva, dark yellow urine, weakness.

REHYDRATION RECIPE

To make a rehydration drink at home for anyone older than 12, mix 1 quart of water with 1 teaspoon of table salt, ½ teaspoon of baking soda, 4 teaspoons of cream of tartar, and 3 to 4 tablespoons of sugar. **Note:** Don't give to children 12 and under. Use only a store-bought drink such as Pedialyte.

only bottled or boiled water or canned drinks. Don't use ice in drinks. Peel fruits and vegetables. Don't eat foods that have been sitting out.

- See **nausea and vomiting** (page 133) for tips about food-related diarrhea.

FOR MORE HELP

Organization: International Foundation for Bowel Dysfunction, Box 17864, Milwaukee, WI 53217. 414-241-9479, M–F 9–5 CST. Offers support and printed advice.

Diverticulitis

SIGNS AND SYMPTOMS

- Abdominal cramping that is most often worse on the lower left side.
- Nausea.
- Fever.
- Diarrhea, constipation, or thin stools.
- Pain made worse when the sore spot on the abdomen is touched.
- Gas.

Many people develop small pouches in the colon (the major part of the large intestine)—a fairly harmless condition known as diverticulosis.

But sometimes one or more of the pouches gets inflamed. This is diverticulitis. It can range from mild infection to bowel blockage or breaks in the bowel wall.

People who eat mostly low-fiber foods, are constipated, or use laxatives seem to have a greater risk of diverticulitis.

Treatment may include bed rest, changes in diet, and antibiotics or other drugs. The chances of a full recovery are good if you get prompt medical help. If you don't, diverticulitis can lead to serious problems that need surgery.

WHAT YOU CAN DO NOW

- If you have symptoms of diverticulitis, see your doctor.
- Never use an enema for this illness.

WHEN TO CALL THE DOCTOR

Call 911 or go to an emergency room **right away:**

- If you have sharp abdominal pain and swelling, fever, chills, and nausea or vomiting—even if you think your symptoms are getting better. Peritonitis, a life-threatening infection of the abdominal cavity's lining, could be the problem.

Call for a prompt appointment:

- If your stools have blood in them; you may have internal bleeding.
- If severe pain lasts despite treatment; you may have another abdominal illness (see **abdominal pain** chart, page 119).

HOW TO PREVENT IT

- Add whole-grain breads, bran cereals, oatmeal, fresh fruits, and vegetables to your diet. Don't add fiber too fast, though. Too much fiber all at once can create a painful amount of gas.
- Be sure you get enough fluids (at least 8 glasses of water a day). If you eat more fiber, be sure to drink at least this much water.
- Avoid foods that are hard to digest, such as nuts, seeds, corn, and popcorn.
- Heed the urge to have a bowel movement.
- Exercise daily to keep the muscles of your abdomen in good shape. This helps you have regular bowel movements.
- Don't use laxatives unless your doctor advises them. Foods such as prunes, prune juice, and psyllium seed (for sale in drugstores as powder or pills) work well.

- ➤ Don't smoke; smoking can make the problem worse.
- ➤ Avoid caffeine, and if you drink alcohol, don't drink much.

FOR MORE HELP

Information line: Intestinal Disease Foundation, 412-261-5888, M–F 9:30–3:30 EST. Offers telephone support, educational programs and brochures, advice on support groups, and names of doctors near you.

Organization: National Digestive Diseases Information Clearinghouse, 2 Information Way, Bethesda, MD 20892-3570. Write for a free fact sheet or packet on diverticulitis.

Gallstones

SIGNS AND SYMPTOMS

- Intense pain in the upper right side or center of the abdomen, perhaps spreading to the back, chest, or right shoulder.
- Nausea and vomiting.
- Gas and indigestion.
- Fever and chills.
- Yellow-tinged skin and eyes (jaundice).

Gallstones are hard lumps of cholesterol or bile salts that collect in the gallbladder. This small, pear-shaped organ holds bile, a digestive juice. The stones can be as small as a grain of salt or as large as a lime. Most cause no harm and no symptoms.

A gallstone attack occurs when a stone gets trapped in one of the bile ducts (the tubes that carry bile from the gallbladder to the small intestine; see illustration on this page, and color illustration, page 174). You may notice an attack a few hours after a big meal or during the night. Attacks can last several hours. Gallstones may cause jaundice if bile backs up into the liver.

You may get gallstones because of your genes. They are found most often among Native Americans and Mexican Americans.

GALLSTONES

Stones may cause no symptoms if they stay in the gallbladder or travel freely through the bile duct. Trouble occurs when they get stuck in the duct.

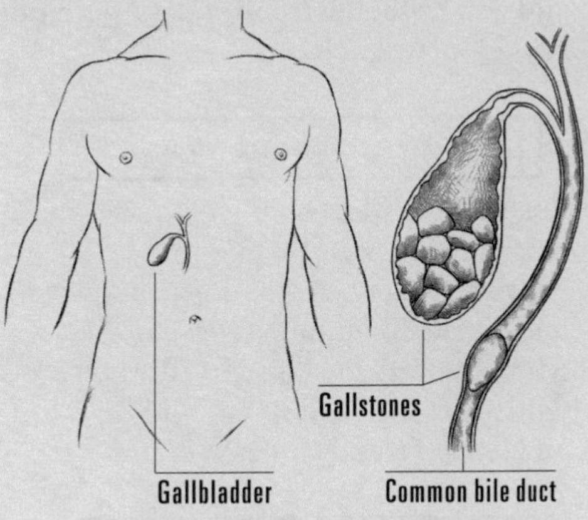

You're more likely to have them if you're obese, eat a lot of fatty foods, or lose a lot of weight quickly. If you're over 40 or a woman between 20 and 60, you're at higher risk. So are pregnant women and women who use birth control pills or estrogen replacement therapy.

Treatment for repeated, painful attacks is often surgery to remove the gallbladder. This procedure is simpler for the patient than it used to be, with less pain and a quicker recovery.

WHAT YOU CAN DO NOW

- ➤ If you have symptoms of a gallstone attack, get medical help right away.
- ➤ In the meantime, do not eat or drink.

WHEN TO CALL THE DOCTOR

Call 911 **right away:**

- ➤ If you have sudden, sharp pain in the upper right area of your abdomen. (If you are also nauseated, sweating, and short of breath, these symptoms may signal a heart attack.)

Call for emergency advice (if you can't get any, call 911 or go to an emergency room):

➤ If you think you are having your first gallstone attack or if you have fever along with the pain.

Call for a prompt appointment:

➤ If you notice a yellow cast to the skin and eyes (jaundice).

➤ If you have been told you have gallstones and you have sharp abdominal pain that lasts more than 2 hours.

HOW TO PREVENT IT

➤ Keep to your ideal body weight (see **maintain a healthy weight,** page 301).

➤ Ask your doctor before trying to lose weight, and diet with common sense.

➤ Some experts say you can cut the risk of gallstones with a diet that is high in fiber and low in fat and cholesterol.

FOR MORE HELP

Organization: National Digestive Diseases Information Clearinghouse, 2 Information Way, Bethesda, MD 20892-3570. Write for a free fact packet about gallstones.

Book: *Indigestion: Living Better With Upper Intestinal Problems From Heartburn to Ulcers and Gallstones,* by Henry D. Janowitz, M.D. Offers a chapter on the causes and treatments of gallstones. Oxford University Press, 1992, $18.

Web access: National Institute of Diabetes and Digestive and Kidney Diseases of the National Institutes of Health. After logging on to the Internet, type: *http://www.niddk.nih.gov/Gallstones/Gallstones.html.* Explores causes and treatment.

Video: *Gallstones at Time of Diagnosis.* Clear overview of causes and treatments, with 4 reports—Understanding the Diagnosis, What Happens Next?, Treatment and Management, and Issues and Answers. Time Life Medical, 1996, $19.95. Sold in many pharmacies; for one near you, call 800-588-9959.

Gas and Gas Pain

SIGNS AND SYMPTOMS

- Burping.
- Passing gas.
- Pain or bloating in the abdomen.

Gas and gas pains are normal. They're often caused by air you swallow if you eat and drink too fast. Gas is also made by food you're digesting. High-fiber foods such as beans, vegetables, fruits, and grains can create lots of gas. So can dairy foods for some people.

When air goes into your stomach, you may get rid of it by burping, which is natural and healthy—though not always polite. Even less polite is passing gas through the anus (flatulence). But what many people think of as lots of gas may be normal. In fact, most adults pass gas from 8 to 20 times a day.

WHAT YOU CAN DO NOW

➤ Try teas made with peppermint, chamomile, or fennel to relieve gas pains.

➤ If you need to release gas, do it—even if you have to leave the room.

➤ If you have severe gas pains, try lying on your back and pulling your legs up to your chest. It's easier to expel the gas this way.

WHEN TO CALL THE DOCTOR

Call for emergency advice. If you can't get any, call 911 or go to an emergency room:

➤ If you have severe pain that starts close to the navel and moves to the lower right area of the abdomen; this could be a sign of **appendicitis** (see page 26).

Call for a prompt appointment:

➤ If you notice pain in the upper right part of the abdomen; this may be a sign of a gallbladder problem (see **gallstones,** page 125) or an **ulcer** (see page 136).

Call for advice:

➤ If you have long-lasting bloating for more than 3 days for no known reason.

- If you have less pain in the lower abdomen after passing gas or having a bowel movement; you may have **irritable bowel syndrome** (see page 132).
- If you have gas often, have lost weight, and have light-colored, bad-smelling bowel movements; you could be unable to digest fat.

HOW TO PREVENT IT

You can most likely avoid too much gas and gas pains simply by changing your diet. Keep in mind, though, that the high-fiber foods that often cause gas are also those most vital to a healthy diet. Rather than cutting down on fruits, vegetables, beans, and whole grains, try these changes:

- Buy dry beans rather than canned. Soak them overnight in water, then pour out the water and replace it with fresh water for cooking. Make sure to cook the beans until they're soft.
- For a good source of protein, try tofu, a soy food; it's easier to digest than many beans.
- Drink plenty of fluids.
- Avoid foods and snacks sweetened with fructose (fruit sugar) or sorbitol (an artificial sweetener). Both can increase gas.
- Eat slowly, chew your food well, and don't overeat. (It may take 20 to 30 minutes to feel full.)
- Take a walk after meals. Mild exercise improves digestion and helps move gas through your system more quickly.
- Avoid carbonated drinks, chewing gum, and drinking through a straw; these may put extra air into your stomach.

FOR MORE HELP

Hotline: Nutrition Hotline of the American Dietetic Association, 800-366-1655, M–F 9–4 CST. Registered dietitians answer questions about gas and give names of registered dietitians near you.

Web access: National Institute of Diabetes and Digestive and Kidney Diseases of the National Institutes of Health. After logging on to the Internet, type: *http://www.niddk.nih.gov/Gas/Gas.html*. Explores the causes of gas and offers advice about eating.

Heartburn

SIGNS AND SYMPTOMS

- A burning feeling just behind the breastbone after eating that lasts from a few minutes to a few hours.
- Chest pain, often after bending over or lying down.
- Burning in the throat; or hot, sour, or salty fluid at the back of the throat.
- Mild pain in the upper abdomen.
- Burping (sometimes).

Heartburn has nothing to do with the heart. Also known as acid indigestion or gastroesophageal reflux disease, heartburn is caused by stomach acid backing up into the lower esophagus (the muscular tube between the throat and the stomach).

It can be triggered by overeating or by too much pressure on the abdomen, often from being overweight or pregnant. A hiatal **hernia** (see page 129) that squeezes part of the stomach up through the diaphragm can also cause it. Eating spicy, acid, or fatty foods can lead to heartburn, as can drinking alcohol. So can certain medicines such as aspirin, ibuprofen, and some antibiotics and other prescription drugs. Smoking also prompts the release of stomach acid.

Heartburn is common. If you have it often, it may cause serious problems, such as bleeding or scarring in the esophagus. It isn't dangerous, though, if it happens only once in a while. Medication or changes in your lifestyle will most likely take care of it.

WHAT YOU CAN DO NOW

Many doctors advise taking over-the-counter aids such as antacids for heartburn that happens now and then. Take them before eating if you get it often. But don't take antacids without first checking with your doctor if you have **high blood pressure** (see page 112), an irregular heartbeat, kidney disease, intestinal problems, chronic heartburn, or any symptoms of **appendicitis** (see page 26).

Pregnant women and nursing mothers should ask their doctor before taking any medication, including antacids.

Try these natural treatments:

- ➤ Drink ginger tea for quick relief.
- ➤ Avoid lying down for 2 to 3 hours after eating. If you must recline, lie on your left side; in this position, your stomach is lower than your esophagus, so the acids are less likely to back up.
- ➤ Don't smoke. Avoid smoky places.
- ➤ Cut down on coffee and alcohol.
- ➤ Practice relaxing to help relieve **stress** (see page 222).
- ➤ Raise the head of your bed 4 to 6 inches by putting something such as bricks or phone books under the legs, or by placing a foam-rubber wedge under your pillows.
- ➤ Ask your doctor whether a medicine that blocks acid secretion might help you.
- ➤ Don't wear tight clothes such as jeans, girdles, or belts.

WHEN TO CALL THE DOCTOR

Call 911 **right away:**

- ➤ If you have sharp chest pain or pain that goes into your arms and shoulders. This could signal a heart attack.

Call for advice:

- ➤ If you've tried the tips above, but your symptoms persist.

HOW TO PREVENT IT

Many of the treatments for heartburn will also help prevent it. In addition:

- ➤ Keep to your ideal body weight (see **maintain a healthy weight,** page 301).
- ➤ Avoid foods and drinks that can set off the problem. These may include tomatoes, citrus fruits, garlic, onions, chocolate, coffee and tea, alcohol, peppermint-flavored food, and carbonated drinks.
- ➤ Cut down on dishes that are high in fats and oils.
- ➤ Eat small meals often (4 or 5 a day) instead of 3 large ones.
- ➤ Avoid eating just before bedtime.
- ➤ Get plenty of rest and exercise.
- ➤ Don't smoke. Nicotine prompts the release of stomach acid, and relaxes a muscle that allows gastric juice to back up from the stomach into the esophagus.
- ➤ Avoid aspirin, ibuprofen, and other nonsteroidal anti-inflammatory drugs. Try acetaminophen (see **pain relief,** page 317).

FOR MORE HELP

Hotline: Nutrition Hotline of the American Dietetic Association, 800-366-1655, M–F 9–4 CST. A dietitian answers questions and lists dietitians near you.

Organization: National Digestive Diseases Information Clearinghouse, 2 Information Way, Bethesda, MD 20892-3570. Write for the packet on heartburn (gastroesophageal reflux disease).

Book: *The Fire Inside,* by M. Michael Wolfe, M.D., and Thomas Nesi. Offers facts and advice on heartburn and reflux disease. W.W. Norton, 1996, $23.

Web access: National Institute of Diabetes and Digestive and Kidney Diseases of the National Institutes of Health. After logging on to the Internet, type: *http://www.niddk.nih.gov/Heartburn/Heartburn.html.* Offers tips for the control of heartburn.

Hemorrhoids

SIGNS AND SYMPTOMS

- Stools with red blood, or blood on toilet paper or in toilet bowl.
- Painful bowel movements.
- Lump near the anus, or a swelling that hurts.
- Itching in or near the anus.
- Mucus coming from the anus.

Hemorrhoids are inflamed or swollen veins either inside or outside the anus. Also known as piles, they may result from straining to pass hard stools during bouts of **constipation** (see page 121). Other causes may include your genes, aging, pregnancy, chronic diarrhea, and the overuse of laxatives. The pain often lingers for many days and recurs. Still, home treatment can help.

WHAT YOU CAN DO NOW

- Try a sitz bath: Sit in warm water for 10 to 15 minutes every few hours. After a bowel movement is a good time.
- Bathe often so your anus stays clean, but be careful when washing the area. Don't scrub the skin. Pat dry.
- Wipe gently. Try cotton balls, alcohol-free baby wipes, or damp toilet paper.
- Many times a day, dab hemorrhoids on the outside of the anus with witch hazel or soothe them with a cold compress.
- To ease painful bowel movements, place a bit of petroleum jelly inside and around the edge of the anus.
- Try an over-the-counter stool softener.
- Use suppositories for pain, but avoid ointments with a local numbing agent (you'll see "-caine" in the name or on the label). These can cause more soreness.
- Don't scratch hemorrhoids. You'll make them worse. Try 0.5 hydrocortisone cream, sold in drugstores, to relieve itching.

WHEN TO CALL THE DOCTOR

- If bleeding persists for more than a few days. You could have a more serious problem, such as **colon cancer** (see page 118).
- If you have lasting or severe pain. You may need outpatient surgery to remove or shrink the hemorrhoids.

HOW TO PREVENT IT

- For soft, easily passed stools, eat plenty of fruit, vegetables, bran cereals, and whole-grain bread. (If you are pregnant, ask your doctor before making changes in your diet.) Also, drink lots of liquids such as water or fruit and vegetable juices (at least 8 big glasses a day).
- Cut back on meat, animal fat, and alcohol.
- Set a regular time for your bowel movements. Sit on the toilet for 5 or 10 minutes at most.
- If you're sitting down all day at work, take breaks and walk a bit. Long periods of sitting reduce blood flow around the anus.
- Don't sit on a "doughnut" cushion; these can trap blood in the swollen veins.

FOR MORE HELP

Hotline: Nutrition Hotline of the American Dietetic Association, 800-366-1655, M–F 9–4 CST. Covers hemorrhoids, and gives names of registered dietitians in your area.

Organization: National Digestive Diseases Information Clearinghouse, 2 Information Way, Bethesda, MD 20892-3570. Write for a free fact sheet about hemorrhoids and a reading list.

Web access: National Institute of Diabetes and Digestive and Kidney Diseases of the National Institutes of Health. After logging on to the Internet, type: *http://www.niddk.nih.gov/Hemmorhoids/Hemmorhoids.html.* (That's how this site spells hemorrhoids.) How to prevent and treat.

Hernia

SIGNS AND SYMPTOMS

- Swelling under the skin in the abdomen or groin. May be tender. May not show when you lie down.
- Fullness or heaviness in the abdomen, sometimes with constipation.
- While lifting or bending, pain or ache in groin or abdomen.
- In severe cases, pain in the abdomen, nausea, and vomiting.
- Chronic heartburn, belching, or stomach fluids backing up into the throat. These could signal a hiatal hernia, which occurs when part of the stomach or lower esophagus squeezes into the chest cavity.

A hernia is a bulge—often visible—caused by a lump of tissue that pokes through a hole or weak area in a nearby muscle. Although hernias can occur in many places in the body, they are most common in the abdominal wall. Pressure on a weak point—from extra body weight, from lifting a heavy object, or from straining during bowel movements—can force a split in an abdominal muscle, or between muscles.

AN ABDOMINAL EXERCISE

Here's a quick and easy exercise you can do every day to strengthen your stomach muscles and help prevent abdominal hernias: Lie down with your knees bent and your feet flat on the floor. Cross your arms over your chest. Raise your shoulders a couple of inches off the floor; hold for a count of 5; lie back down. Repeat 5 times at first, more after a few weeks when you're stronger.

This allows part of an internal organ to push its way through.

Ninety percent of all abdominal hernias occur in men. Some people are born with a weakness in the muscle, which allows a hernia to form. More often, it occurs later in life. Poor diet, excess pounds, smoking, and muscle strain or overexertion can all make hernias more likely.

Most hernias can simply be pushed back into place, by you or by a doctor. But they will protrude again. If the hernia is part of an intestine poking through the abdominal wall, the intestine could become blocked; the result will be pain, nausea, and vomiting. Another danger is a kind of strangling, when tissue around the bulging organ squeezes it and cuts off its blood supply. If the hernia isn't treated, a serious infection can destroy tissue in the bowel.

The 4 types of abdominal hernia that occur most often are: *Epigastric,* between the breastbone and the navel; part of the sheet of fat that covers the intestines pushes through a weak point between muscles. The lump is most often small, but it may be sore. *Paraumbilical,* near the navel. It may or may not be painful. *Inguinal,* in the groin. The main symptom is rarely pain, though you may have a heavy feeling in the groin after standing up for a while. *Femoral,* also in the groin but slightly lower than the inguinal; it may cause no symptoms and give no trouble unless it becomes blocked or strangled.

In many cases, even hernias that aren't serious slowly get worse and may need surgery.

WHAT YOU CAN DO NOW

- Call your doctor if you think you may have a hernia. Some hernias need care right away.
- Don't strain or lift anything heavy.

WHEN TO CALL THE DOCTOR

Call 911 or go to an emergency room **right away:**

- If you have a hernia, and you are nauseated and vomiting, or can't have a bowel movement or pass gas. You may have a blocked or strangulated hernia.

Call for advice:

- If you suspect you have a hernia.

HOW TO PREVENT IT

- If you are overweight, lose some weight to ease the pressure on your abdominal muscles.
- Avoid lifting heavy objects.
- Don't strain when having a bowel movement (see **constipation,** page 121).
- Eat well to avoid constipation.
- Don't smoke. Avoid smoky places. Chronic coughing from smoke or other agents makes a hernia more likely and also can make one recur.
- Do gentle exercises daily to tone and strengthen your abdominal muscles.

FOR MORE HELP

Information line: The Hernia Resource Center, 800-437-6427, M–F 9–5 EST. Sends a brochure on hernias and gives lists of doctors.

Organization: National Digestive Diseases Information Clearinghouse, 2 Information Way, Bethesda, MD 20892-3570. Write for facts on hernias.

Book: *Indigestion: Living Better With Upper Intestinal Problems,* by Henry D. Janowitz, M.D. Covers hernias. Oxford University Press, 1992, $8.95.

Web access: Hernia Resource Center. After logging on to the Internet, type: *http://www.herniainfo.com.* Answers common questions about hernias, covers surgery options, and lists doctors near you.

Inflammatory Bowel Disease

SIGNS AND SYMPTOMS

Most common:
- Abdominal pain (in Crohn's disease, often in the lower right side of the abdomen; in ulcerative colitis, in the left side).
- Stubborn, severe diarrhea.
- Bloody stools or rectal bleeding.

Less common:
- Fever.
- Fatigue and weakness.
- Skin rashes.
- Arthritis-like pains in the joints.

Inflammatory bowel disease (IBD) is the name given to a group of chronic intestinal ailments. They share a number of symptoms and complications. The most common are Crohn's disease and ulcerative colitis.

In Crohn's disease, parts of the digestive tract (see color illustration, page 174) become inflamed, making digestion hard and weakening the body. In ulcerative colitis, tiny sores in the colon flare up and sometimes cause bloody stools or painful attacks of diarrhea. Both can be serious, but only in rare cases are they fatal.

The cause of IBD is unknown. Anyone can get it, including young children; most cases show up before the person is 30. Although there is no known cure, minor changes in diet and the right medication can often control the symptoms. Some serious cases of IBD call for surgery to remove the diseased part of the bowel.

Both the symptoms and the severity of IBD are hard to predict. See your doctor if you suspect you have IBD; proper treatment can keep it from getting worse.

WHAT YOU CAN DO NOW

- If you have many bouts of diarrhea, be careful not to let yourself get dehydrated (see **diarrhea,** page 122).
- Maintain a balanced diet. Diarrhea and poor digestion rob the body of vital fluids and nutrients.
- Avoid foods that irritate the colon. If you suspect a food, don't eat it for 10 to 30 days. Then try it. If your symptoms flare up, stay away from that food. (Common irritants are spicy or high-fiber foods, dairy products, eggs, and wheat.)
- Avoid alcohol.
- Avoid aspirin.
- Because you may be at greater risk of **colon cancer** (see page 118), talk about routine screening with your doctor.
- Reduce **stress** (see page 222).

WHEN TO CALL THE DOCTOR

Call for a prompt appointment:
- If you have a sudden attack of abdominal pain, fever, and the urge to pass gas or to have a bowel movement. You may be in the first stages of **appendicitis** (see page 26).
- If you have rectal bleeding with clots of blood in your stool; this could be a severe stage of colitis.

Call for advice:
- If diarrhea lasts more than 48 hours. You may be at risk of dehydration.
- If you have the most common signs of IBD. These could point to other ailments as well, such as the less serious **irritable bowel syndrome** (see the next entry).

HOW TO PREVENT IT

There is no known way to prevent Crohn's disease or ulcerative colitis. But it may help to stay away from foods that have given you trouble (see What You Can Do Now, above).

FOR MORE HELP

Information line: Intestinal Disease Foundation, 412-261-5888, M–F 9:30–3:30 EST. Provides telephone support, educational programs and readings, advice on support groups, and lists of doctors.

Organization: Crohn's and Colitis Foundation of America, 800-343-3637. Ask for a

DO YOU HAVE A PARASITE?

Parasitic illnesses such as giardiasis or amoebiasis can cause symptoms much like those of IBD. So can certain bacterial illnesses. Parasites and bacteria often enter the body through bad food or water. If you have been traveling, camping, or drinking untreated water, or have another reason to suspect an intestinal parasite, ask your doctor about a stool test.

free fact packet or advice on support groups.

Book: *Your Gut Feelings,* by Henry D. Janowitz, M.D. Covers intestinal problems, including inflammatory bowel. Oxford University Press, 1994, $11.95.

Web access: National Institute of Diabetes and Digestive and Kidney Diseases of the National Institutes of Health. After logging on to the Internet, type: *http://www.niddk.nih.gov/NIDDK_HomePage.html.* Scroll to *Information on Diseases,* then click on *Digestive Diseases.* Click on *Crohn's* or *Ulcerative Colitis.* Offers advice on treatment and lists other resources.

Irritable Bowel Syndrome

SIGNS AND SYMPTOMS

Symptoms of irritable bowel syndrome (IBS) can differ greatly from one person to another but may include:

- Diarrhea or constipation, or both back and forth over a few months.
- Abdominal cramps or pain.
- Lots of gas or bloating.
- Nausea, most often after eating.
- Headaches, fatigue, feeling anxious or depressed.
- A feeling that bowel movements aren't complete.

As you digest your food, your intestinal tract moves it along with waves of muscle contractions. Irritable bowel syndrome occurs when these movements lose their rhythm and upset the process. IBS, also called spastic colon, is the most common digestive ailment, affecting at least 10 to 15 percent of adults at some time. It does not lead to any fatal bowel diseases. It can be hard to treat, though, because no one is sure what causes it. Some experts think it is brought on—or made worse—by **stress** (see page 222) or a poor diet.

WHAT YOU CAN DO NOW

If you have symptoms of IBS, see your doctor. He or she may want you to have some tests, such as a barium enema and X-ray, to rule out more serious ailments (see **abdominal pain** chart, page 119). In the meantime, self-care can help:

- If you have **diarrhea** or **constipation,** see pages 122 or 121.
- Keep a record of what you eat and note which foods seem to cause problems. Avoid those foods if you can.
- Change your diet. Cut down on fatty foods. See if it helps to avoid items that can cause problems, such as eggs, dairy foods, spicy foods, coffee, and diet foods with sorbitol (an artificial sweetener).
- Try slowly adding more high-fiber foods to your diet (raw fruits and vegetables, bran, whole wheat, and dried beans). Some find this helps, but other people find it can make the problem worse.
- Eat smaller meals 4 or 5 times a day to make digestion easier.
- Don't smoke. Avoid smoky places.
- Include exercise and relaxation in your daily life.
- Seek therapy or try a stress-reduction program if you suspect that stress is a cause of the problem (see **is stress putting your health at risk?** page 308).

WHEN TO CALL THE DOCTOR

Call for a prompt appointment:

- If you notice pain in your lower left abdomen, with fever and maybe a change in your bowel movement pattern; **diverticulitis** may be the problem (see page 124).

- If you get a fever with diarrhea, or you wake up at night with diarrhea and you have been losing weight. These may be signs of **inflammatory bowel disease** (see page 131).

Call for advice and an appointment:

- If your stools have blood or mucus, if your stools look different, or if you notice a change in how often you have a bowel movement. You may have colon polyps or **colon cancer** (see page 118).
- If any symptoms of bowel trouble get in the way of your normal daily life.

HOW TO PREVENT IT

- The causes of irritable bowel syndrome are unknown, so the best approach is to take care of your health: Eat well and ease the stress in your life.

FOR MORE HELP

Information line: Intestinal Disease Foundation, 412-261-5888, M–F 9:30–3:30 EST. Offers telephone support, educational programs and fact packets, advice on support groups, and names of doctors near you.

Organization: International Foundation for Bowel Dysfunction, Box 17864, Milwaukee, WI 53217. 414-241-9479, M–F 9–5 CST. Offers support and brochures on bowel problems.

Newsletter: *Nutrition Action.* Offers clear, useful advice on good nutrition and diet. From the Center for Science in the Public Interest, 1875 Connecticut Ave. NW, Suite 300, Washington, DC 20009. 202-332-9110, M–F 12–5 EST. $24 per year.

Book: *Your Gut Feelings,* by Henry D. Janowitz, M.D. Facts about intestinal problems, including irritable bowel. Oxford University Press, 1994, $11.95.

Web access: National Institute of Diabetes and Digestive and Kidney Diseases of the National Institutes of Health. After logging on to the Internet, type: *http://www.niddk.nih.gov/IBS/IBS.html.* Explores the causes of irritable bowel and lists other resources.

Nausea and Vomiting

SIGNS AND SYMPTOMS

Nausea and vomiting sometimes happen with:

- Diarrhea.
- Abdominal cramps or pain.
- Fever, weakness, and fatigue.
- Headache.
- Loss of appetite.

Although nausea and vomiting are common and most often are not serious, they can worry you. In children and young adults, they most often result from the viral infection commonly called stomach flu. In these cases, vomiting and diarrhea often go away within 2 to 3 days, but weakness and fatigue may last about a week.

In old people, medicines and ulcers are more often the culprits (see **ulcers and gastritis,** page 136). Less common causes are bacterial and parasitic infections (see box **do you have a parasite?** on opposite page), food **allergies** (see page 86), and drinking too much alcohol.

Another cause is **food poisoning** (see page 36), which you can get from eating food tainted with viruses, bacteria, or chemicals. In this case, you could also have abdominal cramps and diarrhea, headache, dizziness, or fever and chills. The vomiting may leave you dehydrated.

Mild food poisoning lasts only a few hours or at worst a day or two, but some types—such as botulism and certain forms of chemical poisoning—are severe and may be fatal unless you get prompt treatment.

WHAT YOU CAN DO NOW

If you think you might have severe food poisoning or chemical poisoning:

- Call the local poison control center listed in the front of your phone book. Trained staff members can help you decide if you need medical help. (If you can't find the local center in your phone book, call infor-

Rectal Bleeding and Itching

Itching and bleeding in and around the anus often signal an ailment you can cure fairly easily with home care or some help from your doctor. Even blood on the stools doesn't always mean a bad illness. Some bleeding and itching, however, does require prompt medical help.

SYMPTOMS	WHAT IT MIGHT BE	WHAT YOU CAN DO
Bloody stools, painful abdominal cramping and swelling, nausea and vomiting, constipation, weakness or dizziness.	Intestinal obstruction—blockage of small or large intestine. • Scarring from abdominal surgery. • Strangulated hernia (see page 129). • Colon cancer (see page 118). • Diverticulitis (see page 124). • Object in digestive tract.	Call 911 or go to emergency room **right away.**
Bright red bleeding from the rectum after injury, anal intercourse, or putting an object into rectum.	Tear in sphincter muscle or skin around anus.	Call doctor for emergency advice. If you can't get one, call 911 or go to emergency room **right away.**
Watery diarrhea with blood, mucus, or pus; abdominal cramps or pain; nausea and vomiting; fever; muscle aches or pain; rapid dehydration and weight loss.	Dysentery—bacterial infection of intestinal tract. You can catch it from others or pass it on to someone else.	Call doctor for prompt appointment. Drink lots of fluids, and don't take over-the-counter stomach medications.
Painful anal itching at night, often in children; restless sleep and bad temper.	Pinworms—common intestinal parasites.	Call doctor for advice and appointment. If you're given antiworm medication, follow directions closely.
Painful or hard bowel movements, soreness in rectal area, blood or mucus from rectum, abdominal cramps, constipation.	Proctitis—swelling of rectum and anal tissues. • Bacterial or viral infection. • Inflammatory bowel disease (see page 131). • Sexually transmitted disease (see chart, page 225). • Colon cancer (see page 118). • Injury from anal intercourse.	Call doctor for advice and appointment. Take warm baths often to ease pain. Eat high-fiber foods and drink at least 8 glasses of water a day to soften stools.

Rectal Bleeding and Itching

SYMPTOMS	WHAT IT MIGHT BE	WHAT YOU CAN DO
Bloody stools, diarrhea that won't go away, nausea, cramps or pain in lower right side of abdomen.	Crohn's disease.	See inflammatory bowel disease, page 131.
Repeated bouts of diarrhea with mucus and blood, pain in left side of abdomen that lessens after bowel movements.	Ulcerative colitis.	See inflammatory bowel disease, page 131.
Itching in anal area or bright red blood in stool, pain during or after bowel movements.	Inflamed blood vessels in anus (see hemorrhoids, page 128). • Split or tear in skin around anus (anal fissure). • Psoriasis (see page 177).	Take warm baths, especially after painful bowel movements. Include lots of fiber and plenty of fluids in diet (see constipation, page 121). See doctor if it persists.
Itching around anus.	Often no clear cause. In older people, may be dry skin that comes with aging.	After bowel movements, gently clean anal area with moist, undyed tissue or baby wipes. Avoid soap, which can make itching worse.

mation, a local hospital, or 911.)

- For food poisoning, ask others who ate the same food if they got sick. Try to get a sample of the food, which can be tested if your symptoms get worse or don't go away.

If you have mild vomiting and diarrhea:

- Don't take any antinausea or antidiarrhea medication for 24 hours after your symptoms start, unless a doctor advises it. Vomiting and diarrhea are the body's way of getting rid of whatever may be causing the problem. (Children may need medication because they become dehydrated more quickly.)
- Sip clear fluids. Suck on ice chips or Popsicles if nothing will stay down.
- Once you can keep fluid in your stomach, drink clear liquids for about the next 12 hours. Then, for a full day, eat bland foods—such as rice, cooked cereals, baked potatoes, and clear soups—if your stomach will take them.
- Watch for signs of dehydration, especially in infants, children, and older adults. You can lose lots of fluid from repeated vomiting. Symptoms include dry mouth, sticky saliva, dizziness or weakness, dark yellow urine, and sometimes extreme thirst. For advice about replacing lost fluids, see **diarrhea,** page 122. If you can't keep liquids down and are becoming badly dehydrated, you will need to go to a hospital to get enough fluids into your body.
- Get plenty of rest until symptoms are gone.

WHEN TO CALL THE DOCTOR

Call 911 or go to an emergency room **right away:**

- If, along with vomiting and abdominal pain, you have blurred vision, muscle weakness, a hard time speaking or swallowing, or trouble moving or feeling your muscles. These may be signs of botulism, a rare but sometimes fatal type of bacterial food poisoning.

➤ If you have symptoms of chemical food poisoning—vomiting, diarrhea, sweating, dizziness, very teary eyes, great amounts of saliva, mental confusion, and stomach pain—about 30 minutes after eating. Pesticides or tainted food may be to blame. This type of poisoning can be deadly.
➤ If you vomit blood or anything that looks like coffee grounds. These are signs of bleeding in the esophagus or stomach.

Call for a prompt appointment:

➤ If you have bloody or black, tarry stools; this can signal internal bleeding.
➤ If you develop signs of dehydration—dry mouth, sticky saliva, dizziness or weakness, dark yellow urine, and, sometimes, extreme thirst. Dehydration is very serious in infants (see **diarrhea in children** box, page 123).
➤ If you have intense pain or swelling in the abdomen, rectum, or anus; you may have an abdominal disorder (see **abdominal pain** chart, page 119).

Call for advice:

➤ If your symptoms come back after treatment; you may have another problem such as an intestinal **parasite** (see **do you have a parasite?** box on page 132).
➤ If your vomiting and diarrhea are severe and last longer than 2 or 3 days.
➤ If you have a fever of 101.5 or higher.
➤ If you think a prescribed drug might be the cause.

HOW TO PREVENT IT

To avoid catching viral stomach flu:

➤ Keep your immune system strong with plenty of rest, exercise, and a healthy diet.
➤ Wash your hands often.

To prevent food poisoning:

➤ Don't thaw frozen meat on the kitchen counter. Let meat thaw in the refrigerator, or thaw it quickly in a microwave oven and cook it right away. Be sure that frozen food (above all, poultry) is fully thawed or defrosted before cooking. This will help make sure it cooks all the way through so heat will kill any bacteria.
➤ At picnics or anywhere else, don't eat moist foods that have been out 2 hours or more, or long enough to become warm. Avoid raw meat, fish, or eggs. Cook all these foods well.
➤ Using soap and hot water, wash your hands and any countertops, cutting boards, or utensils touched by uncooked meat, fish, or poultry.
➤ Quickly refrigerate food that can spoil. Set your refrigerator at 37 degrees, and never eat dairy foods or cooked meat that have been out of a refrigerator longer than 2 hours.
➤ Be sure that all members of your household wash their hands with soap and water after using the toilet and before fixing food or eating.
➤ Don't eat any food that looks or smells spoiled, or any food in bulging cans or cracked jars—a sign that the contents have gone bad.
➤ Don't eat wild berries, mushrooms, or other plants unless you know what they are.

Ulcers and Gastritis

SIGNS AND SYMPTOMS

- Pain in the upper abdomen.
- Nausea.
- Vomiting.
- No urge to eat.
- Belching or gas.
- Heartburn.
- Dark or bloody stools.

Stomach ulcers are sometimes called peptic ulcers. They are holes or breaks in the lining of the stomach, in the esophagus (the tube between the throat and the stomach), or in the duodenum (the upper part of the small intestine). Experts used to blame most ulcers on stress, but now a prime suspect is a germ—a common bacterium called *Helicobacter pylori.* Overuse of painkillers such as aspirin and ibuprofen can also cause ulcers. Other factors may include:

➤ **Stress** (see page 222).
➤ Smoking and heavy drinking.

- Too much stomach acid.
- Too little mucus to protect the stomach lining.

Stomach ulcers are fairly easy to treat. If bacteria are the problem, antibiotics (sometimes with another drug) will take care of them.

The bacteria that cause ulcers can also cause gastritis—inflammation of the stomach lining. In some people, but not all, gastritis may cause symptoms like those of indigestion, such as upper abdominal pain, nausea, and vomiting.

Although the symptoms are almost the same as those some people get from overeating, or eating fatty or spicy foods, gastritis is not caused by any of these habits.

Your doctor may advise over-the-counter antacids for gastritis that isn't too serious. If he or she suspects bacteria, you will most likely need antibiotics. Untreated gastritis can cause severe damage.

WHAT YOU CAN DO NOW

- Don't take aspirin, ibuprofen, and other nonsteroidal anti-inflammatory drugs. Try acetaminophen instead (see **pain relief,** page 317).
- Drink lots of water and other liquids to prevent dehydration, but avoid milk, which can increase acid.
- Take antacids.
- Eat smaller meals and eat more often. Stay away from any foods that cause symptoms.
- Don't drink alcohol, or don't drink much.
- Don't smoke. Avoid smoky places.
- Do relaxation or stress-reduction exercises (see **relax,** page 309).

WHEN TO CALL THE DOCTOR

Call 911 or go to an emergency room **right away:**

- If you throw up blood or anything that looks like coffee grounds. These are signs of bleeding in the esophagus or stomach.
- If you faint or feel faint, chilly, or sweaty. These may signal blood loss, a cause of shock (see **shock,** page 24).

Call for a prompt appointment:

- If you have sharp back pain with ulcer symptoms. The ulcer may be perforated—making holes or rips in your stomach or upper intestine.
- If you have an ulcer and are weak and pale. You could have anemia from a bleeding ulcer.
- If your stools are deep red or black, or have blood on them. These are signs of internal bleeding.

Call for advice and an appointment:

- If you have sharp stomach pain.
- If you have symptoms of a stomach ulcer or gastritis that last more than 2 weeks.

HOW TO PREVENT IT

- Cut down use of aspirin and ibuprofen.
- Avoid foods that upset your stomach.
- Do what you can to reduce stress.
- To prevent an ulcer from coming back, follow your doctor's advice for any ulcer drugs you are taking.

FOR MORE HELP

Organization: National Digestive Diseases Information Clearinghouse, 2 Information Way, Bethesda, MD 20892-3570. Write for a free fact sheet and packet on gastritis and helicobacter, the bacterium that may cause gastritis and ulcers.

Book: *Indigestion: Living Better With Upper Intestinal Problems,* by Henry D. Janowitz, M.D. Symptoms and treatment of ulcers. Oxford University Press, 1992, $8.95.

Web access: National Institute of Diabetes and Digestive and Kidney Diseases of the National Institutes of Health. After logging on to the Internet, type: *http://www.niddk.nih.gov/StomachUlcers/Ulcers.html.* Causes, symptoms, and treatment.

Video: *Ulcers (Gastrointestinal) at Time of Diagnosis.* Clear overview of causes and treatments, with 4 reports—Understanding the Diagnosis, What Happens Next?, Treatment and Management, and Issues and Answers. Time Life Medical, 1996, $19.95. Sold in many pharmacies; for one near you, call 800-588-9959.

Urinary System

Kidney Stones

SIGNS AND SYMPTOMS

- Sharp pains that come in waves—often on one side of the body—and start in the back below the ribs, then move toward the groin.
- In men, pain in testicles and penis.
- Trouble urinating.
- Urge to urinate often, but trouble passing more than small amounts of urine at a time.
- Dark urine or blood in the urine.
- Nausea and vomiting.

You may have a kidney infection if you also have:

- Fever.
- Pain when you urinate.
- Cloudy urine.

Kidney stones are just that: hard lumps in the kidneys, most often made of excess calcium.

The kidneys filter waste products out of the blood and mix them with water to make urine. Stones that form in a kidney must pass through one of the tubes (ureters) that connect the kidneys to the bladder (see illustration, page 174). From there, the stones can pass out of the body with the urine.

Some stones aren't a problem. But most cause intense pain as they move from a kidney to the bladder—a journey that can take hours, days, or weeks. The pain and other symptoms go away once you pass the stone.

Sometimes a stone gets trapped in one of the tubes leading to the bladder, blocking the flow of urine. Doctors can often destroy such stones with bursts of shock waves that turn the stones into powder, which is washed out with the urine.

Kidney stones tend to run in families. They're also more common in men than in women. People with gout (see **arthritis,** page 184), **irritable bowel syndrome** (see page 132), Crohn's disease (see **inflammatory bowel disease,** page 131), and chronic urinary tract infections (see **painful urination,** page 140) are among the most likely to get them. Kidney stones are also more common in hot climates than in cool ones: When people sweat a lot and don't drink enough liquids, their urine builds up more of the waste products that turn into stones.

WHAT YOU CAN DO NOW

- If you're having a kidney stone attack, drink lots of water—at least 8 to 10 large glasses a day. This will help flush the stone out of your system and help keep new ones from forming.
- Take an over-the-counter painkiller or one prescribed by your doctor (see **pain relief,** page 317).

WHEN TO CALL THE DOCTOR

- If you feel waves of sharp pain in your back, abdomen, or side.

Urinary Problems

Don't ignore these problems. Most can be treated and, with the right care, prevented.

SYMPTOMS	WHAT IT MIGHT BE	WHAT YOU CAN DO
Passing no urine or very little; weight gain and swelling of ankles and face.	Advanced kidney disease. • Kidney failure—when both kidneys stop working. • Blockage of the tubes that carry urine to the bladder.	Call 911 **right away** if you also have chest pains or trouble breathing. Otherwise, call doctor for prompt appointment.
Urge to urinate often, with extreme thirst.	Diabetes (see page 282). • Disorder of pituitary gland, which regulates body's fluid balance.	Call doctor for prompt appointment if you also have fever, chills, nausea, vomiting, low back pain, or extreme thirst. You may also have a kidney infection.
Urge to urinate often, but passing only small amounts of urine.	Infection of bladder or tube that carries urine out of body. • Prostate problem (see page 234). • Kidney stones (see opposite page). • Sexually transmitted disease (see chart on page 225). • Interstitial cystitis—inflamed bladder wall.	Call doctor for prompt appointment if you also have fever, chills, nausea, vomiting, low back pain, or extreme thirst. You may also have a kidney infection. See also painful urination, page 140.
Pain when you urinate.	Infection of bladder or tube that carries urine out of body (see page 175). • Kidney stones (see opposite page) or other kidney disease. • Sexually transmitted disease (see chart on page 225). • Pelvic inflammatory disease (see page 242). • Prostate problem (see page 234). • Vaginal problem (see page 249).	Call doctor for prompt appointment when acute pain starts or when it hurts to urinate. See also painful urination, page 140.
Blood in urine.	Kidney stones (see opposite page) or other kidney disease. • Prostate problem (see page 234). • Bladder infection. • Bladder or kidney cancer. • Injury to kidneys or bladder.	Call doctor for prompt appointment. See also painful urination, page 140.

- ➤ If you have trouble urinating.
- ➤ If you see blood in your urine.
- ➤ If you have fever with your symptoms.

HOW TO PREVENT IT

Kidney stones can come back. To help prevent them:

- ➤ Drink at least 8 glasses of water a day—more in hot weather.
- ➤ Ask your doctor about drugs or diet changes that might help.

FOR MORE HELP

Organization: National Kidney Foundation, 30 E. 33rd St., New York, NY 10016, 800-622-9010, M–F 8:30–5:30 EST. Call or write for a brochure on kidney stones.

Organization: National Kidney and Urologic Diseases Information Clearinghouse, 3 Information Way, Bethesda, MD 20892-3580, 301-654-4415, M–F 9–5 EST. Facts about kidney ailments.

KIDNEY STONES

A kidney stone can hurt when it passes through a ureter, one of the two tubes leading from the kidneys to the bladder.

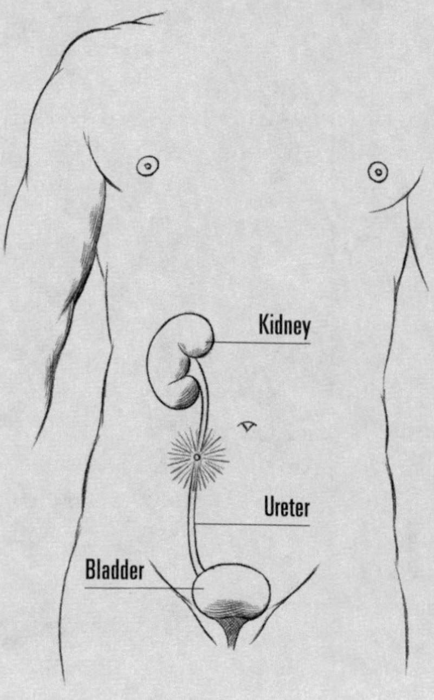

Book: *The Kidney Stones Handbook: A Patient's Guide to Hope, Cure, and Prevention,* by Gail Golomb. Four Geez Press, 1994, $12.95.

Web access: National Institute of Diabetes and Digestive and Kidney Diseases. After logging on to the Internet, type: *http://www.niddk.nih.gov/KidneyStones/kidney.html.* Provides facts about kidney function, advice on treatment, and more resources.

Painful Urination

SIGNS AND SYMPTOMS

- ■ Burning or stinging when urinating.
- ■ Urge to urinate often, but with small amounts passed each time.
- ■ Cloudy, strong-smelling, or bloody urine.
- ■ Yellow discharge from the urinary tube (urethra).
- ■ Pain in the lower abdomen or lower back.
- ■ In women, pain during intercourse.

Many problems can make urination painful, but urinary tract infections are the most common.

Although normal urine contains no bacteria, bacteria always live on your skin and in the anal area. These germs can get into the urinary tract and travel up the tube (urethra) between the bladder and the outside of the body. They grow in the bladder and cause pain, swelling, and redness. This infection is called cystitis. It's the most common urinary tract infection.

The urethra itself can get infected; so can the kidneys if bacteria reach them.

Adult women are more likely than others to get urinary tract infections, and sexually active women are most at risk. That's because the urethra is near the vagina. During intercourse, germs can move into the urethra, and then to the bladder. Women who use a diaphragm may be more likely than others to get these infections because the device can irritate the urethra.

People with diabetes and weakened immune systems also have a higher risk of infection. So do those with kidney stones and other urinary problems, or people who must use catheters (see **diabetes,** page 282, and **kidney stones,** page 138). The risk of a urinary tract infection goes up as you grow older.

Though these infections can be painful, they are easy to cure with antibiotics.

WHAT YOU CAN DO NOW

- Drink plenty of water in the first 24 hours—at least 8 to 10 glasses, more if you can. This will dilute your urine and help wash out the germs. (But don't drink lots of water if you're going to see the doctor. This can dilute any urine samples you may be asked to give. That makes it harder to find the cause of your problem.)
- When you have symptoms, don't drink juices high in acid, such as cranberry juice.
- Stay away from drinks with caffeine or alcohol in them, and foods with lots of spices, such as black pepper or chili powder.
- Take a hot bath or use a heating pad to help relieve pain or itching.
- Don't have intercourse until symptoms are gone.

WHEN TO CALL THE DOCTOR

Call for a prompt appointment:

- If you have a sharp pain that comes in waves, starting in the back below the ribs and moving toward the groin. You may have kidney stones.
- If you have a fever that gets worse quickly, with sudden, intense pain in your back near or above your waistline. You may have a kidney infection.
- If your urine looks bloody or very cloudy.
- If it hurts to urinate and you have any discharge from the penis or vagina that seems strange; you may have a **sexually transmitted disease** (see chart on page 225).
- If you are a woman, it hurts to urinate, and you have: tenderness and a dull ache or pain in your lower back and abdomen; pain during intercourse; and/or you sometimes miss menstrual periods or have very heavy ones. You may have endometriosis (see **menstrual irregularities** chart, page 239) or **pelvic inflammatory disease** (see page 242).

Call for advice and an appointment:

- If you are a man and it hurts to urinate, and you have: a need to urinate often, trouble urinating, painful ejaculation, or pain in the pelvis or lower back. You may have a **prostate problem** (see page 234).
- If it is painful to urinate or you have the other symptoms of a urinary tract infection.
- If your symptoms don't go away or if they come back despite treatment.

HOW TO PREVENT IT

- Drink 8 glasses of fluids—mostly water—each day. Try cranberry juice, too, which can help keep an infection from starting.
- Urinate when you have the urge to go. Empty your bladder every time.
- Wash before and after sex. Ask your partner to do the same.
- Urinate right after sex; this helps flush out bacteria that may have entered the urinary tract.
- Take showers instead of baths.
- Don't use bubble bath or scented soaps. Use a mild, scent-free detergent to wash underwear; scented or harsh products can irritate the skin around the urethra, making infection more likely.
- Wear cotton-crotch underwear and loose-fitting clothes.
- Wash genitals with plain water once a day.

For women:

- If you use a diaphragm, wash it after each use with warm, soapy water, then rinse and dry it. If you have more infections, ask your doctor to see if it fits well. If a different size doesn't help, try using another type of birth control.
- To keep the urinary tract free of bacteria, always wipe yourself from front to back after using the toilet.

FOR MORE HELP

Organization: The American Foundation for Urologic Disease, 300 W. Pratt St., Suite 401, Baltimore, MD 21201. Write for brochures.

Organization: National Institute of Diabetes and Digestive and Kidney Diseases, 301-496-3583, M–F 8:30–5 EST. Covers kidney and urinary tract problems. **Web site:** *http://www.niddk.nih.gov.* Click on *Urologic Disorders* under the *Information on Disorders* heading, then choose 1 of 6 topics.

Organization: Interstitial Cystitis Association of America, Box 1553, Madison Square Station, New York, NY 10159. Send a business-size, self-addressed, stamped envelope for information.

Book: *Overcoming Bladder Disorders,* by Rebecca Chalker and Kristene E. Whitmore, M.D. HarperPerennial, 1990, $12.50.

IF YOU'RE PREGNANT

Urinary tract infections in pregnant women sometimes move up to the kidneys, where they can become dangerous. For this reason, many doctors suggest regular urine testing during pregnancy. If you are pregnant and you're finding it painful to urinate or you have any of the other symptoms listed here, call your doctor for a prompt appointment.

Urinary Incontinence

SIGNS AND SYMPTOMS

- Leaking a small amount of urine when coughing, exercising, laughing, or in any other way putting pressure on the bladder.
- Urge to urinate that you can't control.
- Urinating without knowing it.

More than 10 million people in the United States, mostly older men and women, have trouble holding the flow of urine. This problem is called urinary incontinence. Most of the several types can be helped or cured.

In *stress incontinence,* the muscles that close the tube (urethra) that carries urine outside the body sometimes get weak. When you sneeze, cough, or in any other way put pressure on the bladder, a little urine escapes. Childbirth or being overweight can weaken these muscles and cause this problem.

In *urge incontinence,* also called irritable bladder, you may not be able to control the need to urinate. This problem can be caused by a urinary tract infection, or by **stroke** (see pages 46 and 115), **Alzheimer's disease** (see page 50), or **Parkinson's disease** (see page 59).

With *overflow incontinence,* or an unstable bladder, you no longer feel when it's time to urinate. Rather than being wholly emptied several times a day, your bladder is always a little full. Then urine leaks out in dribbles. This problem may be linked to **diabetes** (page 282), nerve problems, or an enlarged prostate gland that blocks the flow of urine (see **prostate problems,** page 234). In women, it may result from a large fibroid or ovarian tumor.

Sometimes the cause of incontinence is a short-term problem and easy to cure. It may be the first and only symptom of a urinary tract infection (see **painful urination,** page 140), so clearing up the infection will often cure the incontinence. Some drugs, such as sleeping pills, diuretics, and tranquilizers, can make it hard to control your bladder. The problem may go away if your doctor prescribes a different drug.

Incontinence seldom poses a health risk, but you do need to take steps to treat it. Even if it can't be cured, it can almost always be controlled so that it stops being a problem in your daily life.

WHAT YOU CAN DO NOW

- Stay engaged with life and keep on doing the things you like. Don't withdraw from others.
- When you go out, wear underwear that absorbs moisture. But don't wear these garments too long; they can cause rashes.
- Cross your legs when you feel a sneeze coming on. It's a safe, simple way to prevent stress incontinence.

- Don't drink coffee, tea, or other drinks with caffeine. They can irritate the bladder.
- Don't drink a lot of liquid when away from home.
- Wear clothing that's easy to take off.
- Keep a diary—note when you lose control, how much urine is lost, and what you were doing at the time. It will help you and your doctor devise the best treatment plan.
- Try bladder training:
  - Go the bathroom every hour, whether or not you feel the need. Stretch the time between visits by 15 to 30 minutes every 2 days. Slowly work up to 3 or 4 hours between visits.
  - If you need to urinate between visits, relax where you are until the urge is gone, then find a bathroom.
  - Practice "double voiding." Empty your bladder, then relax a moment and try again.

WHEN TO CALL THE DOCTOR

- If you have any bladder control problems.
- If you have signs of an infection, such as fever or pain when you urinate.
- If you think a drug is causing it.

HOW TO PREVENT IT

- Practice Kegel exercises, which tone the muscles that control the flow of urine: As you start and stop the flow, sense which muscles you're working. Later, contract and release them—at least 15 to 20 squeezes, 3 times a day. After some practice, tighten the muscles for at least 10 seconds each time. Kegels are private: You're the only one who will know you're doing them.
- Exercise often and lose extra pounds. Excess body weight puts pressure on the bladder muscles.
- Eat a lot of fresh fruits, vegetables, and whole grains to avoid constipation. Straining can weaken bladder muscles.
- Ask your doctor about biofeedback.

FOR MORE HELP

Hotline: Simon Foundation for Continence, 800-237-4666, 24-hour line. Staff answers questions and sends brochures about incontinence. Call 847-864-3913, M–F 9–5 CST about support groups.

Organization: Help for Incontinent People, 800-252-3337 or 864-579-7900, M–F 8–5 EST. Lists health care providers who treat incontinence.

Booklet: American Foundation for Urologic Disease, 300 W. Pratt St., Suite 401, Baltimore, MD 21201. Write for a copy of "Answers to Your Questions About Urinary Incontinence" or "Incontinence in the Elderly."

Book: *Staying Dry: A Practical Guide to Bladder Control,* by Kathryn L. Burgio, K. Lynette Pearce, and Angelo J. Lucco. Johns Hopkins University Press, 1989, $12.95. Offers step-by-step help.

Book: *Coping With Bowel and Bladder Problems,* by Barbara Doherty King, M.S., and Judith Harke, R.N. Part of the "Coping With Aging" series, written by nurses who work with older people. Singular Publishing, 1994, $18.95.

Skin, Scalp, & Nails

Acne

SIGNS AND SYMPTOMS

- Ongoing outbreaks of reddish blemishes on the face and sometimes on the chest, shoulders, neck, upper back, or buttocks.
- Spots that have a dark, open center (blackheads).
- Bumps under the skin (whiteheads).
- Whiteheads that rupture (pimples).
- Boil-like lumps (nodules).

Acne is an outbreak of pimples, blackheads, whiteheads, or boils. It seems to be linked to too much sebum, the oil that keeps your skin moist. Sebum can plug a hair follicle, forming a whitehead or blackhead. Bacteria that grow behind the plug can cause a pimple or, rarely, a boil or cyst.

Anyone at any age—even newborns—can get acne. You may be prone to it:

- If you have a family history of acne.
- If your male hormones (both men and women have them) increase, chiefly during puberty.
- If you take certain drugs, such as lithium or corticosteroids (anti-inflammatories).
- If you use creams, oils, makeup, or other products that block the skin's pores.
- If you're a woman and you have hormonal changes from menstrual periods, pregnancy, or the Pill.

No matter what people say, stress, poor cleaning habits, and a poor diet don't appear to cause acne, although they can make it worse. You can also get acne-like outbreaks if you have **allergies** to some foods (see page 86).

WHAT YOU CAN DO NOW

- Wash the area twice a day with mild, oil- and scent-free soap. Don't wash too often. Your acne may get worse if you do. Try astringents such as witch hazel if you have very oily skin or an oily "T zone" (forehead, nose, and chin).
- Shampoo your hair often. Oily hair may make the acne worse. Keep long hair off your face and shoulders.
- Shave as seldom as possible. Men with acne should take care to avoid nicking pimples. If you have severe acne, always use a fresh blade to avoid infection.
- Use only hypoallergenic, scent-free makeup made for acne-prone skin. Remove all makeup before going to bed.
- Try an over-the-counter treatment with benzoyl peroxide (a germ-killing agent) or salicylic acid (a mild peeling agent that helps unblock pores).
- After exercising, wipe off your sweat with a moist towel, or take a shower or bath. Do the same if you sweat a lot during the day.
- Wear a sunscreen, but choose one with care. If you have oily skin or sweat a lot, heavy sunscreens with coconut oil and cocoa butter may make your acne worse. Use sunscreen that's "non-comedogenic" (won't clog pores).

Rashes

The causes of rashes range from minor to serious. This chart includes some of the most common, as well as some that could be fatal. If your child has a rash, or if you and your child have the same rash, see the **children's rashes** chart (page 253).

SYMPTOMS	WHAT IT MIGHT BE	WHAT YOU CAN DO
Itchy red bumps anywhere on body; swelling of eyes, lips, and tongue; weakness; shortness of breath; sweating; rapid heartbeat.	Shock from allergy—severe, sudden reaction (that may be fatal) to foods, drugs, or insect bites (see page 24).	Call 911 **right away.**
Fever; stiff neck; headache; light is hard to look at; maybe bumpy, deep red or purplish rash.	Meningitis (see page 57).	Call 911 or go to emergency room **right away.**
Rash that looks like sunburn, often on palms of hands or soles of feet; sudden high fever (above 102); vomiting and diarrhea; headache; weakness; fainting; dizziness; confusion.	Toxic shock syndrome (see page 248).	Call 911 or go to emergency room **right away.** If you are using tampon, menstrual sponge, diaphragm, or cervical cap, remove right away after calling.
Itchy, raised red or pink patches (sometimes with white centers) that may come and go, anywhere on body.	Hives (see page 157).	Call 911 or go to emergency room if you also have wheezing, dizziness, and trouble breathing. This may be shock from allergy (see page 24).
First, rash that often begins at ankles or wrists, then moves to torso, face, and elsewhere. Often with headache, chills, and fever. Next, rash turns deep red, then looks like red pinpricks.	Rocky Mountain spotted fever. Caused by microorganism that enters body through tick bite. Illness gets its name from place where first reported. Now widespread (see tick bites, page 47).	Call doctor for prompt appointment. Can be fatal if untreated. Ask for test for Rocky Mountain spotted fever and also for Lyme disease (see next page of chart).
Butterfly-shaped red rash on cheeks and nose; fever, fatigue, joint pain, swelling.	Lupus (see page 290).	Call doctor for prompt appointment.

(continued)

Rashes *(continued)*

SYMPTOMS	WHAT IT MIGHT BE	WHAT YOU CAN DO
Red rash with bull's-eye shape, spreading several inches from tick bite. Followed within a month by fever, headache, lethargy, and joint pain.	Lyme disease (see page 291). Caused by micro-organism that enters body through tick bite (see tick bites, page 47).	Call doctor for prompt appointment. Get tested for Lyme disease and also for Rocky Mountain spotted fever. If you can find tick, remove with tweezers; don't squeeze or twist it.
Burning or tingling skin followed by painful, blistery red rash; most often on only one side of torso, buttocks, or face.	Shingles (see page 178).	Call doctor for prompt appointment.
Thick patches of itchy red skin anywhere on body; or blisters with severe itching.	Eczema (see page 154). • Dermatitis (see page 151). • Poison oak or ivy (see page 153).	Call doctor for advice and appointment.
Raised patches of itchy pink skin with white scales, often on knees, elbows, and scalp.	Psoriasis (see page 177).	Call doctor for advice and appointment.
Small, pus-filled, pimplelike bumps anywhere on body.	Folliculitis—bacterial infection of hair follicles. May be caused by shaving or by clothing, such as wet sports wear, that rubs against skin.	Use over-the-counter antibacterial soap or cream. If infection gets worse or lasts after 2 weeks of home care, call doctor for advice and appointment.
Itchy, red, flaky, or scaly patches that appear on just one part of body; can affect feet, genitals, skin, and nails.	Fungal infection (see page 155). Could be ringworm—infection that can be caught from another person or even from dog or cat; common in children.	Use over-the-counter antifungal powders and creams. If rash gets worse or lasts after 2 weeks of home care, call doctor for advice and appointment.
Extreme itching (most often at night); rough, red rash in folds of body—between fingers, on wrists, elbows, breasts, buttocks, or waist.	Scabies.	See lice and scabies, page 159.

WHAT IS ROSACEA?

Rosacea (rose-AY-sha) is a rash often thought to be acne. It can cause a swollen, red nose, puffy cheeks, and a lasting blush on other parts of the face. Rosacea occurs when tiny blood vessels enlarge, most often on the cheeks, nose, and forehead. Sometimes red, pus-filled spots appear, but no blackheads or whiteheads. People with rosacea may also get **conjunctivitis** (see page 65), because the bacteria that cause rosacea also grow around the eyes.

Rosacea's cause is unknown. It often affects women over 30. The rash comes and goes, and seems to be made worse by hot or spicy food, alcohol or caffeine, very hot or cold weather or strong sunlight, and rubbing the face.

While rosacea is harmless, it is often ugly and may get worse over time. If you think you have rosacea, see your doctor to check on it and treat it.

- Don't rest your face in your hands while reading, working, or watching TV.
- Avoid propping the phone against your cheek. Try cleaning the receiver often—or buy a headset if you spend long hours on the phone.
- Don't pop, pick, scratch, or squeeze your pimples. This may cause scars.

WHEN TO CALL THE DOCTOR

- If your acne doesn't get better after 2 to 3 months of over-the-counter treatments. You may need further treatment.
- If you have many pimples, if your acne makes you feel shy or ashamed, or if you have signs of scarring. A skin specialist (dermatologist) may give you a drug to keep the acne from getting worse and causing scars.
- If you think you may have rosacea, a rash around your cheeks and nose (see box, this page).

HOW TO PREVENT IT

Doctors believe you can't prevent acne, since it's partly genetic and partly due to hormones.

FOR MORE HELP

Information line: National Institute of Arthritis and Musculoskeletal and Skin Diseases Information Clearinghouse, 301-495-4484, M–F 8:30–5 EST. Staff answers questions and sends facts about acne.

Organization: American Academy of Dermatology, Box 4014, Schaumburg, IL 60168-4014. 847-330-0230, M–F 8:30–5 CST. Send a business-size, self-addressed, stamped envelope for pamphlets on acne and rosacea. Also provides a list of doctors near you.

Book: *SkinWise: A Guide to Healthy Skin for Women,* by Annette Callan. Facts and advice about acne, skin cancer, and other skin problems. Oxford University Press, 1995, $19.95.

Book: *Teenage Health Care,* by Gail B. Slap, M.D., and Martha M. Jablow. Covers teenage growth and a wide range of personal, social, and medical issues. Pocket Books, 1994, $14.

Blisters

SIGNS AND SYMPTOMS

- Sore, fluid-filled bubbles of skin, sometimes in clusters. They can range in size from a pinpoint to a few inches across.
- Sometimes itching, redness, and swelling.

Most blisters form because of friction. Simple movements such as the rubbing of a shovel handle or the pinch of a new pair of running shoes can raise one. Insect bites, viruses, certain skin ailments, such as contact **dermatitis** (see page 151), and some drugs and chemicals can also cause them. You can get blisters from **burns** (see page 28), after you've been in the sun, or in extremes of heat or cold.

WHAT YOU CAN DO NOW

Most of the time no treatment is needed, since new skin forms under the affected area and the fluid is absorbed.

Friction blisters:

➤ Popping a blister makes infection more likely, so it's best to leave a small one alone. To drain a large, painful blister: Clean the area with alcohol. Using a sterile needle, gently pierce one side of the blister. Let it drain. Then apply antibiotic cream and cover it.

➤ Don't pull off or cut away the loose skin from a broken blister. It covers and shields the new skin.

➤ Cover a broken blister to protect it. Use a simple adhesive bandage for a small blister or a gauze pad and adhesive tape for a large one. Change the bandage daily, or more often if it gets wet. Leave the blister uncovered at night to allow it to dry.

Burn blisters:

➤ Flush the affected place right away with lots of cool water or a saline (salt) solution. Don't rub or place ice on burns.

➤ Never pop a burn blister.

WHEN TO CALL THE DOCTOR

➤ If a blister has been caused by a burn, covers a large area, and is very painful. Blisters mean a second-degree burn. Some second- and all third-degree burns need a doctor's care.

➤ If the fluid in the blister isn't clear. White, yellow, or green discharge may signal infection.

➤ If your blisters are the result of a skin ailment or contact with chemicals or other toxic agents.

HOW TO PREVENT IT

➤ Wear gloves for tasks you do only now and then, such as shoveling snow, sweeping, or raking.

➤ Have your feet measured when you buy shoes, and wear only shoes that fit.

➤ Have your shoes repaired often. Worn soles don't protect the feet, and worn linings can chafe the skin.

➤ Keep your feet dry. Wear socks that don't have holes and that soak up moisture. Dust your feet with an antifungal powder if they tend to sweat.

➤ Put petroleum jelly or moleskin pads on areas, such as the heel, where socks are likely to rub. Wear socks that fit well. Socks that bunch up can cause blisters.

FOR MORE HELP

Information line: American Podiatric Medical Association, 800-FOOTCARE, 24-hour recording. Takes requests for free brochures on foot care.

Pamphlet: American Academy of Orthopaedic Surgeons, 800-824-BONES, 24-hour recording. Ask for pamphlet titled "If the Shoe Fits, Wear It."

Boils

SIGNS AND SYMPTOMS

■ Redness, swelling, tenderness, pain, or throbbing of a lump under the skin.

■ A red and swollen lump with a white or yellow pus-filled center under the skin (after a number of days).

A boil may look like a bad pimple. But you get a boil when staph bacteria invade a blocked hair follicle or oil gland. The germs, along with white blood cells and dead skin cells, form pus and cause swelling.

Boils most often appear on the face, neck, scalp, buttocks, armpits, or, sometimes, on a woman's nipple. A cluster of boils is known as a carbuncle—a rarer and more serious form that needs medical help.

Boils are common and most often minor. They can be passed from person to person, though rarely. People with diabetes or immune-system problems and those exposed to some industrial chemicals are the most likely to get them. So are people whose overall health is poor, who lack a clean home or don't wash well, whose diet is poor, or who overuse corticosteroids such as cortisone.

WHAT YOU CAN DO NOW

- Wash the infected area gently with antibacterial soap.
- Apply warm compresses (cloths soaked in hot water and wrung out) to help the boil burst and drain.
- Put an over-the-counter antibacterial cream on the boil to keep the infection from spreading.
- Don't press or prick the boil. This could spread the infection. Most boils will burst on their own after about 10 to 14 days. When one does, hold a warm, clean compress against it to remove all the pus. Next, apply antibacterial cream and cover the boil loosely with a bandage to prevent reinfection.
- Since boils are contagious, wash your hands well and launder towels, clothes, and bed linens in hot water and soap to avoid spreading the infection.

WHEN TO CALL THE DOCTOR

- If you have a boil on your face, a cluster of boils, or boils with a fever. You could get a more serious infection.
- If the pain is severe. A doctor may lance and drain the boil.
- If you get boils often. Your doctor will want to find out what is causing them.

HOW TO PREVENT IT

- Shower or bathe often.
- If you're prone to getting boils, apply an antibacterial cream after shaving.
- Treat minor skin injuries right away.
- Don't share towels or clothes. Clean sports gear well—for instance, straps on helmets and gym machines.
- Eat balanced meals with lots of fresh fruit and vegetables.

Bruises

SIGNS AND SYMPTOMS

- Black and blue or purple skin, turning red or yellow.
- Swelling, or hard lump under the skin.
- Pain.

Bruises are a sign of bleeding and damage to tissues just under the skin, most often from a hard blow. The word comes from the Old English for "crush." A black eye is a classic bruise.

Although the blood under the skin is red, a bruise looks black, blue, or purple because your skin filters out all colors but those. The darker the color, the deeper the bruise. After a few days, it may turn green or yellow as the blood cells begin to break up. This means the bruise is about to fade away.

Most bruises heal on their own, and swift home care can speed the process. But deep bruises, or large ones, may need medical care. They may also be a sign of illness, a blood problem, or a problem with a medication you are taking for another ailment.

WHAT YOU CAN DO NOW

- Ice and cold compresses used right away can hold down the swelling and damage from most bruises. The cold may also keep the bruise from turning deep purple, and it helps dull pain.
- Put a cold compress on the sore place within 15 minutes after an injury. Leave it on for 10 to 20 minutes at a time, then take it off for 30 to 40 minutes. Repeat this many times for the next 3 days.
- Raise the bruised part above the level of your heart, if you can. This holds down fluid buildup and swelling.
- Try not to use the sore area for 1 to 3 days. Use this time to repeat the ice treatment above as often as you can.
- Check your medication: Some drugs in-

Skin, Scalp, & Nails

crease bruising. Or it might be a sign your dose is too high.

- Take an over-the-counter painkiller (see **pain relief,** page 317). Don't take aspirin—it can increase bleeding and make the bruise worse. Never give aspirin to a child under 12 who has chicken pox, a cold, the flu, or any other illness you suspect of being caused by a virus (see box on **Reye's syndrome,** page 96).

WHEN TO CALL THE DOCTOR

- If the bruise doesn't fade or go away after 14 days.
- If it seems infected: The pain gets worse, it swells more, or you have redness, pus, or a fever.
- If you have vision problems with a black eye. The eye may be damaged.
- If you bruise often and easily, for no reason. You may have a blood disease or other illness.
- If an older person or someone with poor circulation gets a bruise on the lower leg but hasn't bumped or hit the leg. This could be a sign of a blood clot.
- If you are taking anticoagulants (they keep the blood from clotting), and you are bruising often or for no reason. Your dose might be too high.

HOW TO PREVENT IT

- Eat a balanced diet with plenty of vitamins C and K, which come in many fruits and vegetables. A lack of C or K can cause bruising (see **the nutrition top ten,** page 304).
- Accident-proof your house to help avoid falls. Light stairways; keep clutter off floors and stairs; use nightlights in bathrooms and hallways (see **be careful out there,** page 305).

Corns and Calluses

SIGNS AND SYMPTOMS

Both corns and calluses are made of thick, hard, dead skin. They differ mainly in where they show up.

Corns:

- On the tops or sides of toe joints or between the toes.

Calluses:

- On palms, soles of feet, or any place that rubs a lot against something hard.

Corns and calluses do your body a service, though they can be painful. Both shield the skin from injury. They're common and seldom cause a problem unless they build up or crack open; then they may hurt.

Most corns and calluses on the feet are caused by shoes that don't fit. Tapered, narrow-toed shoes and open-backed, high-heeled sandals cause the most problems.

WHAT YOU CAN DO NOW

- Place a corn pad on the toe to help ease the pressure on a corn.
- Use a pumice stone or callus file to gently rub dead skin off a callus or hard corn.
- Use a small piece of foot plaster, sold in drugstores, to remove the top layer of skin. Leave on as directed. Then rub the corn or callus lightly with a pumice stone and soak in hot, soapy water.
- Don't cut or burn off corns or calluses.

WHEN TO CALL THE DOCTOR

- If you have constant pain, redness, swelling, or discharge around a corn or callus. You might have an infection.
- If you get corns or calluses and you have diabetes or problems with your circulation. You may get another infection. See a doctor before trying home care.
- If self-care doesn't work, and you think the way you walk is causing the problem.

A foot specialist (podiatrist) may prescribe custom-made shoe inserts (orthotics).

HOW TO PREVENT IT

- Buy shoes at the end of the day, when your feet are largest. Wear only shoes that fit properly. The distance between the front of the shoe and your longest toe needs to be half an inch. Make sure toes can wiggle freely, and avoid pointed shoes and high heels.
- Keep your shoes in good shape by taking them in for needed repairs. Linings shouldn't rub against your skin. Soles shouldn't be so thin that your feet are jarred when you walk. Worn-down heels can't protect the heel bone.
- Keep your feet dry, and make sure they don't rub against your shoes. Wearing socks or nylons and using talcum powder will help. (If wool or manmade fibers make your feet sweat, wear cotton socks.)
- Rub away areas of skin buildup on the feet before they turn into corns or calluses. After bathing, rub the area gently with a pumice stone or callus file, sold in drugstores.

FOR MORE HELP

Information line: American Podiatric Medical Association, 800-FOOTCARE, 24-hour recording. Takes requests for free brochures on foot care.

Pamphlet: American Academy of Orthopaedic Surgeons, 800-824-BONES, 24-hour recording. Ask for pamphlet titled "If the Shoe Fits, Wear It."

Web access: The Center for Podiatric Information. After logging on to the Internet, type: *http://www.infowest.com/podiatry/footcare/index.html*. Click on *Corns, Calluses,* or other foot topics.

Dermatitis

SIGNS AND SYMPTOMS

One or more of these:

- Thick, itchy, dry red patches of skin on any part of the body.
- A pink or red rash anywhere, caused by something such as a chemical.
- Blistered, crusty, or scaly skin in round patches, often on the legs, buttocks, hands, or arms.
- Oily yellow scales on or near the face (nose, eyebrows, ears, scalp).
- Scaly, reddened skin, sometimes with craterlike sores, on lower legs.

Dermatitis is another name for a skin irritation or rash. Dry, red, itchy skin is most often the first symptom; this may be followed by crusty scales or oozing blisters. There are many types of dermatitis. They vary by the kind of rash and where it is on your body.

Contact dermatitis (red bumps and blisters that often weep and crust over) can appear anywhere on the body. It's most often caused by an irritation or allergy to a skin-

ITCHING

Got an itch? Most of the time, it's nothing to worry about. Often the cause is as simple as an insect bite or dry skin. These minor ailments most often clear up on their own or are easily treated at home with lotion or, in more stubborn cases, over-the-counter hydrocortisone cream.

Rarely, itching is a sign of a more serious disorder, such as anemia, kidney failure, or skin cancer. If you have itching with a rash, see the **rashes** chart (page 145). If you have an itch that lasts longer than 10 days and you don't know what's causing it, call your doctor for advice and an appointment.

care product or a plant such as poison ivy or poison oak (see **poison oak and ivy** box on next page). You may get this type of dermatitis when your skin reacts to certain soaps (including bubblebath soap) and detergents, chlorine, and some manmade fibers. Latex or rubber gloves, condoms, and nickel-plated jewelry can cause contact dermatitis. So can leather and new clothing. Be sure to wash new clothes before wearing them for the first time. Perfumes and other items in makeup may also bring it on (see **tips on choosing skin products** box on this page).

Another type, **nummular dermatitis,** is marked by round, red, oozing places, most often on the arms and legs. Stress and other skin problems can bring it on. Older people with dry skin or who live in dry climates often get it. It gets worse if you bathe in very hot water.

Seborrheic dermatitis appears most often on the face and scalp. In infants, a yellow, scaly rash is known as cradle cap. Some experts think it comes from a fungus; it may be made worse by plugged oil glands or by stress. People with immune disorders such as **AIDS** (see page 224) are prone to it.

TIPS ON CHOOSING SKIN PRODUCTS

If you see a rash on your scalp, neck, or face, something you're using for skin care or makeup could be the culprit. Perfume, makeup, shampoo, after-shave lotion, antiperspirants, sunblock, and suntan lotions all can upset the skin.

A scent or preservative is most often the problem, but items labeled "unscented" may cause trouble too. They still may contain fragrances or other chemicals. "Fragrance-free" is a better choice.

Even if a product says it's organic, natural, nonallergenic, or hypoallergenic, your skin may still react. If you have sensitive skin, choose your skin-care products with care. Start with fragrance-free products, and switch brands until you find one that doesn't cause a rash.

Stasis dermatitis is a scaly, dry, reddish rash, usually on the lower legs and ankles. Poor circulation can bring it on.

Extreme, constant itchiness anywhere on the body may be **eczema** (see page 154), also known as atopic dermatitis.

WHAT YOU CAN DO NOW

- For contact dermatitis, seek out the cause and get rid of it. If you find, for example, that nickel-plated jewelry or some type of makeup is the problem, you can simply stop wearing it.
- Test yourself at home if you think your skin reacts to makeup. Apply a small bit of the product to your arm, and cover the spot with a bandage (if you're allergic to these, use gauze and paper tape). If you get a red, itchy rash within 48 hours, the product is the cause, and you'll know to avoid it.
- To ease swelling and itching, toss a half-cup of cornstarch or oatmeal (sold in drugstores—not the type you cook) into a warm (not hot) bath. Soak your skin for only 30 minutes to keep from losing too many of the oils your skin needs. Use a mild, fragrance-free soap or cleanser. Or, use the oatmeal as a compress on your skin.
- For dry or flaky skin, apply petroleum jelly or scent-free body lotion. For an oozing rash, use calamine lotion.
- Shampoo your hair with a tar shampoo if you have dermatitis on the scalp. Your scalp may sunburn more easily for a few hours after using the shampoo, so stay out of the sun. (Never use this shampoo on children—it's too harsh. Use a baby shampoo instead, and wash your child's hair every day.)
- If you have red, oozing sores, apply washcloths that have been soaked in warm, salty water and wrung out. Then use an over-the-counter hydrocortisone cream.
- For stasis dermatitis on the legs and ankles, raise your legs above your hips many times a day. Try wearing support stockings.
- Don't scratch. Cut nails short to keep from breaking the skin.

POISON OAK AND IVY

Poison oak, poison ivy, and poison sumac grow as shrubs or vines throughout the United States except in Hawaii, Alaska, and some Nevada deserts. If you're outdoors just about anywhere else, your skin and the clear, oily sap in these plants' leaves and stems may meet—with nasty results.

The rash you get is a form of contact dermatitis. Symptoms differ from one person to the next, but they often include a line or streak on the skin that may look like insect bites within 12 to 48 hours after exposure. Redness and swelling follow, then blisters and severe itching. In a few days, the blisters begin to dry. Depending on how your skin reacts, the rash can take from 10 days to 3 weeks to go away.

You can't pass the rash to another person, or spread the rash to another part of your body. But if the oily poison is still on your clothes or gets in your home and touches your skin, the rash may return.

To prevent:

- ➤ Learn what poison oak, ivy, and sumac look like in all seasons, and stay away. The sap can remain active for months and, in dead plants, for years.
- ➤ Cover up. Wear long pants, long sleeves, and boots. Also wear cotton or leather gloves, if possible.
- ➤ Rinse sweat off skin with water—not with a cloth, which may spread any poison. Wear a bandanna, scarf, or hat to catch sweat from your brow.
- ➤ Don't let pets run through woods. The poison may come back on their fur.
- ➤ A new barrier lotion shows promise. It uses a substance already used in some deodorants. Look for "bentoquatam 5 percent" on the label. A decade ago, some forestry firefighters noticed their armpits escaped the rash that covered their bodies after battling poison-oak brushfires.

If you've been exposed:

- ➤ Clean the oil off exposed skin as soon as you can. If you have rubbing alcohol handy, splash it on, straight from the bottle. It will remove the oil as it runs off. Rinse with plenty of running water. Air dry your skin or pat dry with a towel. Don't rub. This can spread any remaining poison.
- ➤ If you don't have alcohol, get to a cold, running stream, a lake, or a garden hose quickly. Rinse thoroughly. Don't use soap.
- ➤ Or try gently covering exposed skin with sand or even dirt (make sure there aren't any poison oak or ivy leaves in it). This will help absorb the oil. Rinse off with plenty of water.
- ➤ At the end of a day in the woods, rinse all exposed skin with alcohol. Use a garden hose to rinse your clothes, shoes, gear, and pets.

If you have a rash from poison oak or ivy:

- ➤ To ease itching, use calamine lotion, sold in drugstores.
- ➤ Soak often in cool or lukewarm water with ½ cup baking soda or oatmeal (sold in drugstores). Don't scratch the rash or blisters.
- ➤ If your symptoms are severe or if you're getting new outbreaks after 10 days, call your doctor.

- ➤ Try an over-the-counter hydrocortisone cream.

WHEN TO CALL THE DOCTOR

- ➤ If your skin hasn't improved after 2 or 3 weeks of home care, over-the-counter creams, or medicated shampoos.
- ➤ If you have signs of an infection, such as sores with pus.

HOW TO PREVENT IT

- ➤ If you know you've been exposed to a

Skin, Scalp, & Nails

chemical agent, wash your skin with a mild cleanser and water as soon as you can.

- To keep the air around you moist, Use a humidifier at home and work (see box on **humidifiers and vaporizers,** page 93).
- If your skin is prone to dermatitis, choose untreated cotton or other natural-fiber fabrics for clothing. Make sure clothing isn't too tight.
- Don't wear nickel-plated earrings and other jewelry. Choose surgical stainless steel, sterling silver, or gold instead.
- Avoid contact with anything you suspect will upset your skin.
- When washing dishes or handling chemicals, wear thin cotton gloves under rubber gloves to protect your hands.
- After bathing, replace lost moisture in your skin with a lotion that has no scents or preservatives.

FOR MORE HELP

Organization: American Academy of Dermatology, Box 4014, Schaumburg, IL 60168-4014. 847-330-0230, M–F 8:30–5 CST. Send a business-size, self-addressed, stamped envelope for pamphlets on dermatitis. Also gives list of doctors near you. **Web site:** *http://www.aad.org/pip.html.* Select *Contact Dermatitis, Seborrheic Dermatitis,* or *Poison Ivy.*

Eczema

SIGNS AND SYMPTOMS

- Itchy, red, dry, scaly, blistered, or swollen patches of skin, usually on the scalp or face, hands and wrists, and knee and elbow creases.
- Oozing, crusting, thickening, or odd color of the affected skin area (sometimes).

Eczema (atopic dermatitis) tends to run in families and often has something to do with allergies, asthma, and **stress** (see page 222). It can also be triggered by chemical agents, weather extremes, sweating, and infections. Infants are prone to eczema, although many grow out of it before they turn 2. If it lasts after that age, a child is likely to have chronic eczema.

Eczema is rarely a dire health problem, but its symptoms can be stubborn and annoying.

WHAT YOU CAN DO NOW

- Don't scratch. Soothe skin and keep it moist by taking warm (not hot) baths daily. Use just a little mild cleanser or fragrance-free soap and don't scrub or towel your skin too hard. Apply a fragrance-free body lotion after bathing to restore moisture.
- For an older child or an adult, apply over-the-counter hydrocortisone cream. Avoid lotions with scents, oils, or preservatives. These may make your eczema worse.
- Try an oral over-the-counter antihistamine to relieve itching. Don't use antihistamine cream or antiseptic sprays.
- Wear loose, cool clothing; sweating can make eczema worse. Avoid manmade and wool fabrics, which may irritate the skin.
- Wash clothes with mild, fragrance-free laundry soap. Rinse twice. Don't use fabric softener.
- Trim nails short. Wear soft cotton gloves or mittens to bed to limit scratching. This is helpful for children.
- Ease tension with a quick walk or other exercise.
- Use a humidifier at home and work to keep from breathing dry air.
- Don't eat foods that seem to make your eczema flare up; some people report problems from cow's milk, eggs, wheat flour, nuts, and citrus juices.

WHEN TO CALL THE DOCTOR

Call for a prompt appointment:

- If the affected skin gets a crust, often yellow or brown, or blisters with pus. You may have a bacterial infection that needs treatment with antibiotics, or a rare ailment—caused by a herpes virus—that may be serious.

Call for advice and an appointment:

- ➤ If your skin doesn't get better after a week or two of home care, or if the eczema keeps coming back. Your doctor may suggest further treatment.
- ➤ If you develop an itchy rash that seems to have no cause, and eczema or asthma runs in your family.

HOW TO PREVENT IT

- ➤ To keep skin from getting dry, take short, warm (not hot) showers or baths, then apply a lotion to put moisture back in your skin right away. Don't use soap every time you bathe.
- ➤ To keep your hands from getting dry and chapped, wear mittens or gloves in cold weather. Wear cotton gloves under wool or manmade-fiber gloves to help protect your skin. Use cotton-lined rubber gloves when you are cleaning clothes and dishes.
- ➤ Avoid skin irritants and allergy-causing agents. These include soaps, detergents, perfumes, dust, pet hair, and tobacco smoke.
- ➤ Learn to spot stressful times, and do relaxation techniques, such as yoga or meditation (see **relax,** page 309).

FOR MORE HELP

Information line: National Eczema Association, 810 River Rd., Fair Haven, NJ 07704. 800-818-SKIN, 24-hour line. Sends facts about eczema.

Organization: American Academy of Dermatology, Box 4014, Schaumburg, IL 60168-4014. 847-330-0230, M–F 8:30–5 CST. Send a business-size, self-addressed, stamped envelope for a pamphlet on eczema. Also gives list of doctors near you. **Web site:** *http://www.aad.org/ pip.html.* Select *Atopic Dermatitis and Eczema* or *Hand Dermatitis and Eczema.*

Book: *Eczema & Psoriasis: How Your Diet Can Help,* by Steven Terrass. A nutrition guide to skin problems. HarperCollins, 1995, $9.

Fungal Infections

SIGNS AND SYMPTOMS

Athlete's foot:

- ■ Itching, scaling, and redness that often starts between the toes.
- ■ Dryness, flaking, or blisters on the toes or soles of the feet.
- ■ Toenails that thicken and become layered or scaly and yellowish.
- ■ Odor, in severe cases.

Jock itch:

- ■ Itchy red bumps in the groin and on the genitals of men. Rash may extend to the buttocks and inner thighs.

Yeast infection:

- ■ Thick, white, cheesy discharge from the vagina.
- ■ Itching, pain, or tenderness around the genitals (men or women). In men, the head of the penis may be inflamed.
- ■ Pain or soreness during sex.
- ■ Urge to urinate often. Urine may sting or burn.
- ■ Creamy yellow or white coating in the mouth or on the tongue that can be easily scraped off and may be painful (thrush).
- ■ A red, itching rash with flaky white patches on moist skin areas, such as around the genitals, between the buttocks, or under the breasts.

More people get **athlete's foot** (tinea pedis) than any other fungal infection. It can be vexing, but it's easy to control if treated right away.

The fungus that causes **athlete's foot** is like those that cause jock itch and yeast infections. It breeds in closed, damp places and feeds on dead skin cells. Walking barefoot in the shower at a gym and around pools may increase your chance of getting athlete's foot. Moisture, sweating, and shoes that don't let your feet breathe are likely to make it worse.

Jock itch (tinea cruris) is a fungal infection in the groin that most men get sometime. The culprit in women is a *yeast infection*, which occurs when a fungus that's already in the body displaces the helpful bacteria that keep it under control. It begins in the vagina and may spread if left untreated. If you are pregnant or taking oral antibiotics or birth control pills, you are more likely to get the infection. Men, too, can get yeast infections, which irritate the penis.

Thrush is a yeast infection in the mouth. It makes a white or yellow coating on the cheeks or tongue that may look like milk and is easy to scrape away, exposing raw red skin. Babies often get thrush. So do people with AIDS and others with weak immune systems, such as people being treated with chemotherapy for cancer. Taking large doses of antibiotics may bring on thrush. So can the steroid inhalers many people use for asthma.

Other people who are prone to fungal infections include those who perspire a lot or who are overweight and likely to have folds of skin that rub together.

Athlete's foot, jock itch, and yeast infections can most often be cured quickly.

WHAT YOU CAN DO NOW

Athlete's foot:

- Wash twice a day, and dry well between the toes after showering or swimming.
- Apply an over-the-counter antifungal powder or cream to your feet, and sprinkle some powder in your shoes every day.
- Wash sports shoes at least once a week.
- Wear clean cotton socks, and don't wear the same shoes each day. Fungi take 24 hours to die.
- Take your shoes and socks off at home to give your feet plenty of air.

Jock itch:

- Use an antifungal powder, cream, or spray 2 or 3 times a day until the rash goes away. Keep using the medication for at least a week after that, to make sure the fungus is dead.
- Don't wear tight pants or underwear. Try boxer shorts.
- Change your underwear and jock strap daily. Wash them in hot water.
- Dry your groin well after showering. You can even use a hair dryer set on low.

Yeast infection:

- Use condoms or stop having sex until you get treatment if you have a yeast infection in the vagina (it can be passed on to others).
- If you're sure it's yeast, use an over-the-counter yeast medicine. Read the label and follow the steps.
- Wear clean cotton underwear, and avoid panty hose and tight jeans and pants.
- Eat plain yogurt if you get a yeast infection after taking antibiotics for some other ailment. The bacteria in the yogurt will help keep the yeast in check.
- For thrush, try a gentle mouthwash to loosen the white coating.

WHEN TO CALL THE DOCTOR

Athlete's foot:

- If your foot has an odor that doesn't go away after treatment at home—a sign that you have a severe case.
- If your rash starts to spread or isn't better after 2 weeks of self-care. Once athlete's foot spreads, it is hard to get rid of and often returns.
- If the infection has reached your nails. This is hard to clear up. It also makes your nails more prone to bacterial infection because moisture gets trapped in the cracks.

Jock itch:

- If over-the-counter treatments fail to work after a couple of weeks.
- If you develop an open sore that oozes pus. This is a sign of a secondary infection.
- If the rash spreads, gets worse, or keeps coming back.

Yeast infection:

- If you suspect you have one and you aren't better after using an over-the-counter medicine. Your doctor can prescribe antifungal suppositories, creams, or tablets for you (and maybe your sexual partner).
- If you see signs of thrush. Your doctor may prescribe antifungal creams, pills, or suppositories.

HOW TO PREVENT IT

- Bathe daily and dry your body well.
- Avoid tight shoes and underwear, most of all in hot weather.

Athlete's foot:

- Wear sandals when you can, and go barefoot at home to air your feet. Wear plastic sandals or thongs in public dressing rooms and showers.

Jock itch:

- Change your clothes as soon as you finish working out, and don't share towels at the gym. Jock itch is mildly catching.

Yeast infection:

- Don't use feminine hygiene sprays or douches, which may kill the helpful bacteria in the vagina that can ward off a fungus.
- Don't wear nylon underwear. It doesn't let air near the skin and gives fungi a chance to grow. Avoid noncotton workout clothes as well.
- Wash your workout clothes in hot water after each use.
- If you have repeated bouts of the infection and you take the Pill, ask your doctor about changing your birth control method.

Thrush:

- If you use a steroid inhaler for asthma, be sure you rinse your mouth well after each use to prevent thrush (see **asthma,** page 89).

FOR MORE HELP

Information line: American Podiatric Medical Association, 800-FOOTCARE, 24-hour recording. Ask for pamphlets on athlete's foot.

Organization: National Women's Health Network, 514 10th St. NW, Suite 400, Washington, DC 20004. 202-347-1140, M–F 9–5:30 EST. Send an $8 check for a packet on yeast infections.

Web access: American Academy of Dermatology. After logging on to the Internet, type: *http://www.aad.org/AthletFoot.html* for facts about athlete's foot.

Hives

SIGNS AND SYMPTOMS

- Itchy, raised, red or pink swellings on the skin (called wheals). Each may range in size from smaller than a pea to the size of a dinner plate.
- Wheals that occur in groups.
- A wheal with a whitish center, rimmed by a red rash.
- Wheals that itch or burn and sting. New ones may appear as the old ones fade.
- Swelling on the lips, tongue, eyelids, or genitals. Swelling may also occur on the backs of the hands and feet.

When an irritant invades your body, your immune system sends chemicals, including histamine, to fight it. This sudden jump in histamine levels can cause an outbreak of hives. Many people—about 1 in 5—get hives at some point.

Milk, eggs, nuts, shellfish, berries, food additives, and medicines such as penicillin and aspirin can all prompt hives in some people. So can insect bites, sunlight, extreme heat or cold, pressure on the skin, and sometimes infections. **Stress** can make hives worse (see page 222).

One form of hives, known as angioedema, is a deep swelling in skin tissues such as the lips, tongue, eyelids, or genitals. It often lasts 24 hours or more. Most other hives go away on their own within a few days or weeks. If they last longer than 6 weeks, you and your doctor will need to find the cause.

WHAT YOU CAN DO NOW

- Take an antihistamine to reduce your body's response and relieve pain.
- Soothe your skin with cold compresses or calamine lotion.
- Take a cool bath with a few tablespoons of cornstarch (the kind sold in drugstores) added.

- Relax with a book, some music, or a movie on videotape—tension tends to make hives worse (see **relax,** page 309).

WHEN TO CALL THE DOCTOR

Although most often harmless, hives can signal more serious, and sometimes fatal, conditions. Call 911 or go to an emergency room **right away:**

- If you have hives with hoarseness, wheezing, cold sweats, nausea, dizziness, or trouble breathing after a bee sting, insect bite, eating, or taking a medicine; you may have **shock from allergy** (see page 24). If you have a first-aid kit, give yourself an epinephrine shot. **Caution:** Don't take epinephrine if you're older or have heart trouble.
- If a burning feeling or itchy hives shows up in your throat.

Call for advice:

- If you get hives after taking medication; you may be having an allergy attack.
- If you have hives that keep coming back for a month or more.

HOW TO PREVENT IT

Find the cause of your outbreak. If you are reacting to a food, you will feel the hives begin within 2 hours after you start eating. To find the food:

- For a few days, eat foods that you think won't make you break out. (Some doctors advise lamb and rice.)
- Slowly add other foods back into your diet, watching for a response.
- Look for a pattern. Keep a list of what you eat as well as what you do each day and the products you use. You'll need this list to talk over with your doctor.

FOR MORE HELP

Information line: American Academy of Allergy and Immunology, 800-822-2762, 24-hour line, 365 days a year. Ask for brochures on subjects that tie in with allergies and hives, as well as lists of allergists near you.

Organization: Food Allergy Network, 800-929-4040, M–F 9–5 EST. Provides fact sheets, support, and a newsletter for people with food allergies.

Ingrown Toenails

SIGNS AND SYMPTOMS

- Swelling, pain, and redness at the side of a toenail, most often on the big toe.

Ingrown toenails occur when the sharp corners or sides of the nail push into your skin, mostly because the toenails are cut too short or because tight shoes or stockings press the nail into the flesh. Jamming your toes into the ends of shoes day after day doesn't help matters. Ingrown toenails also seem to run in some families.

Ingrown toenails sometimes become inflamed or infected, but they're easily treated at home. You can treat infections with antibiotics, and badly ingrown nails can be cut away by a doctor using local anesthetic.

WHAT YOU CAN DO NOW

- Cut the nail straight across. Push a small wad of sterile cotton between the nail and the skin. Use a new piece of cotton every day until the nail has grown out.
- If there's redness, clean the area with hydrogen peroxide, then apply an over-the-counter antibacterial cream. Cover the nail with a bandage.
- Soak your foot in warm water or apply a warm compress if your toe aches from the ingrown nail.
- If it hurts a lot, take an over-the-counter painkiller (see **pain relief** box, page 317).

WHEN TO CALL THE DOCTOR

- If redness or swelling around the nail comes with severe pain or discharge.
- If you cannot trim the ingrown nail.
- If you have diabetes and an ingrown toenail becomes infected.

HOW TO PREVENT IT

- Using nail trimmers, cut straight across, but not too short. Leave some of the white nail at the end. If your nails are very hard, soften them by soaking your feet first.
- Wear stockings and shoes that fit well (you should be able to wiggle your toes).
- When you buy new shoes, do it at the end of the day, when your feet are at their largest (they tend to swell during the day).
- Don't wear pointed shoes.
- Don't expect to break in new shoes that pinch. They should feel good when you try them on.

FOR MORE HELP

Information line: American Podiatric Medical Association, 800-FOOTCARE, 24-hour recording. Sends free brochures on foot care.

Pamphlet: American Academy of Orthopaedic Surgeons, 800-824-BONES, 24-hour recording. Ask for pamphlet titled "If the Shoe Fits, Wear It."

Lice and Scabies

SIGNS AND SYMPTOMS

Both lice and scabies:
- Severe itching.
- Marks and sores on the body from scratching (sometimes).

Head lice:
- Itchy scalp.
- Small, grayish-white, oval eggs (nits) clinging to hairs close to the scalp.
- Crusty infection on the scalp.
- Grayish insects (lice) as long as an eighth of an inch, sometimes visible at the nape of the neck or behind the ears.

Body lice:
- Raised, red bumps (bites) on the shoulders, trunk, and buttocks.
- Nits found on clothing, often in the seams of underwear.
- Headache, fever, and sick feeling with swelling and infected bites (in severe cases).

Crab lice ("crabs"):
- Itching around the genitals.
- Tiny crablike insects (the size of a flake of dandruff or smaller) on the skin in the crotch.
- Small dark specks (crab feces) on underwear.

Scabies:
- Itching anywhere that gets worse just after you go to bed.
- A rough, red, grainy rash with itchy, raised bumps, mainly on the wrists, elbows, breasts, genitals, around the waist, and on the webs between the fingers.
- Dotted lines or wavy gray ridges like pencil marks on the skin.
- Large areas of crusty, thick, itchy skin (Norwegian or crusted scabies).
- In adults, itching from the neck down only. (Babies and young children may have itching on the face.)

As much as they dislike the itching caused by lice and scabies, people are more often upset by the shame they feel at having these tiny pests. But lice and scabies can infest anyone, anywhere. In fact, in recent years there has been a rash of head lice outbreaks in the United States, with 6 to 12 million cases reported yearly.

Lice are wingless insects that feed on human blood. Three types move onto either the scalp, the body, or the pubic region. Lice are found most often from August through November, and they are easily spread by skin-to-skin contact or by sharing clothes, combs, and bedding. Crab lice, the kind that infests your pubic region, are often spread by sex, but you can also get them from a toilet seat because they live away from the body for up to 3 days.

Scabies is an allergic response caused by a burrowing mite that lays eggs in tunnels under the upper layer of human skin. You may not realize you have scabies until you start to itch, and that doesn't happen until about 2 weeks after infestation. Scabies is most often spread through close contact with other people, including sex, and through sharing clothes and bed linen.

While rapid treatment can get rid of lice and scabies, it doesn't always kill them all on the first try. You may have to reapply treatments a few times, maybe more, before the pests are gone.

WHAT YOU CAN DO NOW

The best way to rid yourself of lice and scabies, many experts say, is to cover the affected part of the body with an over-the-counter shampoo or cream that contains permethrin, pyrethrin, or pyrethrum.

Caution: Because all lice and scabies removers are poisons, you must wait at least 10 days between treatments. Your skin may still itch long after the mites and lice are dead. The chemical lindane, used in some treatments for lice and scabies, is no longer prescribed for children, since it has been known to cause convulsions and other problems. For kids, use something else. Lindane has shown no such problems in adults, but tell your doctor if you prefer to use a lotion without lindane.

For all lice and scabies:

- For itching, try cool soaks, calamine lotion, an oral antihistamine, or pain relievers (see **pain relief,** page 317).
- Don't try drastic home care such as scrubbing with harsh soaps or dousing your skin or hair with kerosene.
- On the day you start treatment, vacuum well, and wash sheets, towels, and clothes worn in the last week in hot water; set the dryer on high. Iron or dry-clean clothes that can't be washed. Seal stuffed animals and pillows that can harbor lice in plastic bags, and keep them out of the reach of children for at least 20 days.

Head lice:

- Cover the scalp with a shampoo or creme rinse containing 1 percent permethrin, pyrethrin, or pyrethrum. Follow package directions.
- None of these products kills the nits (eggs), though. If just a few live through the treatment, they can start a new outbreak. To soften and remove nits, shampoo hair in warm water and then comb the nits out with a special fine-tooth comb (sold at drugstores) while the hair is still wet. (Give haircuts to young children to make the process easier.)
- Boil combs, curlers, and brushes.
- If your child has repeated bouts of head lice and you don't want to keep using toxic treatments, some doctors advise this: Mix 50 drops of tea tree oil (sold in health food stores) in 2 ounces of warm olive oil; apply to the hair and scalp. Cover with a shower cap and a hot, moist towel for 2 hours. Then rinse the hair well and comb out the nits with a fine-tooth comb.

Body lice:

- Bathe with soap and water.
- Apply an antilouse cream to the entire body.
- Vacuum floors, and wash clothes and linens as directed for head lice.

Crab lice:

- Use an antilouse shampoo. Follow package directions.
- Ask your doctor to test you for other sexually transmitted diseases.
- Be sure that your sexual partner is treated.

Scabies:

- Call your doctor for a prompt appointment. The most effective, safe treatment (a lotion containing 5 percent permethrin or pyrethrin) is given only by prescription.
- Wash clothing and linens as for head lice.
- Be sure all family members and people with whom you've been in close contact are treated at the same time.
- Try an over-the-counter antihistamine for relief from itching.

WHEN TO CALL THE DOCTOR

Call for advice and an appointment:

- If you suspect you have any form of scabies.
- If you are unsure of the cause of your itching. Other rashes and problems can mimic the signs of scabies.
- If the pests come back after treatment.
- If your sores become infected and ooze.
- If you have lice on your eyelashes. Your doctor may need to remove the pests.
- If a baby or young child is infested.

(continued on page 177)

The Body Illustrated

Each part of the human body works with other parts to keep the whole system in good repair—most of the time. Sometimes, as you can see in the striking illustrations starting on this page, something breaks down: Thinning cartilage in a joint can lead to arthritis, for example; thickening artery walls to a heart attack; or aging of the eye's lens to cataracts.

A NEW LENS FOR CATARACTS

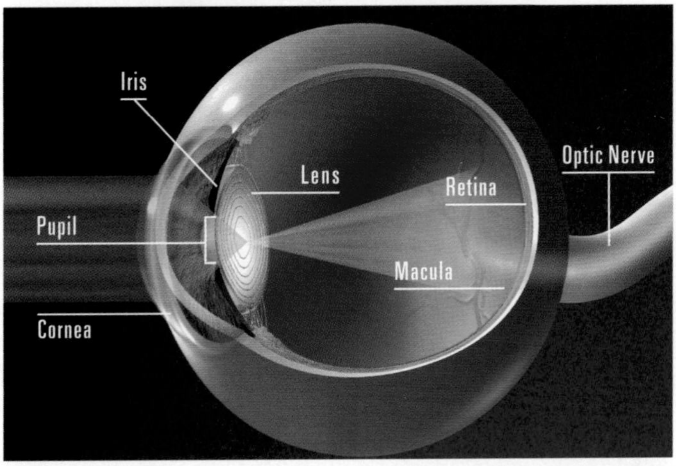

The healthy eye acts like a camera. The cornea and the lens focus light on the retina; from there, signals travel through the optic nerve to the brain, where they are turned into images. A cataract—clouding of the lens—distorts the focus, blurs vision, and can cause blindness.

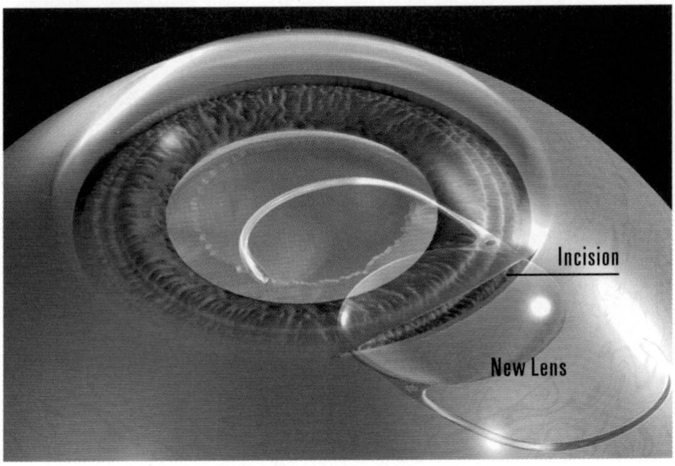

Surgeons can repair a severe cataract by making a small cut in the cornea, popping out the cloudy lens, and slipping a clear plastic lens into the pouch where the original sat. They most often stitch the cut with special thread that does not have to be removed.

Every year, half of all Americans get pains in the back. The lower back (lumbar region) supports 70 percent of the body's weight and often suffers chronic pain. Even sitting at a desk can cause back pain.

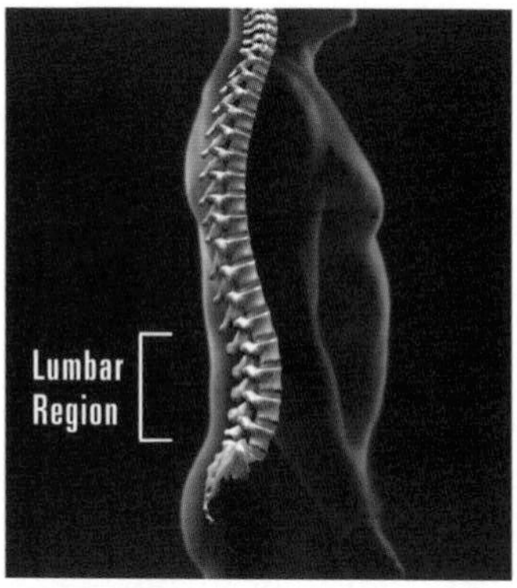

The spine is a column of 26 bones, the vertebrae. The spinal cord, a thick cable of nerves, runs from the brain through the column.

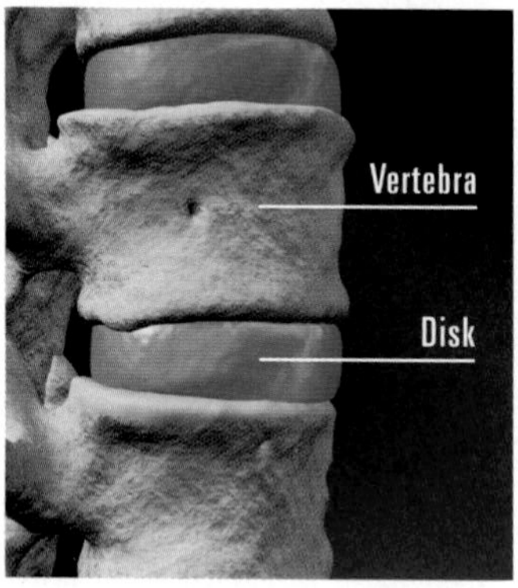

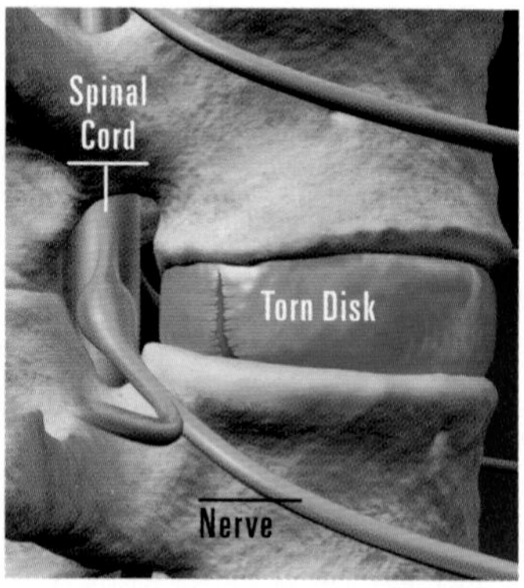

Disks between the vertebrae let the spinal column move. They absorb shock and cushion the impact of walking and other motion. Their tough outside shell protects a soft gel-like center. Aging and stress on the spine can cause the shell of a disk to bulge and tear.

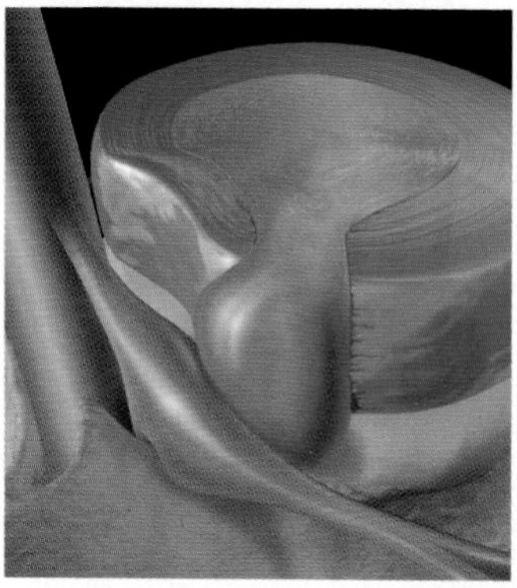

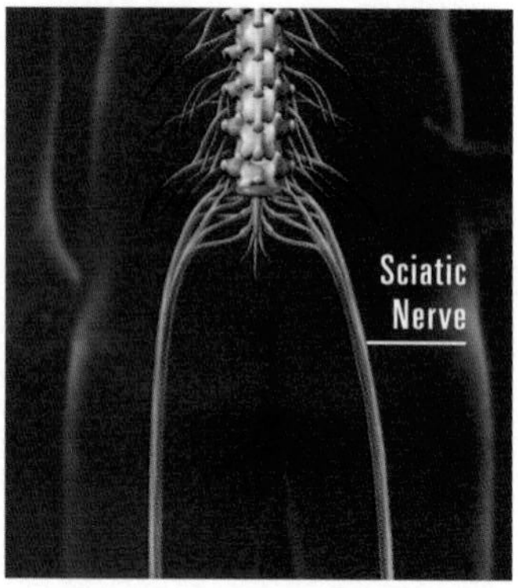

The bulging disk, which sometimes leaks its contents, may press on a nerve. When that happens to the sciatic nerve, you may feel pain and numbness in the legs. That's because the sciatic nerve, which starts at the base of the spine, carries nerve impulses down the legs to the feet.

Arthritis is a name for many kinds of swelling, stiffness, and pain in the joints. Nearly 16 million of us have a touch of the wear-and-tear type (osteoarthritis), which is most common in people over 45.

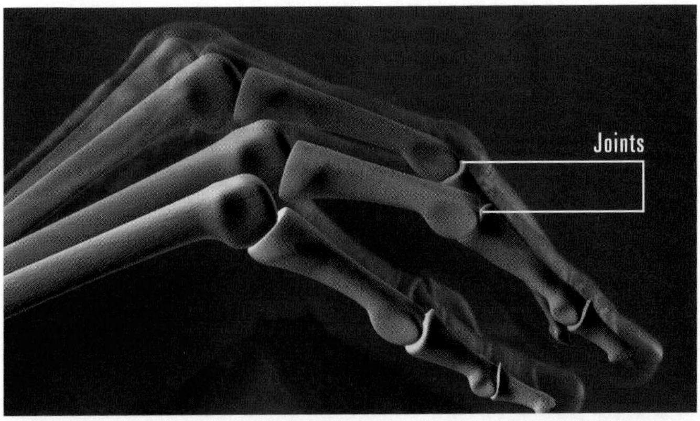

The highly mobile joints of the hands are often the first to feel stiff and painful. Other joints that often become arthritic are in the neck, knees, hips, spine, and big toes. Here's how osteoarthritis comes on:

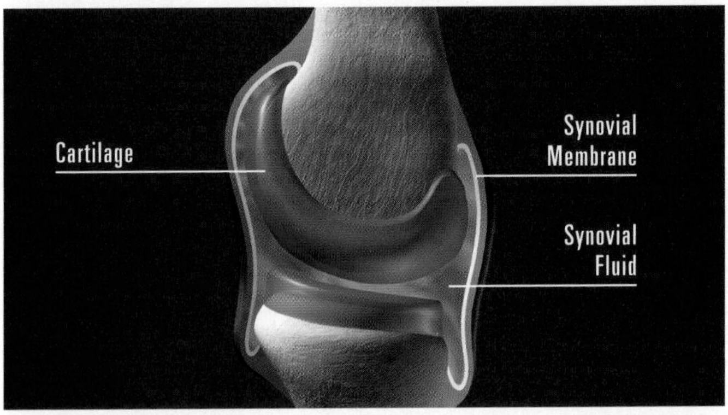

In a young joint, a layer of smooth cartilage cushions the place where the two bones meet. The joint itself is sealed in a capsule filled with synovial fluid—a thick lubricant that looks like egg white.

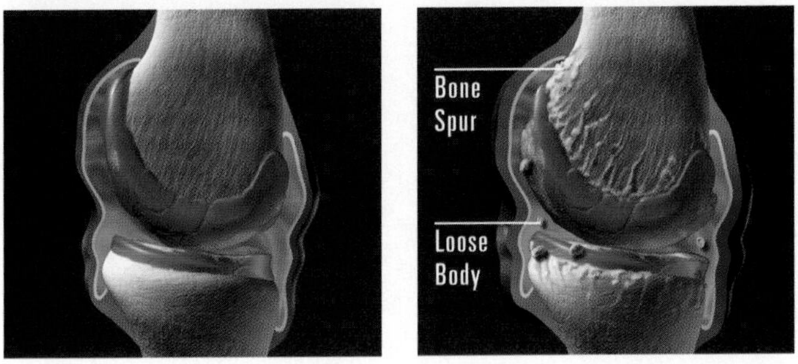

With age, the cartilage becomes pitted and frayed. Exposed, rough surfaces of bone rub against each other. They may also grow small bumps—spurs—that cause pain. Bits of bone and cartilage, called loose bodies, may break free and float in the joint space, causing more pain and making it hard for the joint to move.

Though it looks hard and solid, bone is built around a porous core, which keeps it both light and strong. Osteoporosis, the slow breakdown of the bone core, affects 25 million Americans, most of them women.

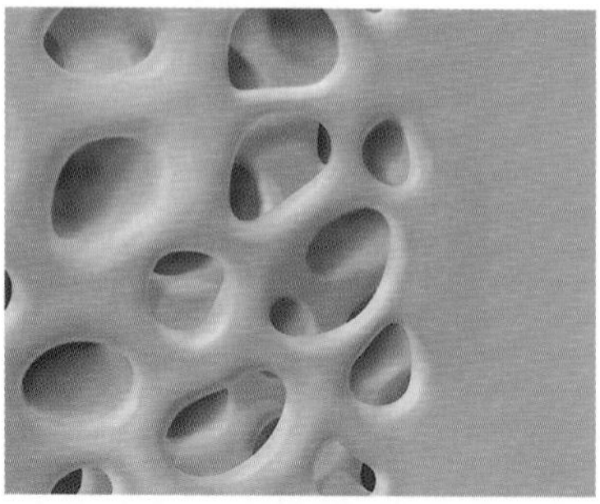

The center of a bone is honeycombed with open spaces. A hard, compact layer surrounds and protects this core. In both, special cells are always tearing down and building up calcium stores.

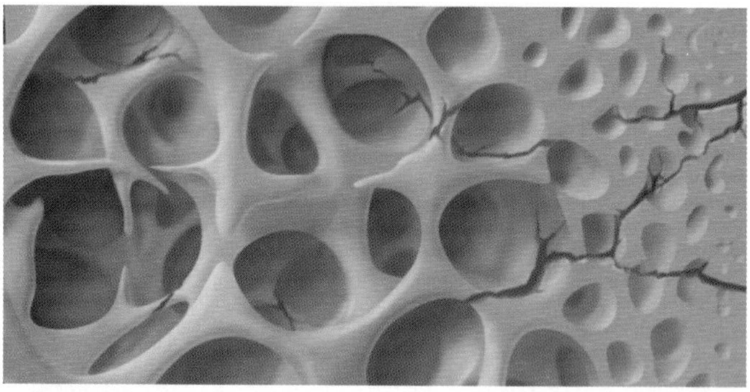

If more calcium goes out than comes in, more bone is torn down than rebuilt, and osteoporosis begins. The bridges of bone between the open spaces become thin and brittle, and break easily.

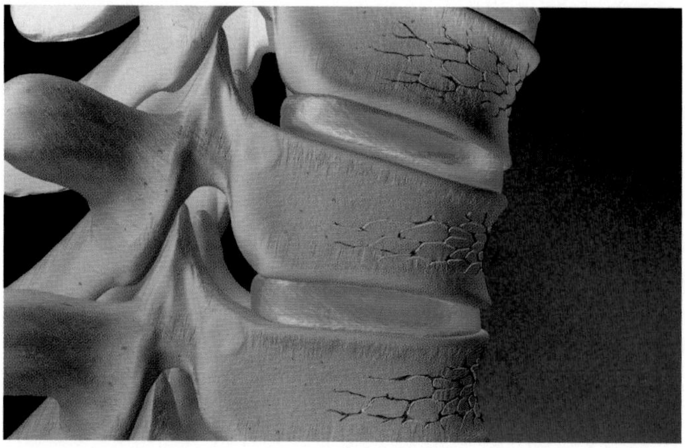

When osteoporosis weakens the bones of the spine, even the pressure of normal body weight can cause networks of tiny cracks called crush fractures or spinal compression fractures.

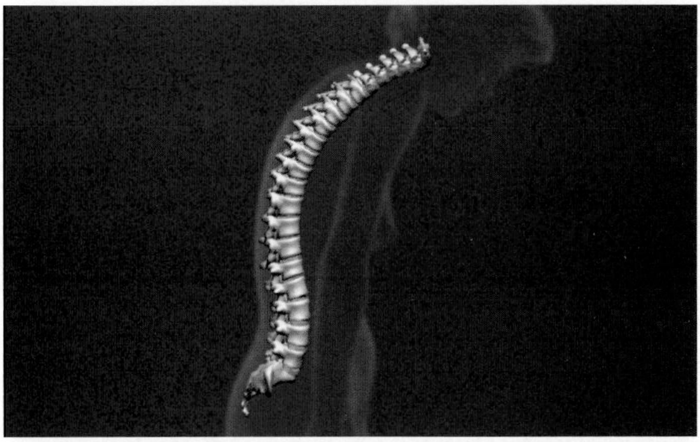

Over time, these small fractures can lead to chronic back pain, loss of height, and the curving upper spine known as dowager's hump.

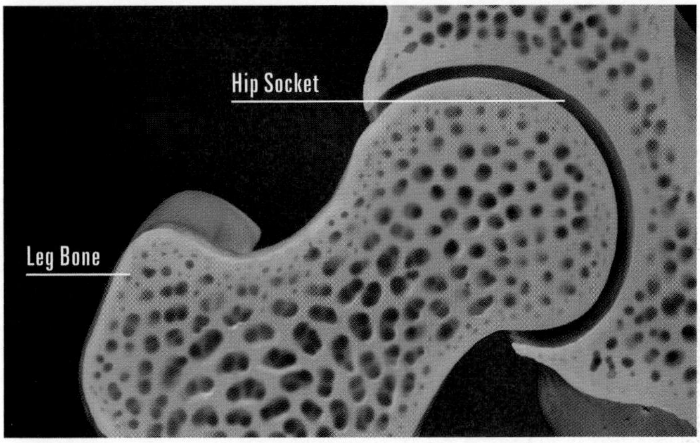

Sometimes the first symptom of osteoporosis is a bone that breaks for no clear reason. Bones with large porous areas, like the bones of the hip joint, are the most subject to fractures.

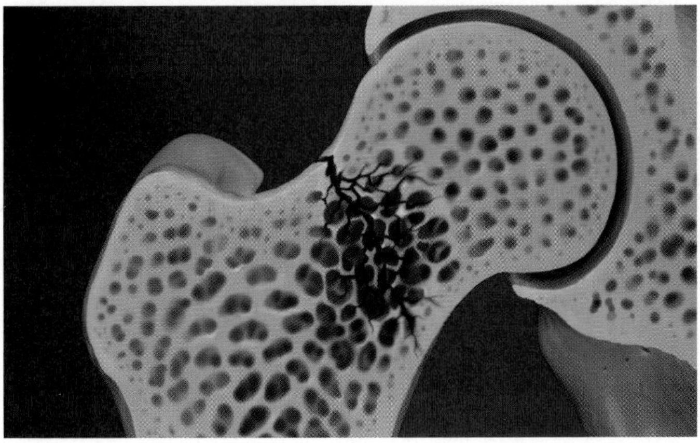

Minor falls and jolts that wouldn't hurt a younger person—even sitting down too quickly— can damage and break weakened bones.

Skin cancer affects 1 in 6 people in this country. Most skin cancers are caused by ultraviolet (UV) rays from the sun. You can protect yourself from skin damage by staying out of the sun and wearing sunscreen.

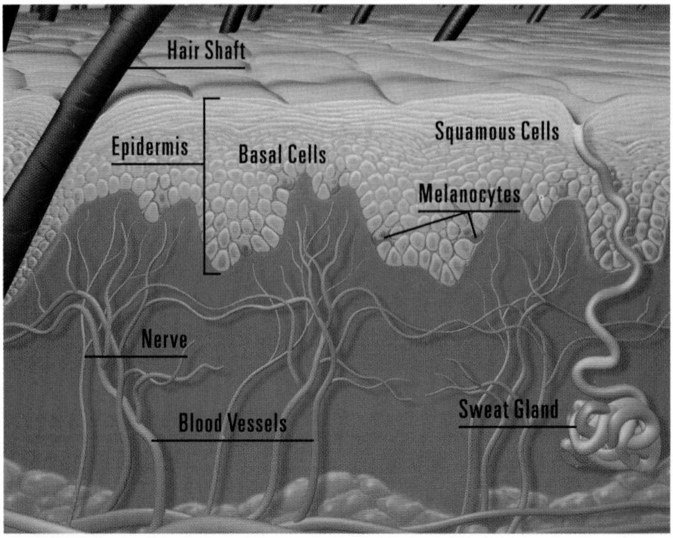

The top layer of the skin (the epidermis) is made of 3 kinds of cells: squamous cells, basal cells, and melanocytes. Cancer occurs when skin cells begin to grow out of control, forming tumors.

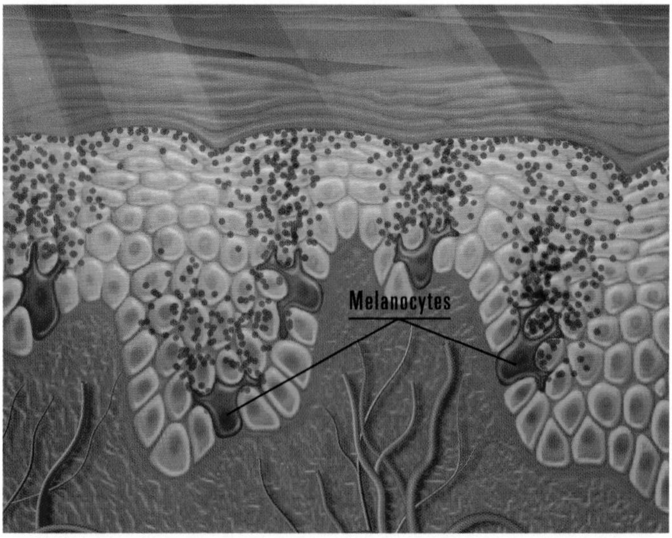

A tan is the skin's emergency response to UV rays from the sun. When UV light hits, melanocytes try to repair the damage by putting out more melanin, a dark pigment, and multiplying faster than usual. Also, over time, stretchy tissues in the lower layer begin to sag.

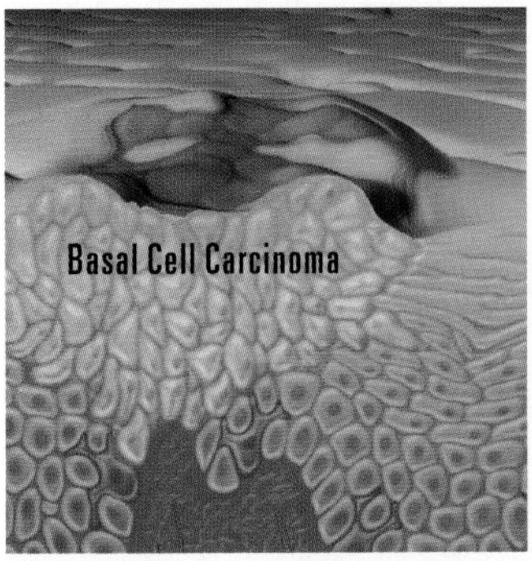

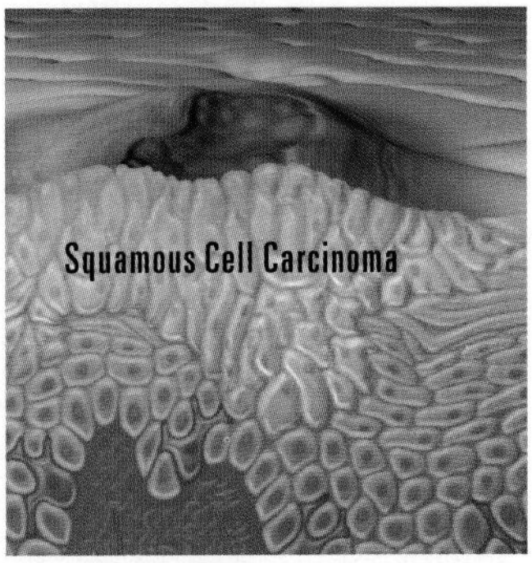

When a basal cell becomes cancerous, it produces a cluster of cells—called a carcinoma—which may look like a shiny, waxy pimple. When a squamous cell becomes cancerous, it forms a rough, thick carcinoma that may have a hard crust on its surface.

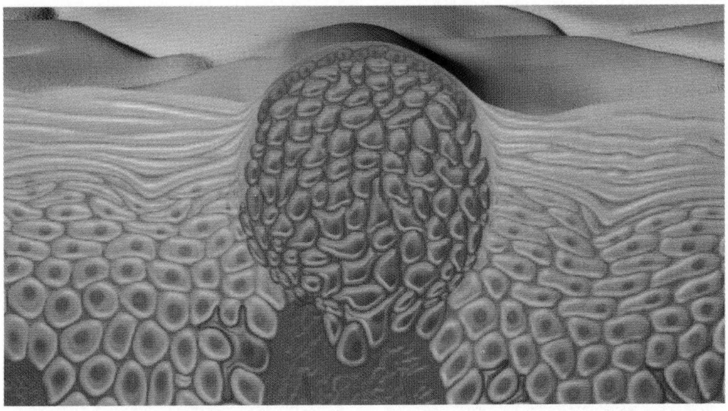

Sometimes a closely knit cluster of melanocytes pushes to the surface of the skin, forming a dark and compact, but harmless, mole.

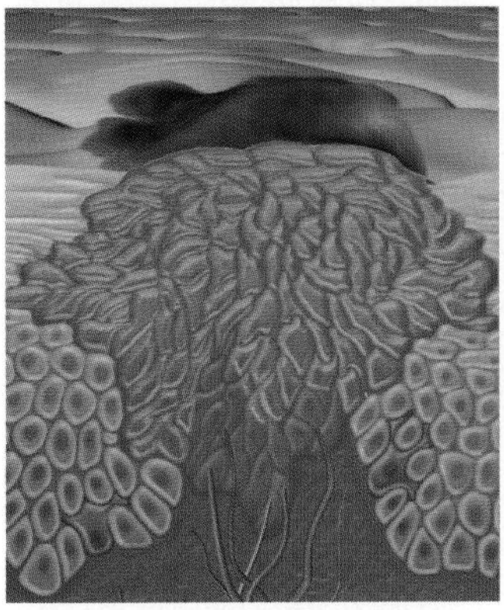

Sun exposure can push the melanocytes to grow wildly into a cancerous tumor known as a malignant melanoma. Sometimes cells from a melanoma break away and form cancerous tumors in other parts of the body.

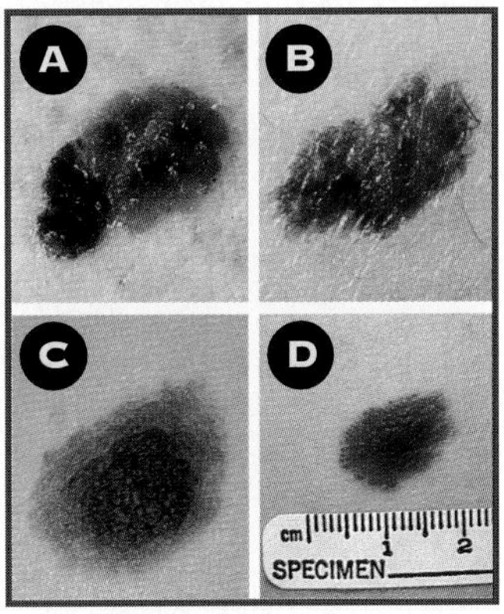

These signs help you tell a melanoma from a normal mole:

Asymmetrical shape.
Borders are blurry.
Color varies within mole.
Diameter larger than a pencil eraser.

Most of the 12 million people with asthma feel as if they can't get enough air into their lungs during an attack. The reason is that they can't get "old" air out of their lungs when the airways narrow and clog.

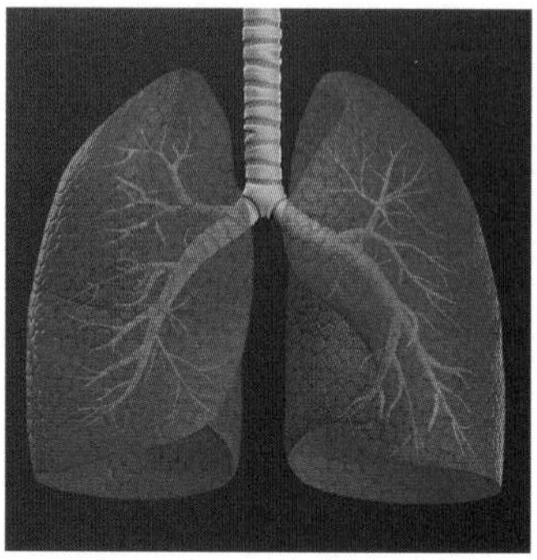

When you breathe in, air travels into each lung through bronchial tubes that branch like tree limbs into smaller and smaller airways.

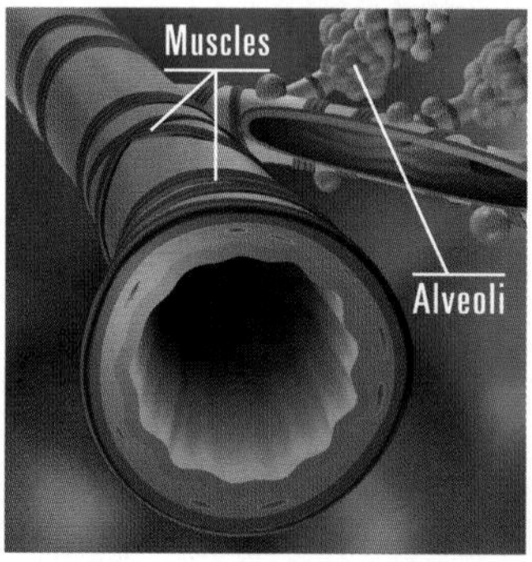

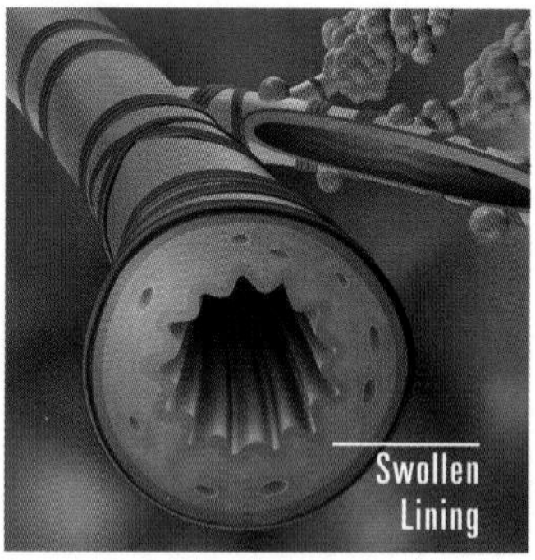

Finally, air reaches the tiny, grapelike alveoli, which pass oxygen from the air into the bloodstream. When a person with asthma inhales dust, pollen, or any other allergy-causing substance, the lining of the bronchial tubes swells. The person may wheeze when breathing.

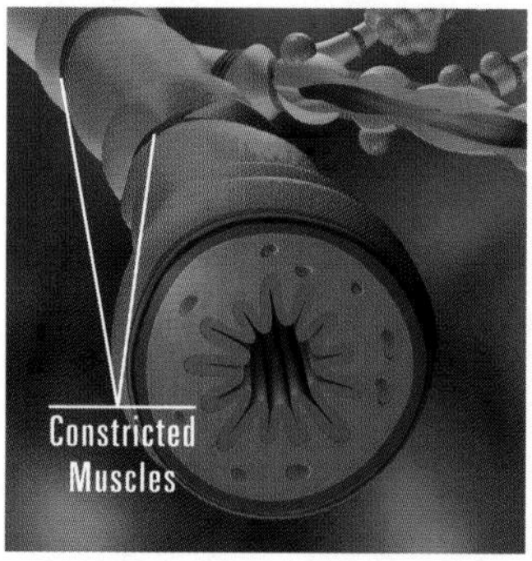

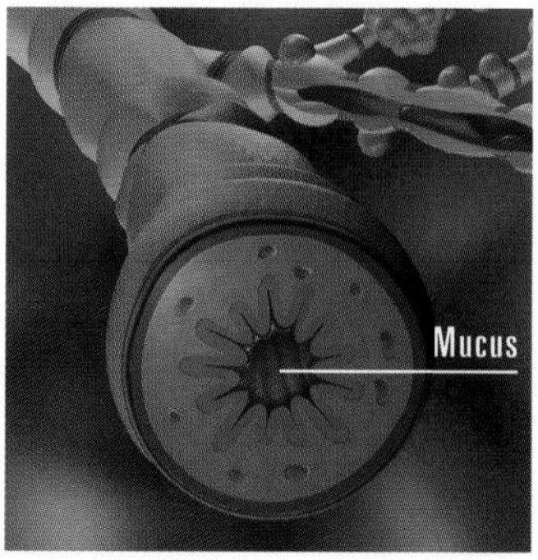

The muscles around the bronchial tubes can also start to tighten, making breathing even harder. People with asthma may use as much as 25 times more effort to take a breath than people without it. In a severe attack, the lining of the tubes produces sticky mucus, so there is even less room in the lungs, and the person can manage only a weak cough.

In atherosclerosis, the arteries slowly grow thicker and harder. The process can start as early as childhood and can go on without symptoms for decades until the buildup causes a heart attack or stroke.

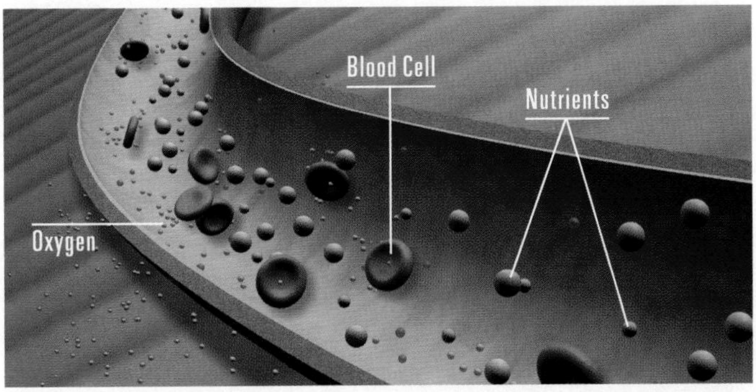

The arteries carry blood rich in nutrients, oxygen, and other substances, including cholesterol, from the heart and lungs to the body.

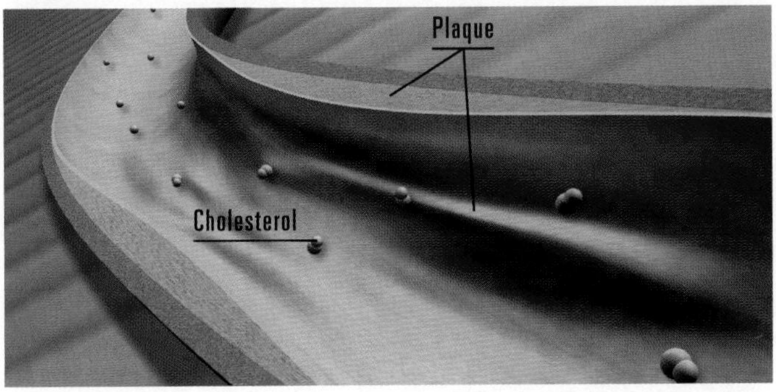

Over time, the walls of an artery may collect dense streaks of minerals and fats. (Cholesterol is shown here without other blood factors.) These streaks, which bulge from the wall, are called plaque.

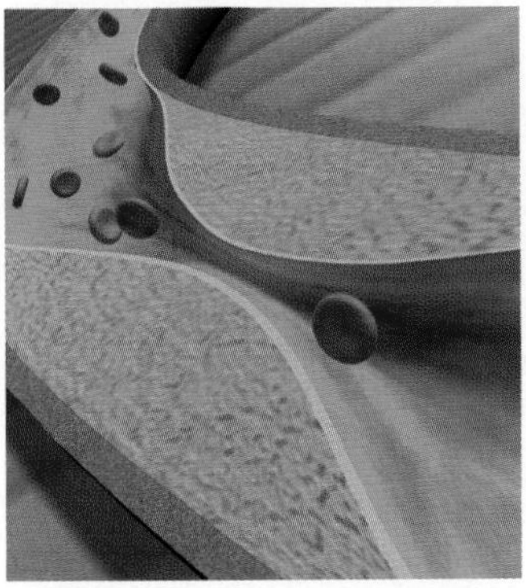

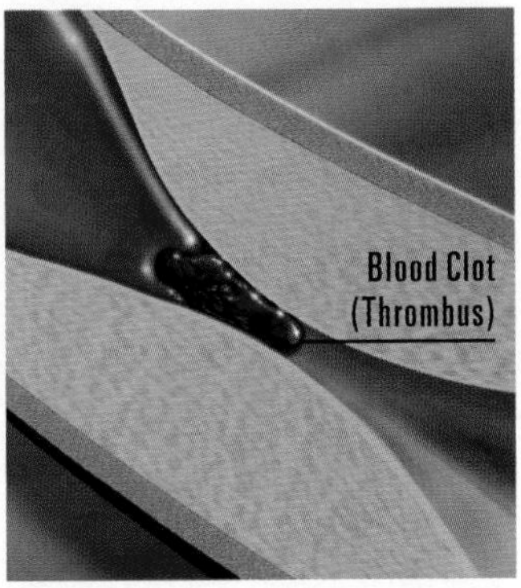

As plaque builds up and narrows an artery, it restricts the amount of blood that can flow through. The bulges and rough spots on its surface allow clots to form easily. A clot that wedges in a narrowed spot and blocks the flow of blood can cause a heart attack or stroke.

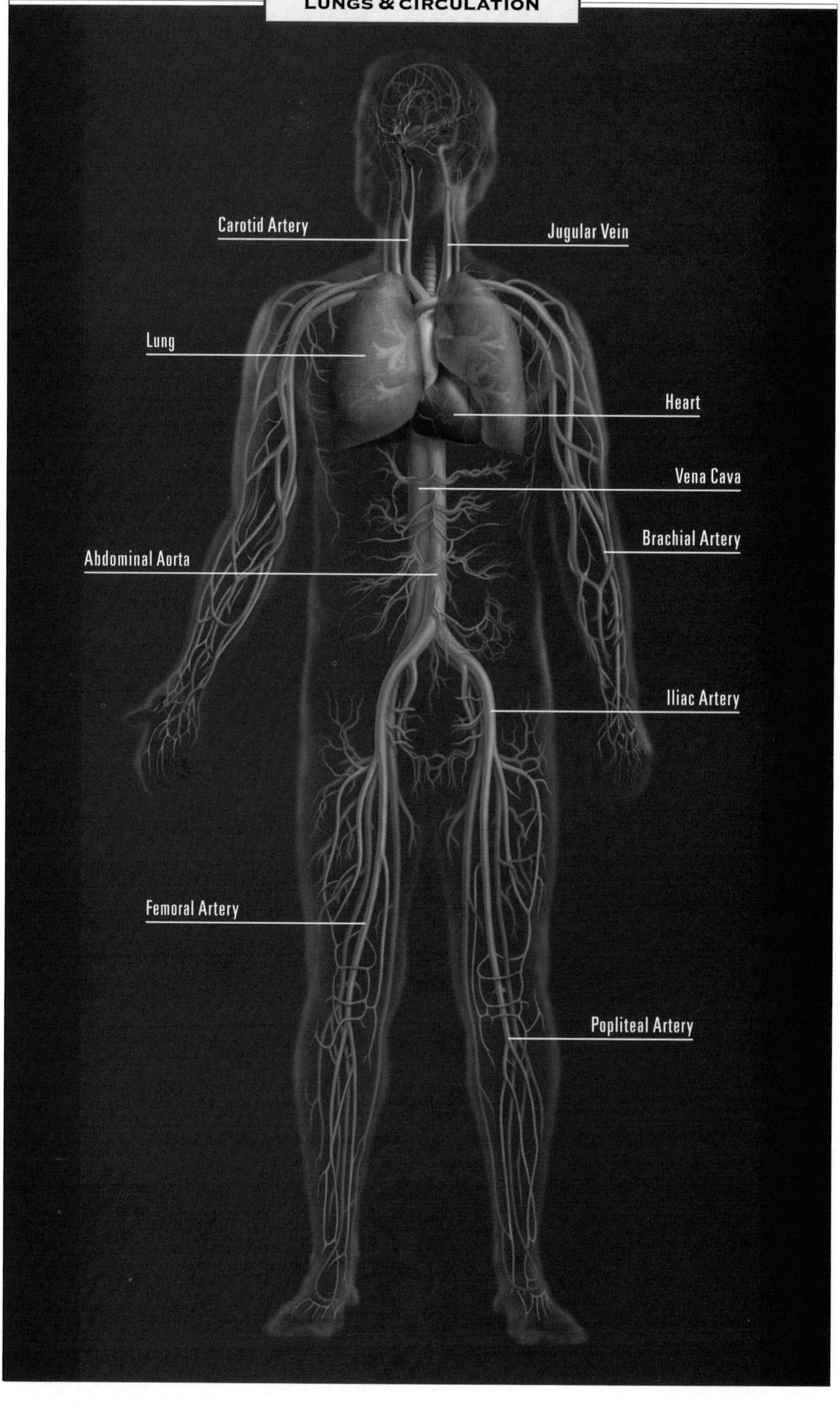
Carotid Artery
Jugular Vein
Lung
Heart
Vena Cava
Brachial Artery
Abdominal Aorta
Iliac Artery
Femoral Artery
Popliteal Artery

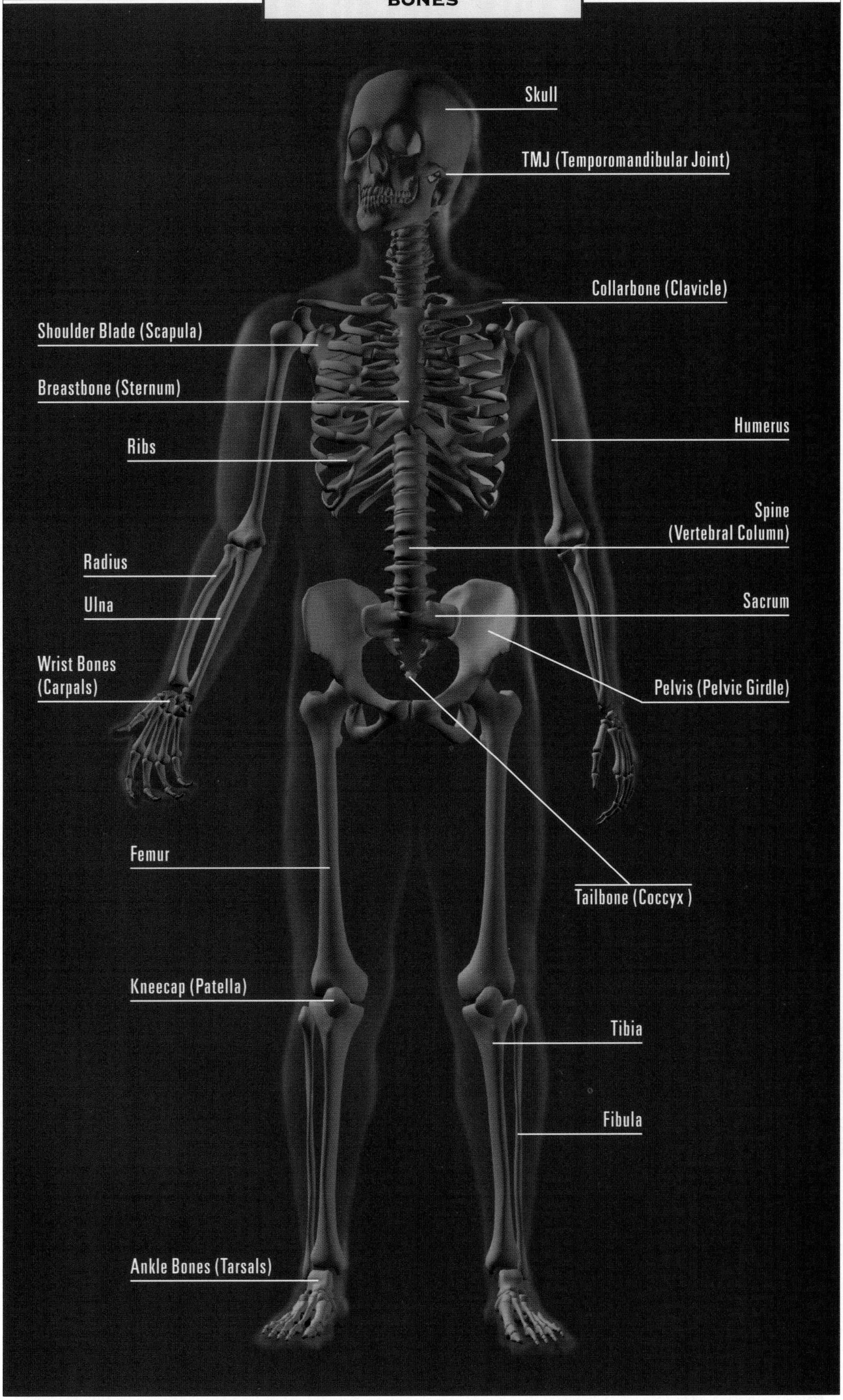
Skull
TMJ (Temporomandibular Joint)
Collarbone (Clavicle)
Shoulder Blade (Scapula)
Breastbone (Sternum)
Humerus
Ribs
Spine
(Vertebral Column)
Radius
Ulna
Sacrum
Wrist Bones
(Carpals)
Pelvis (Pelvic Girdle)
Femur
Tailbone (Coccyx)
Kneecap (Patella)
Tibia
Fibula
Ankle Bones (Tarsals)

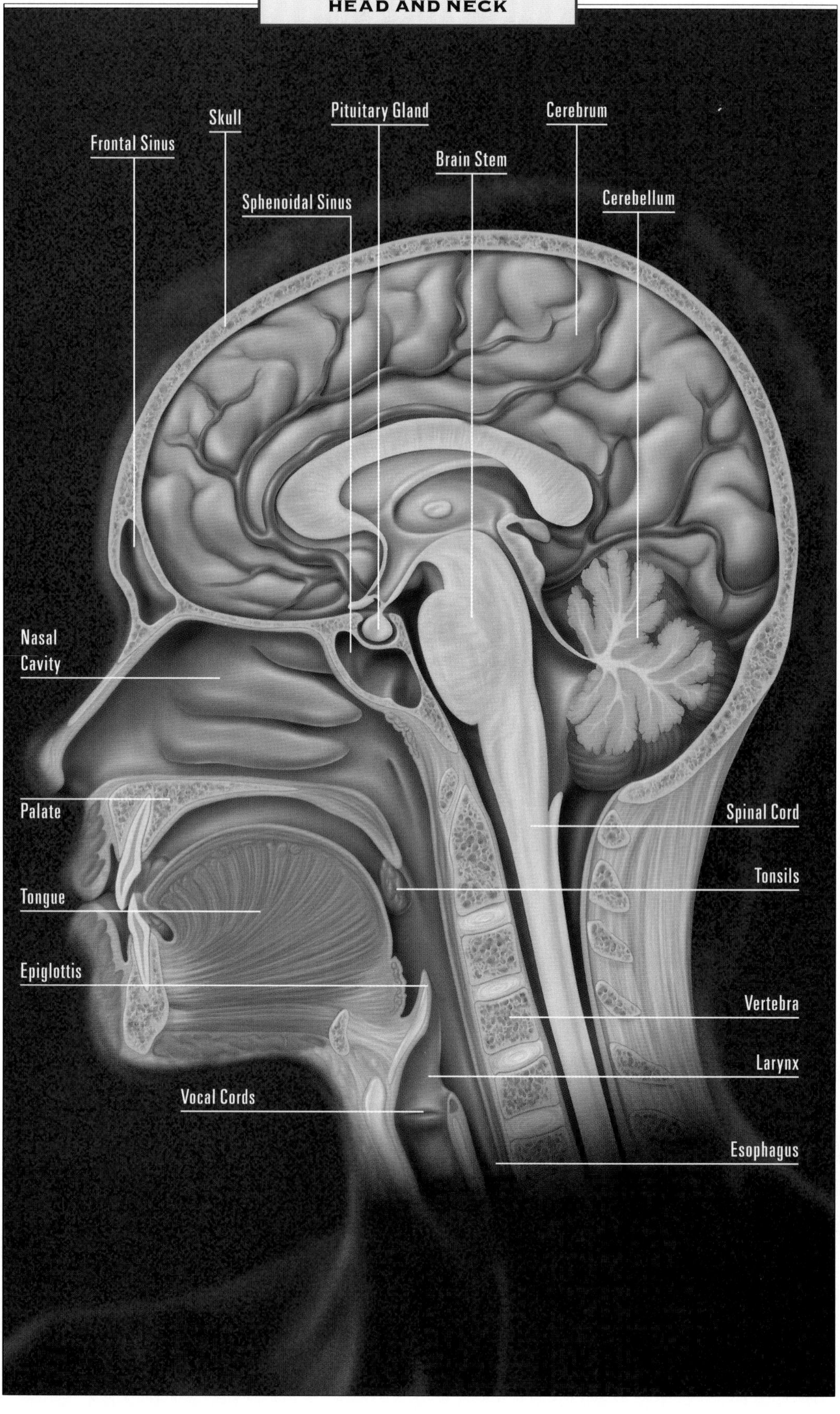
Frontal Sinus
Skull
Pituitary Gland
Cerebrum
Brain Stem
Sphenoidal Sinus
Cerebellum
Nasal Cavity
Palate
Spinal Cord
Tonsils
Tongue
Epiglottis
Vertebra
Larynx
Vocal Cords
Esophagus

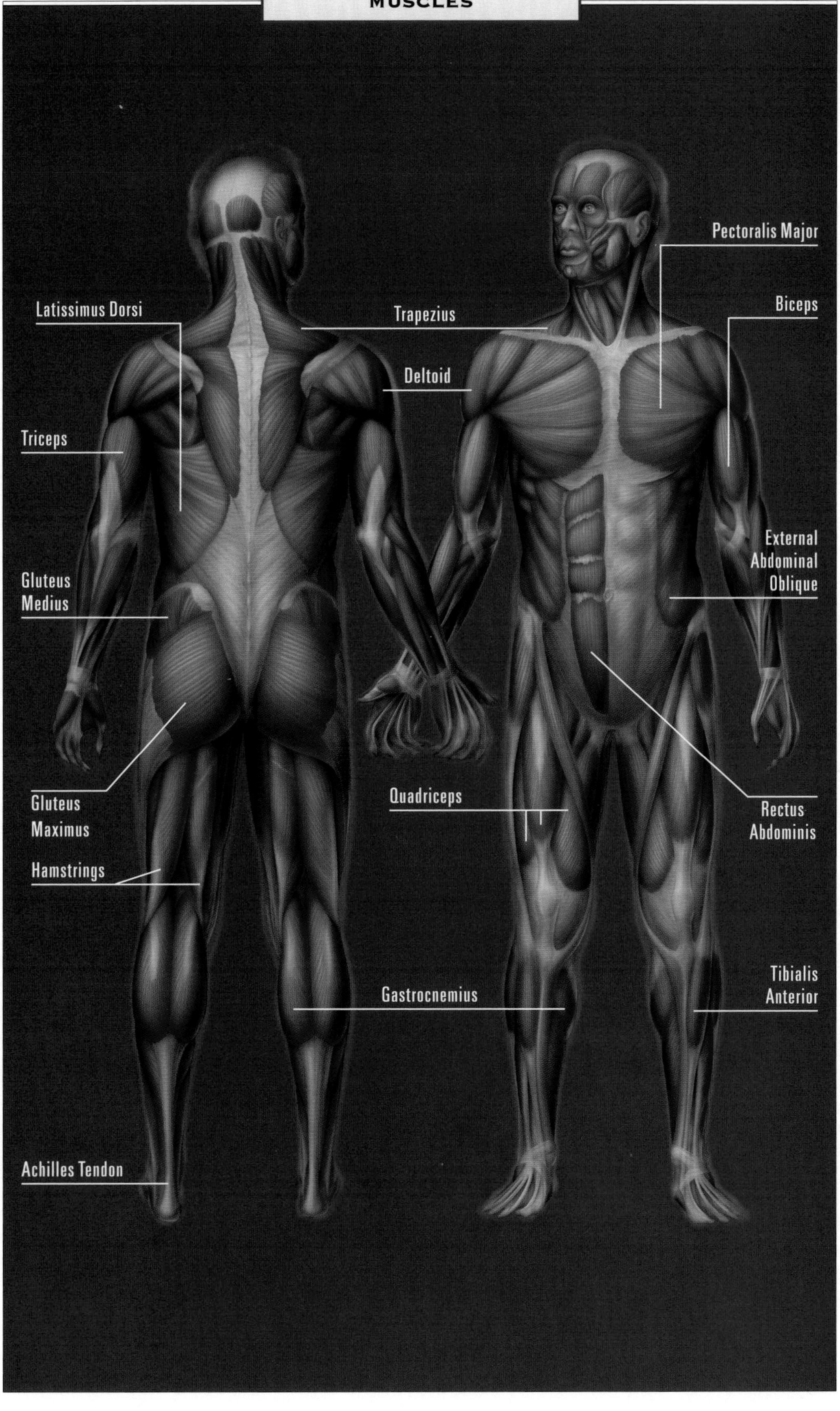
Latissimus Dorsi
Trapezius
Pectoralis Major
Biceps
Deltoid
Triceps
External Abdominal Oblique
Gluteus Medius
Gluteus Maximus
Quadriceps
Rectus Abdominis
Hamstrings
Gastrocnemius
Tibialis Anterior
Achilles Tendon

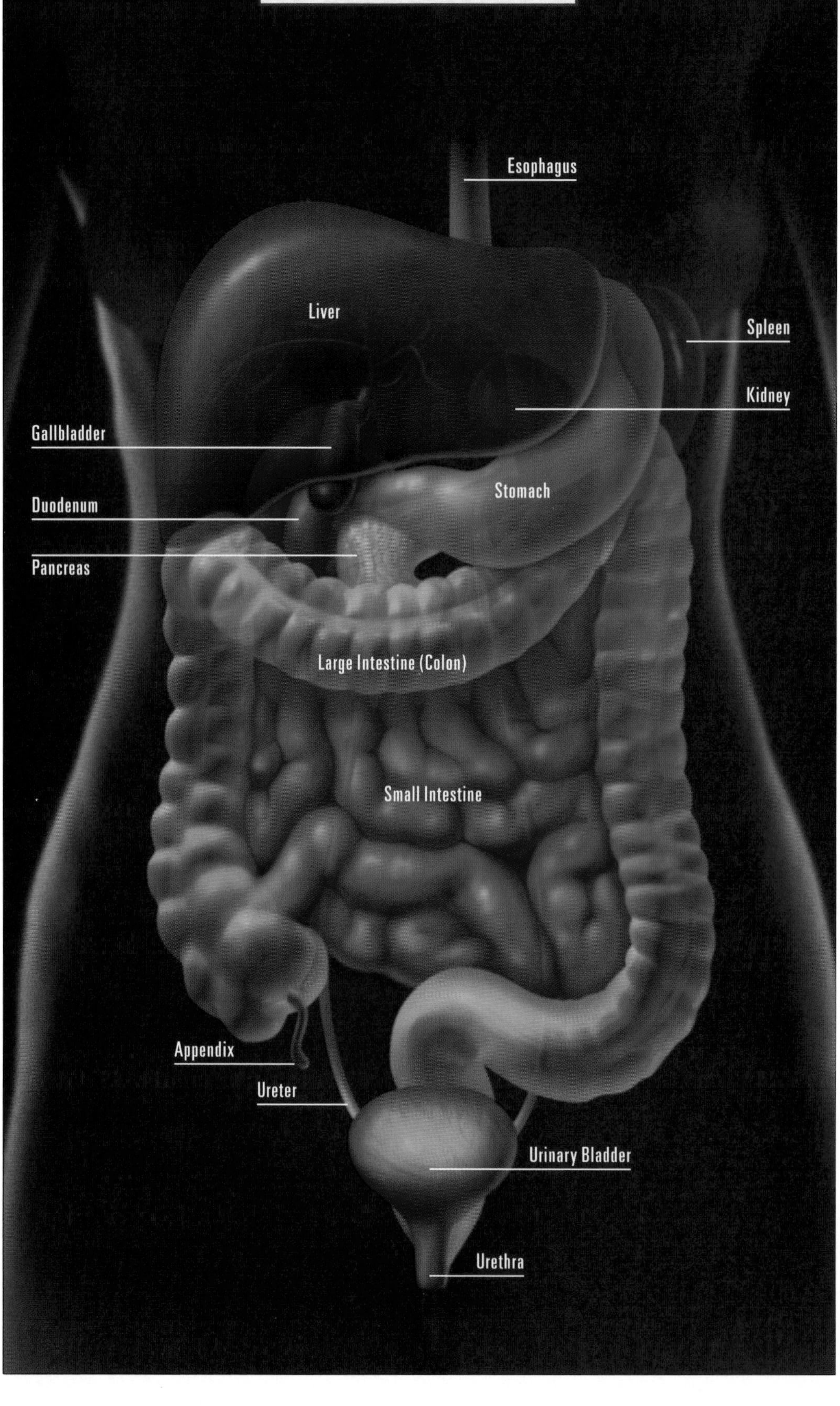
Esophagus
Liver
Spleen
Kidney
Gallbladder
Stomach
Duodenum
Pancreas
Large Intestine (Colon)
Small Intestine
Appendix
Ureter
Urinary Bladder
Urethra

The male and female reproductive systems produce and store the cells that combine to make new human beings. When a woman's egg and a man's sperm cell join, the fertilized egg is a tiny speck weighing less than one-twentieth of a millionth of an ounce.

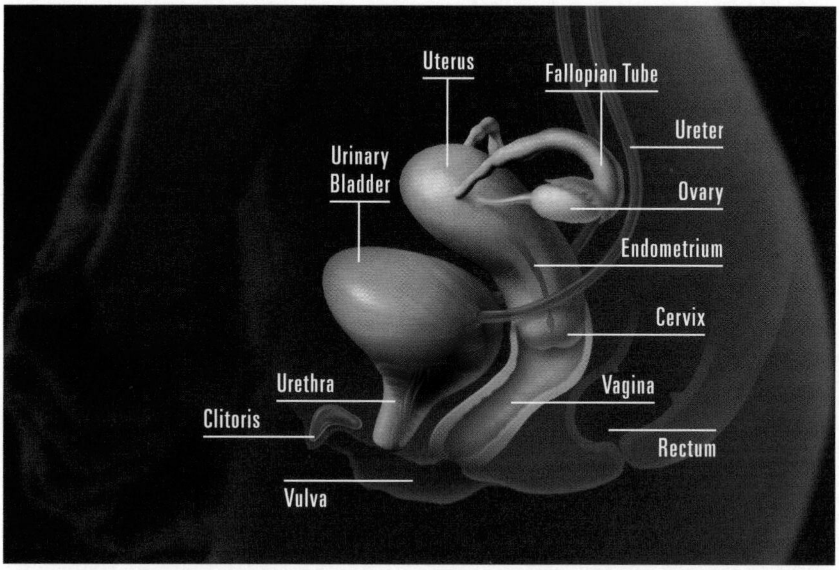

Six months before a girl is born, her ovaries contain all the eggs she'll ever have—200,000 of them. As she reaches her teens, her ovaries begin to release one or more of the eggs every month into the fallopian tubes, which carry them to the uterus. If an egg is not fertilized, the lining of the uterus (endometrium) will shed during menstruation. Sometimes fragments of endometrial tissue grow outside the uterus (the problem is called endometriosis) and cause painful menstruation.

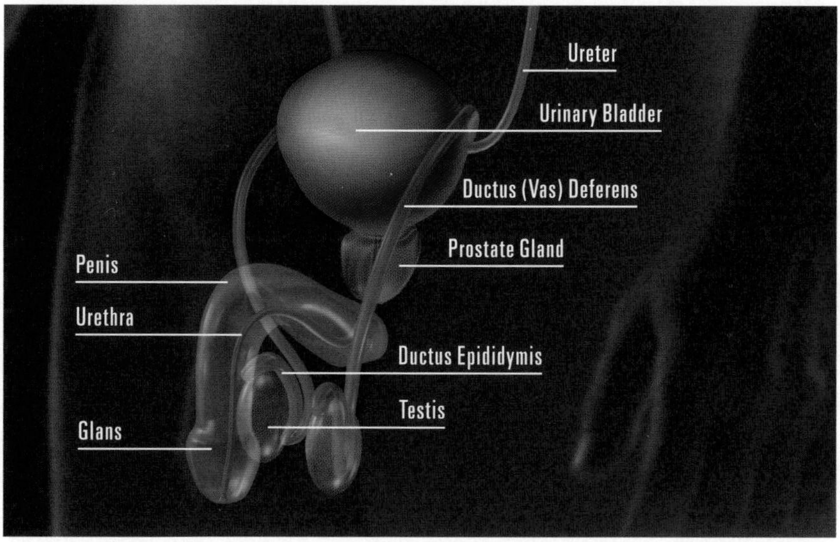

Sperm produced in a man's testes move on to the ductus epididymis, where they mature. When a man ejaculates, he releases 300 to 500 million sperm cells. The prostate gland, which produces fluid that makes sperm more active, often becomes enlarged as a man grows older. The enlarged gland may squeeze the urethra and make urination harder.

Referred pain: Ever wonder how it can be that a person having a heart attack sometimes feels pain not in the heart but in the shoulder, chest, and left arm? The answer is referred pain. Pain from an internal organ is sometimes referred to—that is, felt in—other places served by nerves from the same part of the spinal cord as the organ.

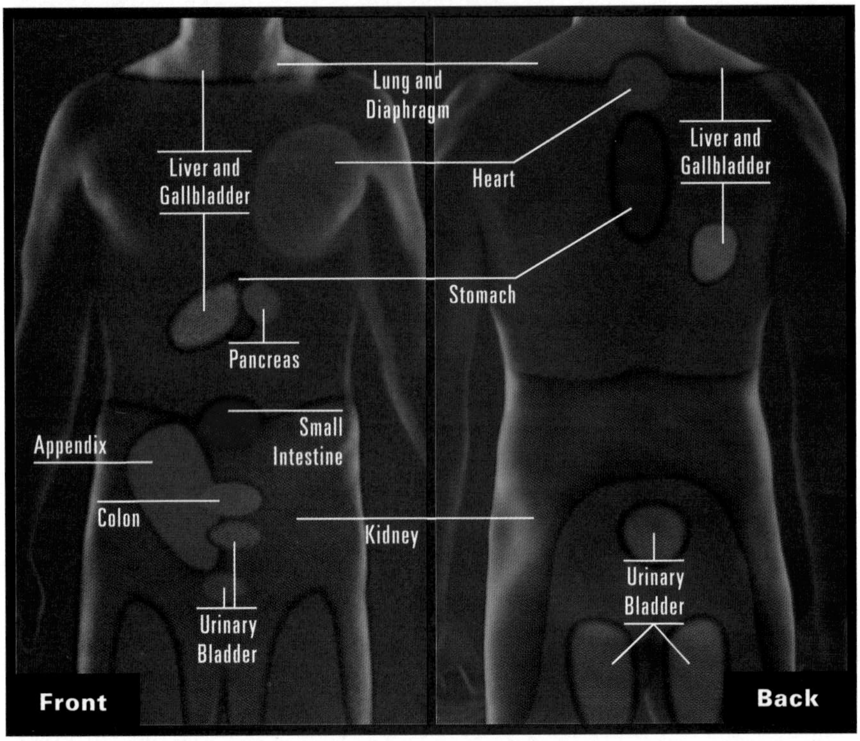

Pain from an internal organ often shows up on or just under the skin, in spots over the organ, or sometimes far from it. For example, pain from liver and gallbladder trouble (green) may be felt in the right side of the neck, the front of the chest, or the right shoulder blade; and from the stomach (orange), high in the abdomen and between the shoulders.

Pain in the face (the shaded areas) often signals a deeper problem.

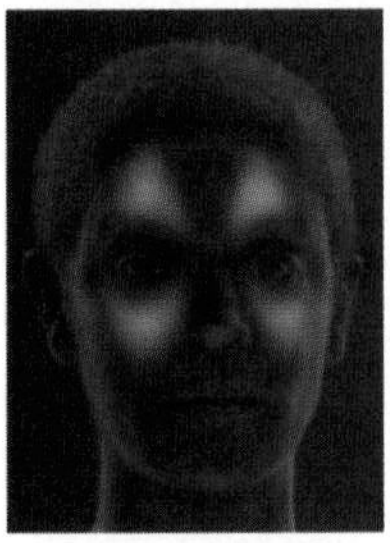

If pain gets worse when you bend your head forward, you may have a sinus infection.

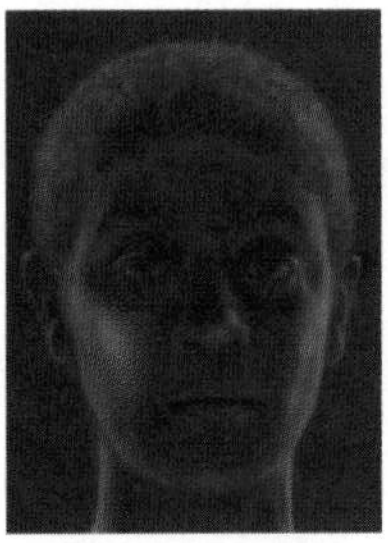

If throbbing pain gets worse at night, you may have a tooth abscess.

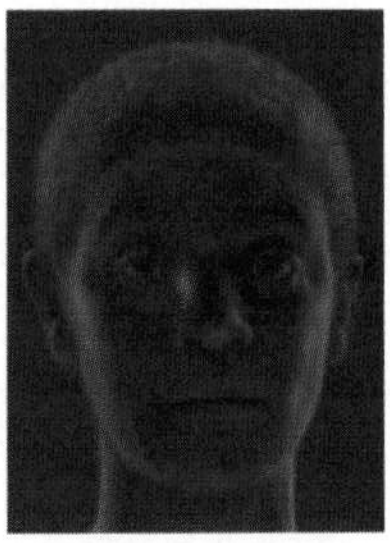

If your nose and one eye are runny and you have a headache, you may have a migraine.

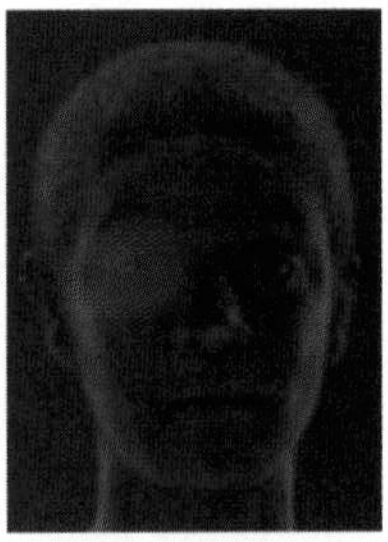

If your eye is bloodshot, vision blurry, and pain intense, you may have acute glaucoma.

(continued from page 160)

- If the itching is driving you crazy.
- If you develop a rash or have a seizure after using a medicated lice or scabies treatment.

HOW TO PREVENT IT

Head lice:

- Use a flashlight to check your children for lice, especially from August through November. Look for bites, nits, or lice at the nape of the neck and behind the ears.

All infestations:

- Wash clothes after 1 or 2 wearings.
- Wash towels and linens often.
- Bathe or shower daily.
- Don't share hats, combs, headphones, and other such items.
- If you have a new sexual partner, trade news about any lice or scabies either of you has had.

FOR MORE HELP

Information line: National Pediculosis Association, Box 610189, Newton, MA 02161. 617-449-6487, M–F 9–4 EST. Ask for information on screening programs, educational materials, and the latest lice and scabies treatments.

Organization: American Academy of Dermatology, Box 4014, Schaumburg, IL 60168-4014. 708-330-0230, M–F 8:30–5 CST. Send a business-size, self-addressed, stamped envelope for a pamphlet on scabies, and names of doctors near you. **Web site:** *http://www.aad.org/scabies.html.*

Web access: North Carolina State University, Department of Entomology. After logging on to the Internet, type: *http://www.ces.ncsu.edu/depts/ent/notes/Urban/lice.html.* Offers a survey of head, body, and pubic lice, and treatment.

Psoriasis

SIGNS AND SYMPTOMS

- Pink, raised skin flaked with white scales. Sometimes itchy or painful. Most often on scalp, knees, and elbows, less often in armpits, under breasts, on genitals, and around the anus.
- Rough, pitted fingernails that may crumble or come off.
- Raised areas on the hands and feet that may crack or form blisters filled with pus.
- Stiffness and inflamed flesh in fingers and toes, from a form of arthritis found in 10 percent of psoriasis.
- Small, scaly patches along with a sore throat and strep infection (mostly in teens and young adults).

The scales of psoriasis are dense piles of dead skin formed when cells in the outer layer (the epidermis) grow faster than they can be worn away. Those who get psoriasis may have it in their genes. You can't catch it from a person who has it. Psoriasis shows up most often in people between the ages of 10 and 30.

Injuries to the skin and infection may be causes. Stress may also be a culprit, though some experts say it isn't. Often, the ailment itself brings on feelings of low self-esteem and depression—so dealing with the emotions is a vital part of the treatment.

Some people keep psoriasis in check by using moisturizers. Others, especially those who have it on the hands and feet or on more than 30 percent of the body, may need to use stronger measures.

Psoriasis can't be cured, but home care combined with medical help often keeps it under control. Some common medical treatments include steroid creams, ultraviolet light, and oral medications, including methotrexate, an anticancer drug.

WHAT YOU CAN DO NOW

- Follow your doctor's skin-care advice well, even though it may take a lot of time.
- Don't pick at scales. New ones may form.
- Use warm (not hot) water to soak the scaly spots. When the scales are plumped up with water, gently remove whatever will come away easily with a loofah sponge or pumice stone.
- Shampoos and lotions made with tar may help psoriasis or even get rid of it for up to 2 years. If your psoriasis is on your scalp, a dandruff shampoo may help.
- Use lotions to keep your skin moist. Petroleum jelly and cooking oil don't cost much and they will do the job.
- Sunlight helps clear up the skin. The trick is to stay in the sun until just before you burn. Talk with your doctor about finding the right balance. Use a sunscreen on skin without psoriasis. If you're using tar products, your skin may be less able to handle the sun.
- If you suspect your flare-ups are triggered by stress, learn to reduce it. Techniques such as yoga or meditation may help (see **relax,** page 309).

WHEN TO CALL THE DOCTOR

Call for a prompt appointment:
- If you get pus-filled blisters or your whole body is red and scaly; you may need treatment right away.

Call for advice:
- If psoriasis flares up whenever you have a sore throat; ask your doctor for medication to combat a sore throat at the first sign of illness.
- If home care doesn't improve or control your psoriasis.

HOW TO PREVENT IT

There is no known way to prevent psoriasis.

FOR MORE HELP

Information line: National Psoriasis Foundation, 800-723-9166, M–F 8–5 PST. Staff answers questions about causes and treatments, and gives names of doctors near you. They also send pamphlets and a newsletter. **Web site:** *http://www.psoriasis. org.*

Information packet: National Institute of Arthritis and Musculoskeletal and Skin Diseases Information Clearinghouse, 301-495-4484, 24-hour line. Request a packet of recent articles on psoriasis.

Book: *Eczema & Psoriasis: How Your Diet Can Help,* by Steven Terrass. A guide to nutrition and skin problems. HarperCollins, 1995, $9.

Web access: American Academy of Dermatology. After logging on to the Internet, type: *http://www.aad.org/Psoriasis.html.* Explores causes and treatments.

Shingles

SIGNS AND SYMPTOMS

The first symptoms of shingles vary widely from person to person and can mimic other sources of pain, including muscle strain or a heart attack. Watch for:

- Puzzling pain (sometimes pulsing or unbearable) and tingling, itching, or extreme tenderness in an area of skin on only one side of the body or face.
- Fever and headache.
- A red, blistering rash in a band on one side of the body. This rash may show up 1 to 3 days after the first symptoms. If confined to one side of the body, it almost always means shingles. In rare cases, the rash may appear on both sides.
- Fluid-filled blisters that scab over, most often in 2 to 3 weeks.
- Pain and tenderness that may last longer than the blisters.

Thought chicken pox was behind you? Think again. Anyone who has had chicken pox has a chance of getting shingles as an adult. That's because chicken pox and the painful blisters of shingles are caused by the same herpes virus. Instead of going away when the chicken pox sores dry up, the virus hides in the nerve cells near the spine, sometimes for decades. Later, perhaps because the immune system is weakened or stressed, the virus comes back in its new form, inflaming certain nerve pathways.

Shingles is most common in adults over 50, and half of people over 85 have had it. People with immune systems weakened by AIDS, Hodgkin's disease, leukemia, or some kinds of drugs are also more likely to get shingles.

You can't catch shingles from a person who has it. But if you've never had chicken pox, there's a small chance that you will get chicken pox if you come into contact with fluid from the broken blisters of someone with shingles. That risk is highest for newborns.

In its worst form, which happens in 10 to 15 percent of cases, the ailment can cause intense shooting, burning pain (postherpetic neuralgia) for a month or more after the blisters are gone. But antiviral drugs can halt the disease. Prompt treatment reduces the chances of having this type of pain.

Shingles may also involve the nerves to the iris of the eye. This can lead to glaucoma and even blindness. Watch for blisters on the nose—they're the first sign the eyes may be affected. In those with other diseases, shingles may affect skin all over the body, and even the internal organs.

Most people who get shingles get over it in a few weeks, and the disease rarely recurs.

WHAT YOU CAN DO NOW

Call your doctor for advice if you notice the first signs of shingles. There are medicines that fight the virus. In mild cases, you may not need drugs—but if you do, the sooner you take them, the better your chance of avoiding the pain of shingles.

- Soothe the pain with cool compresses or ice packs.
- Take an over-the-counter painkiller (see **pain relief,** page 317).
- Relieve the itching with calamine lotion.
- Ask your doctor about using over-the-counter capsaicin cream, made from the fiery substance in chili peppers, to help reduce the severe pain of postherpetic neuralgia. Use it only after the blisters are healed.
- Put a few tablespoons of cornstarch or oatmeal (sold in drugstores) in your bathwater.
- Cut nails short. Do not scratch. The blisters can become infected or leave scars.
- Wear gloves at night so you won't scratch in your sleep.
- If you have severe pain that won't go away, join a chronic pain support group.

WHEN TO CALL THE DOCTOR

Call your doctor for emergency advice (if you can't get any, call 911 or go to an emergency room):

- If you have eye pain or a fluid-filled blister on your face. You may be at risk of getting herpes in your eye, which can lead to blindness.

Call for a prompt appointment:

- If you have a fever over 101 degrees or swelling, redness, and pus. This can signal a system-wide infection or a bacterial infection in the blisters.
- If you can't stand the pain.

Call for advice:

- If you have symptoms of shingles.

HOW TO PREVENT IT

There is no known way to prevent shingles. A vaccine for chicken pox is now in use, but its effects on shingles are unknown.

FOR MORE HELP

Information line: National Institute of Neurological Disorders and Stroke, 800-352-9424, M–F 8:30–5 EST. Ask for facts about shingles and postherpetic neuralgia.

Information line: American Chronic Pain Association, Box 850, Rocklin, CA 95677. 916-632-0922, 24-hour line. Ask for facts about shingles and advice on support groups for those with chronic pain.

Web access: American Academy of Dermatology. After logging on to the Internet, type: *http://www.aad.org/Zoster.html*. Explores causes and provides advice on treatment.

Skin Cancer

SIGNS AND SYMPTOMS

Basal cell carcinoma:

- A pearly or shiny skin growth, often with a dent in the center and raised edges, that expands over time.
- A patch of skin that itches, bleeds, hurts, or forms a scab.
- An open sore that fails to heal in one month or that closes and reopens.

Squamous cell carcinoma:

- Reddish or brownish rough, scaly patches on skin that has been exposed to sunlight.
- A stubborn, scaly patch that sometimes crusts or bleeds.
- A raised growth that looks like a wart and sometimes bleeds.
- A firm, fleshy lump that gets bigger and bigger.

Malignant melanoma:

- A mole that changes the way it looks. It may become scaly or ooze, bleed, or enlarge.
- A dark area of the skin that feels itchy, or the sudden growth of a "bubbly" mole.
- Dark spots or moles that have these "ABCD" traits: Asymmetrical, Border blurry, Color uneven, Diameter larger than a pencil eraser.

About half the people in the United States who live to 65 will get skin cancer at least once. (See color illustrations, page 166.) The 3 main kinds are:

Basal cell carcinoma. The most common kind in Caucasians; often found on the face. It develops slowly and most of the time doesn't send cancer cells to other parts of the body.

Squamous cell carcinoma. Most often found on the face, lips, or rim of the ear. It grows more quickly than basal cell and can form large masses. If ignored, it can spread to other parts of the body.

Malignant melanoma. The most harmful type of skin cancer. A cancer of the dark-pigmented cells that produce melanin, it often spreads to other parts of the body and can be fatal if left untreated.

People who had even one bad sunburn as children have a greater chance of getting skin cancer later in life than those who didn't get burned. The risk rises for people who live in Sun Belt states; work outside; have 2 or more relatives who have had skin cancer; or have light-colored eyes, red or blond hair, and skin that freckles easily. If you have brown or black skin, you are less likely to get skin cancer, but you still run a risk.

The good news is that skin cancer can nearly always be cured if caught in time. And because sunlight is the main cause, skin cancer can be prevented.

WHAT YOU CAN DO NOW

- ➤ See a doctor promptly if you suspect you have skin cancer. The earlier it's caught, the better your chances that treatment will cure it.

WHEN TO CALL THE DOCTOR

Call for a prompt appointment:

- ➤ If you have an itchy mole or a dark spot or bump that changes color, bleeds, or oozes (see color illustrations, page 167).

Call for advice:

- ➤ If you see any of the signs of skin cancer.
- ➤ If what looks like a pimple crusts over, doesn't go away, and gets bigger.
- ➤ If you develop a lump on or beneath an area of your skin that is often exposed to the sun and it doesn't go away after 2 weeks of home treatment with warm compresses.

HOW TO PREVENT IT

Since sunlight causes 90 percent of skin cancers, the best way to prevent them is to avoid the sun as much as you can.

- ➤ Apply a sunscreen of SPF 15 or higher 30 minutes before you go outside, and wear a hat, long-sleeved shirt, and long pants. (Ultraviolet rays can get through haze.) Avoid being outdoors between 10 A.M. and 2 P.M. (or if possible, 4 P.M.), when the sun's rays are most intense.

SIMPLE STEPS TO SAVE YOUR SKIN

- Standing in front of a mirror, look at your front and, using a hand mirror, your back. Look for any strange lumps or new growths (see color illustrations, page 167).
- Raise your arms and turn to the right and left as you examine your sides and underarms.
- Bend your arms and inspect them from fingertips to shoulders, including the undersides.
- Sit down and use a hand mirror to look at the backs of your legs; also look at the tops of your feet and the spaces between your toes.
- Use the hand mirror to check the back of your neck and your scalp, or ask someone to check these areas for you.

- ➤ Don't go to tanning salons; they use harmful ultraviolet light.
- ➤ Don't use suntan oil; it doesn't protect your skin.
- ➤ Do a skin self-exam every month (see box above). If you are light-skinned, have freckles, burn without tanning, or have a family history of skin cancer, visit your doctor for a checkup and help in learning the danger signs.

FOR MORE HELP

Information line: Cancer Information Service, 800-422-6237, M–F 9–4:30 your time. In English and Spanish. Offers brochures, treatment advice, access to a database of clinical trials, and names of cancer-related resources near you.

Information line: American Cancer Society, 800-227-2345, M–F 9–5 your time. Offers brochures and lists of classes and events.

Pamphlet: American Academy of Family Physicians. For a copy of "Skin Cancer," send a self-addressed, stamped business envelope to AAFP, 8880 Ward Parkway, Kansas City, MO 64114.

Book: *Saving Your Skin,* by Barney Kenet, M.D., and Patricia Lawler. Complete guide to guarding against skin cancer. Four Walls Eight Windows, 1994, $14.95.

Web access: American Academy of Dermatology. After logging on to the Internet, type: *http://www.aad.org/SkinCancerNews.* Offers advice on spotting symptoms early, safe sunning, and new treatments.

Video: *Skin Cancer at Time of Diagnosis.* Clear overview of causes and treatments, with 4 reports—Understanding the Diagnosis, What Happens Next?, Treatment and Management, and Issues and Answers. Time Life Medical, 1996, $19.95. Sold in many pharmacies; for one near you, call 800-588-9959.

Sunburn

SIGNS AND SYMPTOMS

- Red, "burned" skin (even in dark-skinned people).
- Pain and (sometimes) blisters.

Not too long ago, a suntan—or even a slight burn—was seen as a sign of good health. Now we know it's the body's attempt to protect itself from the sun, and a sign of skin damage.

That's because some rays of sun—called ultraviolet A and B (UVA and UVB)—damage skin cells. If you're out in the sun year after year, even if you never sunburn, the result is wrinkles and perhaps **skin cancer** (see opposite page and illustrations, pages 166–167).

A sunburn raises the risks. People of all skin colors can get a sunburn, but those with fair skin are the most likely to get long-term skin damage or skin cancer from it.

WHAT YOU CAN DO NOW

- ➤ Soothe the skin with a cool bath or a compress.
- ➤ Try ice for pain. Take one cube and melt it slightly so it has no rough edges. Glide it over the burn until it melts, keeping it mov-

ing to avoid skin damage. Repeat every hour as needed for pain.

- ➤ Try lotions or gels with aloe vera to soothe pain and speed healing.
- ➤ Use an over-the-counter painkiller (see **pain relief,** page 317). Aspirin works best because it blocks a chemical the body makes in response to burns. (Never give aspirin to a child under 12 who has chicken pox, flu, a cold, or any other illness you suspect of being caused by a virus; see box on **Reye's syndrome,** page 96.)
- ➤ Consider a lotion or spray that contains benzocaine for pain relief. **Caution:** It may cause an allergic response. Don't use these if you have skin allergies or if allergies run in your family.
- ➤ Watch for signs of dehydration—dry mouth, sticky saliva, dizziness or weakness, and dark yellow urine—especially if the sunburned person is a child. Give water to drink or a **rehydration** drink (see box on page 124).
- ➤ Watch for **heat stroke** and **heat exhaustion** (see page 40). **Caution:** If you suspect heat stroke, don't give anything to drink.

Later:

- ➤ If skin peels, use a lotion to add moisture and ease itching. Lotions with aloe vera are soothing at any point.
- ➤ If you must go back into the sun, keep the burn from getting worse by using sunscreen with an SPF (sun protection factor) of at least 15.

WHEN TO CALL THE DOCTOR

- ➤ Call 911 or go to an emergency room **right away** if you see signs of heat stroke.
- ➤ Call for advice if the skin blisters. Don't cover the blisters.

HOW TO PREVENT IT

- ➤ Wear a hat with a 4-inch (or wider) brim and protective clothing. Dark colors shield you better than light ones. But you can get a sunburn through most clothes—they don't block harmful rays. The average T-shirt has an SPF of 9 at most, and that drops to 3 if the shirt is wet. So you may need to apply sunscreen all over. You can also get special clothing that blocks UV rays.
- ➤ Apply sunscreen if you plan to be out more than a few minutes, even in winter or when it's overcast: Clouds don't stop all UV rays. **Caution:** Don't put sunscreen on babies younger than 6 months—it can get in their eyes or mouth. Keep infants out of the sun.
- ➤ For best results, put on sunscreen at least 30 minutes before you go out (to give it time to bond to the skin), and put on more every 2 hours. **Caution:** If you have allergies or tender skin, test some on a small spot to see if you react. You might want to avoid sunscreens with PABA, or try a product with titanium dioxide.

FOR MORE HELP

Information line: National Institute of Arthritis and Musculoskeletal and Skin Diseases Information Clearinghouse, 301-495-4484, 24-hour recording. Request the "Sun and Skin" packet.

Organization: American Academy of Dermatology, Box 4014, Schaumburg, IL 60168-4014. 847-330-0230, M–F 8:30–5 CST. Send a business-size, self-addressed, stamped envelope for the pamphlets "Sun and Your Skin" and "Sun Protection for Children." **Web site:** *http://www.aad.org.*

Warts

SIGNS AND SYMPTOMS

Common warts:

- ■ Small, hard, rough, raised growths that most often appear on the skin of the hands and fingers.

Plantar warts:

- ■ Same hard growths as common warts but on the soles of the feet, sometimes making walking painful.

Flat warts:

- ■ Small, flat growths, clustered in groups of many hundreds. Often found on the hands, wrists, forearms, knees, face, neck, and chest.

Filiform warts:

- Slim, stringlike growths that take root on the face or neck.

Genital warts:

- Itchy, small bumps, round or flat, sometimes in groups, that appear on or near the genitals. Can be passed from person to person.

In folklore, warts come from handling frogs or toads. But the real source is any one of about 70 types of the human papilloma virus.

You pick up the virus by coming into contact with skin shed from a wart (either your own or someone else's). It enters through a cut or nick in the skin, causing skin cells to grow quickly, creating a new wart. But this doesn't happen easily, except for genital warts.

Children, young adults, and people with weakened immune systems are most likely to get warts. In children, warts nearly always go away on their own within a year or so, but in adults they may take longer, or may need to be removed.

WHAT YOU CAN DO NOW

If you don't mind your warts, relax. They're harmless, and can go away by themselves. If they bother you, you can often remove them at home. If you're over 45 and a new wart appears, check with a doctor before trying home care.

- If you have genital warts, see your doctor.
- You can remove warts, when they are not on the face or the genitals, with an over-the-counter product that contains salicylic acid. It gently peels the surface of the wart away. You may need to apply the acid many times.
- Sit quietly, close your eyes, and create an image of the wart shrinking and vanishing. Do it for 5 or 10 minutes 2 or 3 times a day for several days. Strange as it may seem, some experts think this mental process really makes warts shrink.
- Don't cut or burn a wart.
- Plantar warts often extend below the surface of the skin. You may need a skin doctor's help to remove them. Padded insoles in your shoes may reduce pain, or use a doughnut-shaped pad to relieve pressure.

WHEN TO CALL THE DOCTOR

- If you or your partner have genital warts, which can be passed on to others and also may be related to cervical cancer in women (see **sexually transmitted diseases** chart, page 225).
- If you are over 45 and you find a new wart. Your doctor will want to check it to make sure it's not **skin cancer** (see page 180; see also color illustration, page 167).
- If you want a wart on your face removed.
- If you have a wart that does not respond to home treatment, above all if it bleeds, changes color, or looks infected.

HOW TO PREVENT IT

- Don't scratch warts—you could make them spread.
- When shaving, use an electric razor to avoid the small nicks and scratches that may allow viruses to enter.
- Don't touch other people's warts.
- When using public showers, wear sandals or other footwear.

FOR MORE HELP

Organization: American Academy of Dermatology, Box 4014, Schaumburg, IL 60168-4014. 847-330-0230, M–F 8:30–5 CST. Send a business-size, self-addressed, stamped envelope for facts about warts and a list of doctors near you. **Web site:** *http://aad.org/warts.html.*

Muscles, Bones, & Joints

Arthritis

SIGNS AND SYMPTOMS

Osteoarthritis:
- Joint pain that movement makes worse.
- Stiffness in the morning.
- Knobby growths on finger joints.

Rheumatoid arthritis:
- Painful, red, swollen joints that may feel warm.
- Low fever, loss of weight and appetite; feeling "sick all over."
- Morning stiffness.
- Skin lumps, often on the elbows, fingers, or buttocks.
- Dry eyes and mouth.

Gout:
- Severe, sudden pain in a joint, often the wrist, big toe, or knee.
- Redness, swelling around joint.
- Fever.

Arthritis is a name given to lots of joint problems that cause swelling, pain, and stiffness. The more than 100 types of arthritis range from mild to crippling. The 3 most common types are:

Osteoarthritis: It's caused by chips and cracks in the smooth cartilage that lines the joints (see color illustration, page 163). The bone ends may also rub together and grow bumps called spurs. Osteoarthritis affects about half of those over 65, most often in the hands or in large weight-bearing joints such as the knee and hip.

Rheumatoid arthritis: In this type, the lining of the capsule around a joint becomes inflamed and thickened, causing swelling, pain, and stiffness. Rheumatoid arthritis can also inflame the eyes and lungs. Some experts think it's the result of a problem with the body's immune system—the body turns on itself and attacks its own tissues. It most often affects people between 20 and 50, and more women than men.

Gout: It most often affects men over 40 and is caused by high blood levels of uric acid, one of the body's waste products, which forms crystals in the joints. The body's immune system reacts to these crystals as if to a foreign invader, and the joint becomes inflamed and painful. Symptoms of each attack go away in about a week.

Treatment of arthritis depends on the type and how bad it is. Most can be treated with gentle exercise to keep the bones and muscles strong, and drugs to reduce pain, swelling, and stiffness. Gout can be treated with drugs to reduce uric acid in the blood. In more severe cases of osteoarthritis and rheumatoid arthritis, surgery may smooth rough joint surfaces or replace a damaged joint.

WHAT YOU CAN DO NOW

➤ For rheumatoid arthritis, take aspirin, or the anti-inflammatory painkiller your doctor suggests. If these upset your stomach,

Neck Pain

Neck pain is most often a sign of simple muscle strain that you can take care of at home, but it can be a symptom of more serious problems.

SYMPTOMS	WHAT IT MIGHT BE	WHAT YOU CAN DO
Severe headache, then neck pain and stiffness; sometimes with nausea, drowsiness, or trouble seeing in bright light.	Meningitis—infection of tissue around brain (see page 57).	Call 911 or go to emergency room **right away.**
Severe pain and/or swelling in neck after injury; numbness, weakness, or paralysis below injured spot; lack of bladder or bowel control; shock.	Spinal cord injury (see head, neck, and back injuries, page 38).	Call 911 **right away.** Never attempt to move someone who may have a spinal cord injury.
Bad neck pain, worse when moving head; or tingling, numbness, or weakness in one arm.	Protruded disk pressing on a nerve (see low back pain, page 192).	With sudden numbness or weakness, call doctor for advice and appointment **right away;** if you can't get one, call 911 or go to emergency room. Take painkillers (see box, page 317), and rest.
Pain and stiffness that begin in neck and move to shoulders, upper arms, hands, or back of head; numbness or tingling in arms, head, and fingers; weakness in arms and legs.	Cervical spondylosis—breakdown of joints in neck that may press on nerves and muscles.	With numbness and tingling, call doctor for prompt appointment. Otherwise, call for advice and appointment. Apply moist heat. Sleep with thin pillow under head and thin, rolled-up towel under neck.
Pain and soreness in front of neck, fever, swelling.	Thyroiditis (see thyroid problems, page 294).	Call doctor for prompt appointment.
Stiff neck that may come with pain or swelling in other joints.	Arthritis.	See arthritis, page 184.
Pain with swelling on back or side of neck.	Swollen lymph nodes from infection.	See infections, page 286.

(continued)

Neck Pain *(continued)*

SYMPTOMS	WHAT IT MIGHT BE	WHAT YOU CAN DO
Neck pain or stiffness that starts within 24 hours of a jolt (such as car stopping suddenly); sometimes with dizziness, headache, vomiting, or trouble walking.	Whiplash—also known as cervical acceleration/deceleration injury.	Call doctor for prompt appointment. Wear soft, padded collar to hold neck still. Sleep with thin pillow under head and thin, rolled-up towel under neck. Apply ice pack, and take painkillers (see box, page 317).
Stiff neck or pain on waking, or when sitting or standing.	Strained neck muscles or joints from sleeping or sitting in awkward way.	Sleep with thin pillow under head and thin, rolled-up towel under neck. If stiffness or pain lasts more than 24 hours, call doctor for advice and appointment.

try an "enteric-coated" brand. Or ask your doctor about drugs that can reduce the risk of ulcers.

- For osteoarthritis, use acetaminophen. If you have gout, don't take aspirin. Take aspirin, ibuprofen, or naproxen separately; never combine them (see **pain relief** box, page 317).
- Apply cold packs to swollen, painful joints, or warm packs for stiffness without other symptoms for 10 minutes every hour.
- Apply an over-the-counter lotion that contains capsaicin or an over-the-counter cream containing methyl salicylate for pain relief.
- Twice a day, put each joint gently through a full range of motion to prevent stiffness.
- Take a warm shower or bath to get started in the morning—this helps relieve stiffness.
- Enroll in an arthritis self-help program or join a support group with other people going through the same things you are.
- To ease the strain on painful joints, use electric can openers and enlarged grips for pens or tools.
- Don't grip objects tightly for a long time.
- Get lots of rest.

WHEN TO CALL THE DOCTOR

- If you have joint pain or stiffness that gets in the way of normal activities.
- If you have fever or chills along with other arthritis symptoms. You may have infectious arthritis, caused by bacteria.
- If you get the painful symptoms of gout.
- If your arthritis doesn't get better with self-care.

HOW TO PREVENT IT

Osteoarthritis:

- Exercise gently and often to keep your bones and muscles strong. Swimming, biking, and low-impact or water aerobics are ideal.
- If you weigh more than you should, lose those extra pounds. Too much weight puts added pressure on the joints.
- Try not to do the same movements over and over—for instance, typing or hammering.
- Stand up straight to ease strain on joints.

Rheumatoid arthritis:

There's no known way to prevent rheumatoid arthritis.

Gout:

- Control your weight, but don't fast; fasting can raise levels of uric acid.

- If you drink, drink moderately—no more than 2 drinks a day if you're a man, 1 if you're a woman. A drink is 1.5 ounces of hard liquor, a 5-ounce glass of wine, or a 12-ounce beer.
- Avoid protein-rich foods such as organ meats, shellfish, and dried beans—all can cause gout.
- Drink plenty of water—at least 10 big glasses a day. The water will help flush out the uric acid.

FOR MORE HELP

Organization: Arthritis Foundation, 1330 W. Peachtree St., Atlanta, GA 30309. 800-283-7800, 24-hour recording, or 404-872-7100 M–F 9–5 EST. Provides basic facts about arthritis and tips on exercise and pain control. Also lists support groups near you. Membership starting at $20 includes *Arthritis Today* magazine. **Web site:** *http://www.arthritis.org.*

Book: *Arthritis: What Exercises Work,* by Dava Sobel and Arthur C. Klein. Exercises that help arthritis. St. Martin's Press, 1993, $19.95 hardcover, $10.95 paperback.

Book: *The Arthritis Helpbook,* by Kate Lorig, R.N., Dr.P.H., and James F. Fries, M.D. How to live with arthritis. Addison-Wesley, 1995, $14.

Web access: University of Birmingham, Department of Rheumatology. After logging on to the Internet, type: *http://rheuma.bham.ac.uk:80/primer.html.* Covers the basics of rheumatoid arthritis.

Video: *Arthritis at Time of Diagnosis.* Clear overview of causes and treatments, with 4 reports—Understanding the Diagnosis, What Happens Next?, Treatment and Management, and Issues and Answers. Time Life Medical, 1996, $19.95. Sold in many pharmacies; for one near you, call 800-588-9959.

Bunions and Hammertoes

SIGNS AND SYMPTOMS

Bunion:
- A lump on the side of the joint that connects the big toe to the foot.
- A big toe that points in or out.
- Pain, swelling, or stiffness in the joint.

Hammertoe:
- A toe (often the second one) bent in a clawlike position.
- A corn at the top of the toe.
- Pain in the toe.

One in 6 people in the United States has a foot problem, and among the most common complaints are bunions and hammertoes. Both tend to run in families, but shoes that don't fit well can cause them or make them worse.

Bunions are most often harmless, but they can hurt. A bunion may become inflamed when a tight shoe rubs against it. Long-term pressure can cause **bursitis** (see page 189).

A hammertoe occurs when the tendons in the toe tighten and bend it down so it can't straighten. Where the toe rubs against shoes, a painful **corn** (see page 150) can develop. For some people, the pain may interfere with walking and standing.

These problems can be prevented or helped with shoes that fit well (you should be able to wiggle your toes in them). Severe cases can be fixed with surgery.

WHAT YOU CAN DO NOW

Self-care won't get rid of a bunion or hammertoe, but it can ease the pain.
- Wear shoes that are wide enough to relieve pressure on the foot.
- For relief around the house, wear old shoes with a hole cut out for the bunion.
- To relieve the pain of a hammertoe, buy

Shoulder Pain

Most shoulder pain results from injury or overuse. Rest and self-care are often all that's needed.

SYMPTOMS	WHAT IT MIGHT BE	WHAT YOU CAN DO
After injury, severe pain and tenderness, worse when moving; numbness, tingling in arm; joint may be misshapen.	Shoulder dislocation (see fractures and dislocations, page 37).	Call doctor for advice right away. If you can't get one, call 911 or go to emergency room.
Sudden joint pain with flu or other infection.	Side effect of infection.	Take over-the-counter painkillers (see box, page 317). If temperature is over 101, call doctor for prompt appointment.
Pain and swelling around shoulder, painful movement, fever (sometimes).	Bursitis (see page 189).	If temperature is over 101, call doctor for prompt appointment; bursa may be infected.
Pain and stiffness that begin in neck and move to shoulders; numbness or tingling in arms, hands, and fingers; weakness in arms and legs.	Cervical spondylosis—a breakdown of joints in neck that may put pressure on nerves and muscles.	With numbness and tingling, call doctor for prompt appointment. Otherwise, call for advice. Apply moist heat. Sleep with thin pillow under head and thin, rolled-up towel under neck.
Severe pain during movement, trouble moving arm, ache when not being used.	Frozen shoulder—inflamed shoulder joint from lack of use (often because of injury).	Call doctor for advice and appointment. Use RICE treatment (see box, page 200).
Pain or dull ache in shoulder, trouble raising or lowering arm, weakness in shoulder.	Rotator cuff injury—inflammation of tendons that hold shoulder in place.	Call doctor for advice and appointment.
Pain and stiffness in shoulders (or other joints).	Arthritis.	See arthritis, page 184.
Pain in distinct spot, worse with movement, after injury, exertion, or heavy lifting.	Strained or torn tendon, ligament, or muscle.	See sprains and strains, page 46.
Pain and tenderness, often worse at night; muscle spasms.	Tendinitis.	See tendinitis, page 204.

toe caps (padded sleeves that go around the top of a toe).

- Try a "contrast soak"—soak your foot in cold water for 1 minute, then warm water for 5 minutes, then another minute in cold water. Repeat 3 or 4 times. Ice packs and heating pads also work well.
- Put a small sponge or pad between your big toe and second toe to help align them with the other toes.
- Cushion the sore area with moleskin or foot pads to prevent rubbing.
- Take over-the-counter painkillers (see **pain relief** box, page 317).

WHEN TO CALL THE DOCTOR

- If redness, pain, or swelling lasts long.
- If your feet hurt so much that you find it hard to walk, wear shoes, or go about your normal activities.
- If you have diabetes or poor blood flow in your limbs and notice irritated skin over a bunion or hammertoe; it can become infected and lead to problems such as gangrene (tissue death).

HOW TO PREVENT IT

- Wear roomy, low-heeled shoes that don't pinch your toes.
- Fit new shoes to your larger foot. Most people's feet are not exactly the same size.
- Feet tend to swell during the day, so shop for new shoes at the end of the day, when your feet are largest.
- If you have early signs of a bunion or hammertoe, ask your doctor or podiatrist about orthotics, custom-made shoe inserts that can reduce the risk of foot problems.

FOR MORE HELP

Information line: American Podiatric Medical Association, 800-FOOTCARE, 24-hour recording. Ask for free brochures on 40 topics related to feet.

Organization: American Academy of Orthopaedic Surgeons, 800-824-BONE, 24-hour recording. Ask for brochures on how to choose shoes and how to exercise without injury.

Bursitis

SIGNS AND SYMPTOMS

- Pain and swelling in or near a joint.
- In bursitis of the shoulder, pain moving into the neck, arms, or fingers.
- Fever, if infection is present.

Where your bones, tendons, and ligaments move against each other, they are cushioned by small fluid-filled sacs called bursae. These sacs help joints move smoothly. Bursitis occurs when a bursa becomes inflamed—often from too much pressure, overuse, infection, or injury.

Athletes and people who do heavy lifting or the same motions again and again, such as hammering, tend to get bursitis. Working for a long time in an odd posture can also bring it on. Calcium deposits near bursae at the joints can make it worse. Bursitis can also be an early sign of arthritis.

Bursitis is seldom serious and often gets better in 1 to 2 weeks, as long as you take a break from whatever caused the problem. Bursitis may come back, though, and can become chronic—meaning it may last a long time, with symptoms that come and go.

Bursitis responds well to rest, self-care, and gentle exercise that helps restore normal movement and prevent stiffness. In the worst cases, a doctor may need to drain fluid from the bursa, inject drugs to reduce pain and swelling, or surgically remove the bursa.

WHAT YOU CAN DO NOW

- Rest the sore joint.
- Change any movements that cause pain, if you can.
- Take aspirin, ibuprofen, or naproxen to ease pain and reduce swelling (see **pain relief** box, page 317).
- Hold an ice pack on the sore joint for 20 minutes at a time, 3 or 4 times a day, for 2 days, to reduce pain and swelling. A bag of frozen peas wrapped in a washcloth works well. After 2 days, if pain returns,

apply warmth for 15 to 20 minutes 3 or 4 times a day. Use a washcloth soaked in warm water and wrung out.

- Exercise the tender joint twice a day: Move the joint gently as far as you can through its range of motion. Let pain be your guide; stop when it hurts.
- As you get better, begin to add gentle strength training to build muscle around the joint. This will help protect the joint and prevent future problems.

WHEN TO CALL THE DOCTOR

Call for a prompt appointment:

- If your temperature is over 101 or if the skin around the joint turns red and swollen; you may have an infected bursa.

Call for advice and an appointment:

- If pain or swelling lasts for more than 2 weeks despite rest and home care; you may have chronic bursitis or early arthritis.

HOW TO PREVENT IT

- Warm up before exercise; cool down afterward (see **overuse injuries,** page 199).
- Wear padding when you're playing contact sports.
- Avoid doing the same movements over and over, such as hammering or kneeling on a hard surface.
- If you can't avoid such things, change your position often and take 5- to 10-minute breaks every hour.
- To prevent bursitis in the feet, don't wear high heels or badly worn running or walking shoes.
- To avoid bursitis in the hip, sit on cushioned chairs. Get up often.
- Stretching or yoga can help.

FOR MORE HELP

Organization: Arthritis Foundation, 1330 W. Peachtree St., Atlanta, GA 30309. 800-283-7800, 24-hour recording, or 404-872-7100, M–F 9–5 EST. Offers brochures. Also lists support groups near you.

Organization: American Chronic Pain Association, Box 850, Rocklin, CA 95677. 916-632-0922, 24-hour line. Lists support groups for those with chronic pain.

Web access: American College of Rheumatology. After logging on to the Internet, type: *http://www.rheumatology.org/patient/tendin.htm.* Covers bursitis and lists doctors near you.

Carpal Tunnel Syndrome

SIGNS AND SYMPTOMS

- Numbness and tingling in the first 3 fingers.
- Shooting pain in the hand, wrist, and sometimes forearm.
- Pain that may be worse at night, causing trouble sleeping.
- Weakness in the hands and fingers (in severe cases).

The pain and numbness of carpal tunnel syndrome (CTS) come from repeated use of the wrists in the workplace, often when using a keyboard, or in sports. It happens when a nerve that runs through a narrow channel of ligaments and wrist bones (called carpals) is squeezed by fluid or inflamed tissue in the carpal tunnel.

CTS is also common in women when pregnancy or menopause causes fluid buildup. **Arthritis** (see page 184), **diabetes** (see page 282), and hypothyroidism (see **thyroid problems,** page 294) may also cause the problem.

CTS is easy to treat if it's caught early; left untreated, it can damage nerves and muscles. Injections in the wrist may help reduce the worst pain and swelling. As a last resort, pressure on the nerve can sometimes be eased by surgery in the doctor's office.

WHAT YOU CAN DO NOW

- Stretch and exercise your wrists every day (see next page).
- Rest the hand and wrist when possible.
- If you have trouble sleeping, wear a wrist

splint at night to reduce pressure on the nerve. Most drugstores carry splints.

- At work, wear a wrist splint if it relieves your pain. Try to change movements that cause the pain.
- Cut salt from your diet; this may help reduce swelling.
- Drink plenty of water—at least 8 large glasses a day.
- Take ibuprofen, naproxen, or aspirin to reduce pain and swelling (see **pain relief** box, page 317).
- Apply a cold pack, 10 minutes on, 10 minutes off, for an hour. A bag of frozen peas wrapped in a washcloth works well.

WHEN TO CALL THE DOCTOR

- If pain and other symptoms persist or get worse despite a month of home care.

HOW TO PREVENT IT

- Change your hand position often when working, and take a 5- to 10-minute break each hour.

STRETCHES TO HELP YOUR WRISTS

Try these exercises 3 times a day.

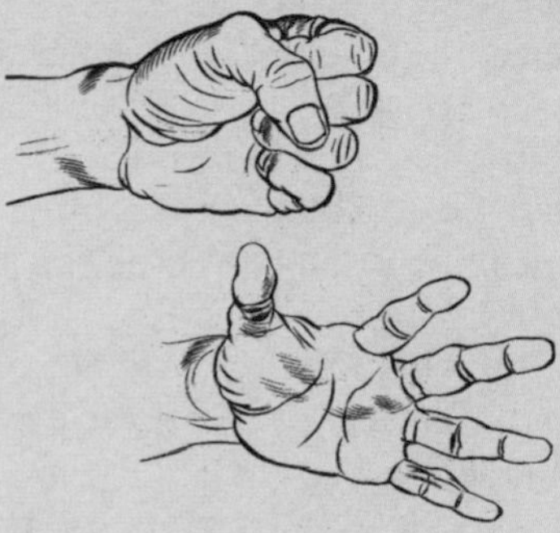

❶ Close your fist tightly, then release, spreading fingers wide. Repeat 5 times.

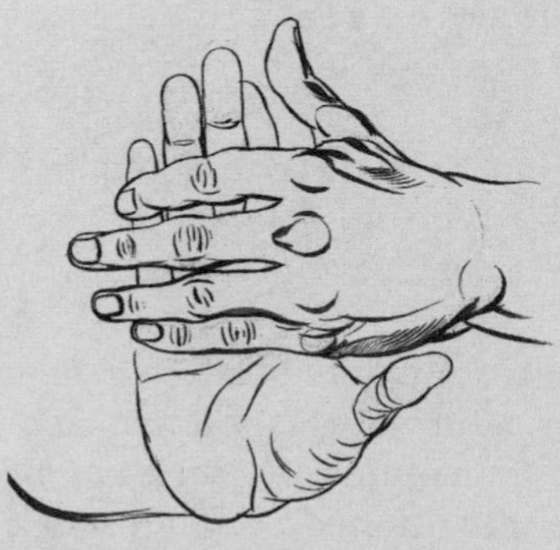

❷ Keeping your shoulder relaxed and low, extend your arm in front of you, palm out, fingers up. Use your other hand to pull back on your knuckles (not fingertips). Hold for 10 seconds.

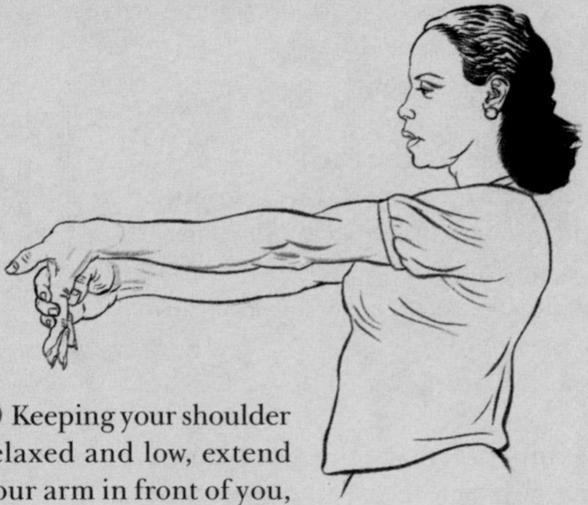

❸ Keeping your shoulder relaxed and low, extend your arm in front of you, fingers down. Gently pull knuckles (not fingertips) toward your body with other hand. Hold for 10 seconds.

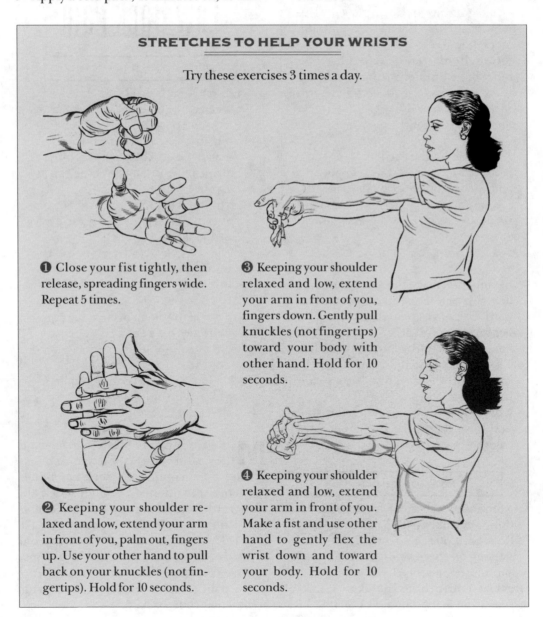

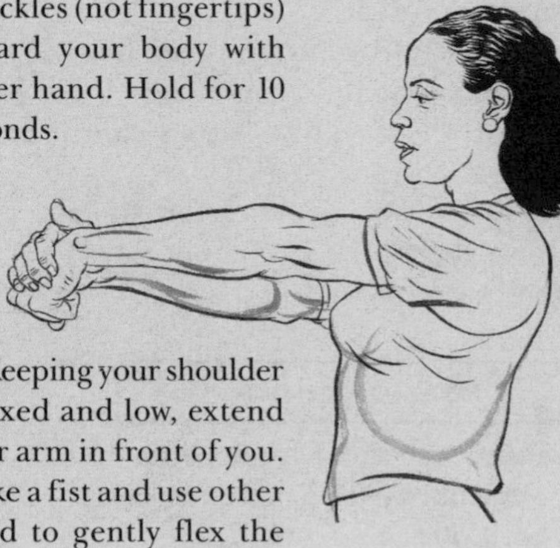

❹ Keeping your shoulder relaxed and low, extend your arm in front of you. Make a fist and use other hand to gently flex the wrist down and toward your body. Hold for 10 seconds.

OTHER HAND AND WRIST PAIN

Fracture: pain that worsens with pressure; swelling, bleeding, or bone showing through skin (see **fractures and dislocations,** page 37). Call your doctor for prompt advice. If he or she isn't available, call 911 or go to an emergency room **right away.**

Dislocation: joint swelling, pain, trouble moving the joint (see **fractures and dislocations,** page 37). Apply an ice pack for swelling, and use a splint to prevent movement. Call your doctor for a prompt appointment.

Ganglion: a round, soft or hard cyst under the skin, often on the wrist, sometimes with pain or soreness. It's harmless, but call your doctor for advice if it hurts or swells. Your doctor can drain or remove it.

Osteoarthritis: cartilage worn away in one or more joints. Causes pain, may limit movement (see **arthritis,** page 184).

Rheumatoid arthritis: joint pain, swelling, redness, and stiffness (see **arthritis,** page 184).

➤ As you work, make sure your hands are in line with your forearms, not cocked backward. Use a wrist pad when you type. Office supply stores carry them.

➤ Some people find that vitamin B6 helps. Take no more than the recommended daily amount, though; high doses can be harmful.

➤ Ask your employer to check with an expert in workplace design about ways to ease wrist strain on the job.

FOR MORE HELP

Organization: Association for Repetitive Motion Syndromes (ARMS), Box 514, Santa Rosa, CA 95402. 707-571-0397, 24-hour answering machine. Staff sends fact packet and answers questions.

Organization: Arthritis Foundation, 1330 W. Peachtree St., Atlanta, GA 30309. 800-283-7800, 24-hour recording, or 404-872-7100, M–F 9–5 EST. Sends free brochures on CTS, exercise, and pain management.

Book: *Repetitive Strain Injury: A Computer User's Guide,* by Emil Pascarelli, M.D., and Deborah Quilter. A guide to preventing and treating these injuries. John Wiley & Sons, 1994, $14.95.

Web access: University of Nebraska/Lincoln. After logging on to the Internet, type: *http://engr-www.unl.edu/ee/eeshop/rsi.html.* Offers advice and other on-line help.

Low Back Pain

SIGNS AND SYMPTOMS

- Pain low in the back; may be severe. It can come on quickly or slowly; it may be constant or occur only at certain times or when you are in a certain posture; it may be confined to one place or move to other parts of your back.
- Numbness, tingling, or a shooting pain in your legs or buttocks, often on one side only.
- Pain made worse by coughing, sneezing, or twisting.
- Stiffness.

Call a doctor right away if you also have these symptoms of nerve damage:

- Numbness or weakness, especially numbness around your groin or rectal area.
- Bladder or bowel control trouble.
- Weakness in one or both legs.

Most of us get a bit of back pain now and then, most often in the lower back.

The spinal column is a series of bones (vertebrae) cushioned by small shock absorbers (disks) and held up by muscles and ligaments. (See color illustrations, pages 171 and 173.) Most low back pain comes from muscle or ligament strain, disk problems, stress, or sometimes all of these. In most cases, the pain goes away on its own, though for some it may come back.

Disks break down somewhat with age or

from a lot of bending and twisting. In some cases, a swollen disk may press on a nerve in the lower back and send pain down the buttocks or legs. Most disk problems clear up with proper care. In severe cases, surgery to remove the disk or part of it may help.

WHAT YOU CAN DO NOW

- When your back starts hurting, apply an ice pack to hold down pain and swelling. Leave it there 10 to 15 minutes every hour. After 2 days, apply a heating pad or hot towel, or take hot showers. The heat will increase blood flow, bringing healing white cells to the sore spot.
- When pain is bad, lie flat on the floor with your knees bent and your lower legs on a chair or pile of pillows. This helps flatten the lower back and ease the strain.
- Sitting may be hard on a sore back. Stay away from soft chairs. Try a straight-back chair instead, and don't sit for a long time. Don't sit up in bed.
- Walk as much as you can, but only if it doesn't make your pain worse.
- If pain disturbs your sleep, put pillows under your knees when lying on your back.
- If you sleep on your side, bend your knees and put a pillow between them. Don't lie on your stomach.
- Take acetaminophen, aspirin, or ibuprofen for the pain (see pain **relief box,** page 317). Don't bother with prescription drugs for relaxing muscles; they work no better and often have side effects.
- If you think stress could be giving you a pain in the back, learn to spot—and avoid—situations that make you tense. Many people don't realize stress is making them tighten their back muscles.
- Learn some relaxation methods. They may help ease pain. Practice deep breathing or meditation (see **relax,** page 309).

WHEN TO CALL THE DOCTOR

Call promptly for advice (if your doctor is not in, call 911 or go to an emergency room):

- If you have back pain with symptoms of nerve damage, especially loss of bladder or bowel control.

THE SPINE

The curves of the spine give it strength and allow humans to walk upright.

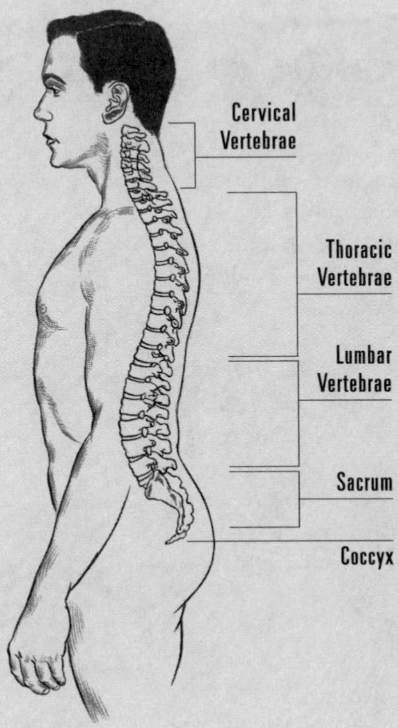

Call for advice and an appointment:

- If back pain is severe or disrupts your normal activities.
- If the pain doesn't go away within a few days or keeps coming back.

HOW TO PREVENT IT

- Exercise often. Avoid twisting or wrenching your body, or anything that seems to make your back pain worse. Walking, swimming, and even walking in a pool are ideal.
- Do exercises to strengthen the abdominal muscles (always do sit-ups with your knees bent). Also, stretch the muscles that run parallel to your spine (lie flat on your back; pull one knee, then the other, toward your chest).
- Try yoga. Doctors and people with back pain like it for building strength and flexibility. It also helps you relax.

Back Pain

Most backaches have no clear cause. Many come from simple strain, because the stacked bones and disks of the spine are not well suited to our upright posture, and gravity takes its toll. Sometimes, though, the pain signals a problem you can trace to another source.

SYMPTOMS	WHAT IT MIGHT BE	WHAT YOU CAN DO
Stubborn pain, often worse at night; numbness, tingling, and weakness that gets worse; in some cases, loss of bladder or bowel control.	Spinal tumor.	With loss of bladder or bowel control, call doctor for advice right away; if you can't get one, call 911 or go to emergency room. Otherwise, call doctor for prompt appointment.
Severe low back pain made worse by twisting, bending, coughing, or lifting (pain may shoot down one leg); in the worst cases, loss of bladder or bowel control.	Bulging disk pressing on a nerve (see low back pain, page 192).	With loss of bladder or bowel control, call doctor for advice right away; if you can't get one, call 911 or go to emergency room. Otherwise, call doctor for advice and appointment, take painkillers (see box, page 317), and rest.
Low back pain that comes and goes (may be worse at night); back or hip stiffness in morning that improves with activity; pain and stiffness in rib area; neck or chest pain; fatigue, weight loss, and poor appetite; fever; eye pain; blurred vision.	Ankylosing spondylitis—a rare form of arthritis that chiefly affects spinal column, usually in men under 40.	Call doctor for advice and appointment. Physical therapy, strength training, massage, and over-the-counter painkillers (see box, page 317) may help.
Numbness, weakness, and/or mild pain in back and legs; worse when walking, eases when sitting.	Spinal stenosis—narrowed spinal canal due to arthritis, thickened ligaments, or bulging disks.	Call doctor for advice and appointment. Weight loss and exercise to strengthen abdominal muscles may help.
Stiffness and pain in back, buttocks, and thighs; trouble moving or bending.	Arthritis.	See arthritis, page 184.
Pain in lower back of women more than 4 months pregnant.	Stress on back from extra weight. • Sign of early labor.	See pregnancy, page 244.

Back Pain

SYMPTOMS	WHAT IT MIGHT BE	WHAT YOU CAN DO
Stiffness and soreness after exertion or injury, or soreness that develops slowly during night; may spread to buttocks and thighs.	Back sprain or strain (see low back pain, page 192).	Rest for a few days; take over-the-counter painkillers (see box, page 317); return to normal activities when comfortable.
Aching, pain, and stiffness in back muscles (also pain elsewhere); points on body feel sore when pressed; fatigue, headaches, and trouble sleeping.	Fibromyalgia.	See box on fibromyalgia, page 282.
Backache; easily broken bones, especially in spine, wrists, and hips; stooped or hunched posture.	Osteoporosis.	See osteoporosis, page 198.

- Wear comfortable, low-heeled shoes.
- If you sit for long periods, make sure your work surface is at the right height for comfort and that your chair provides good lower back support. Walk around for a few minutes every half hour or so. If sitting is painful, try changing your workplace so you can stand while resting one foot on a low block.
- Don't lift and twist at the same time. Lift by bending your legs, not your back, and lift as little weight each time as possible.
- Lose weight if you need to. A big belly puts strain on the lower spine.

FOR MORE HELP

Hotline: Back Pain Hotline at Texas Back Institute, 800-247-2225, M–F 8–5 CST. Nurses call back (often within an hour) to answer questions and send out free literature, including illustrated back exercises. **Web site:** Texas Back Institute. After logging on to the Internet, type: *http://www.texasback.com.* Explains basic anatomy, offers advice, and lists doctors near you.

Organization: National Chronic Pain Outreach Association, 7979 Old Georgetown Road, Suite 100, Bethesda, MD 20814-2429. 301-652-4948, 24-hour recording. Sends fact packet on chronic pain.

Booklet: *Acute Low-Back Problems in Adults,* Agency for Health Care Policy and Research. Covers recent news in back pain research and care. For a free copy, call 800-358-9295.

Book: *Good News for Bad Backs,* by Robert L. Swezey, M.D., and Annette M. Swezey. Advice, exercise tips, and treatment options. Cequal Publishing, 1995, $12.95. To order, call 800-350-2998.

Book: *American Medical Association Pocket Guide to Back Pain.* Offers tips on preventing back pain and describes treatments. Random House, 1995, $4.95.

Video: *Back Pain (Lower Back) at Time of Diagnosis.* Clear overview of causes and treatments, with 4 reports—Understanding the Diagnosis, What Happens Next?, Treatment and Management, and Issues and Answers. Time Life Medical, 1996, $19.95. Sold in many pharmacies; for one near you call, 800-588-9959.

Leg Pain

Most leg pain comes from an injury or overuse. But sometimes it can signal a more serious problem in the blood vessels. If you have leg pain that isn't from an injury or other cause you know of, be sure to talk with your doctor about it.

SYMPTOMS	WHAT IT MIGHT BE	WHAT YOU CAN DO
Severe leg pain, swelling, and tenderness after an injury; you can't move leg.	Bone fracture (see fractures and dislocations, page 37).	Call 911 or go to emergency room **right away.**
Leg pain after injury, but you can move leg.	Strained, inflamed, or torn tendon, ligament, or muscle (see sprains and strains, page 46).	Call doctor for prompt appointment.
Pain and fatigue in muscles of thighs, calves, feet, or hips when active; stops with rest; mostly in older adults.	Peripheral vascular disease (see artery disease, page 106).	Call doctor for prompt appointment.
Pain and burning with redness, tenderness, and itching; hard, cordlike swelling beneath skin along length of a vein in leg (in phlebitis). Swelling, warmth, and redness throughout leg; bluish color in toes (in deep-vein thrombosis).	Phlebitis (also known as thrombophlebitis)—inflamed vein near surface of skin, most often from infection or injury, causing clotting. • Deep-vein thrombosis—blood clots in deep veins.	Call doctor for prompt appointment. Phlebitis is rarely harmful, but deep-vein thrombosis can cause clots that break off and travel to lung. Varicose veins (see page 116) may increase risk of either problem.
In children: pain that comes and goes in leg muscles, most often at night; goes away by morning.	Growing pains—common in children 3 to 12.	Gently massage area. For pain, give acetaminophen with food at bedtime (never aspirin; see Reye's syndrome box, page 96). Call doctor for advice if pain persists or causes trouble sleeping.
Pain in front or side of lower leg that begins during or just after exercise.	Shin splints—inflamed bone, tendon, or muscle in calf or shin.	Rest. Use ice for pain and swelling. Switch from high-impact sports, such as running, to gentler ones such as swimming or bicycling. Call doctor for advice if pain persists.

Leg Pain

SYMPTOMS	WHAT IT MIGHT BE	WHAT YOU CAN DO
Leg muscles tighten for a few minutes, then return to normal.	Leg cramps.	See muscle cramps, page 197.
Pain and sometimes swelling after athletic or other physical activity.	Overuse injury.	See overuse injuries, page 199.
Numbness, tingling, or pain in buttocks or back of one leg.	Disk in spine pressing on sciatic nerve in leg. • Other sciatic nerve injury.	See low back pain, page 192.
Aching or itching in legs, with blue or purple veins; sometimes swelling in feet or ankles.	Varicose veins.	See varicose veins, page 116.

Muscle Cramps

SIGNS AND SYMPTOMS

- A sudden tightening of a muscle, with sharp pain.
- A muscle that is hard to the touch.
- At times, twitching of the muscle.
- Heat cramps: sudden, severe spasms in the arms, legs, and sometimes the abdominal muscles.

A muscle cramp can happen any time—in bed, during a walk, after working in the garden. The muscle contracts with great force and stays this way, most often for about a minute, before relaxing.

Muscle cramps are most common in the legs, often after exercise in the heat, or a long time in an awkward posture. They may also result from an imbalance in minerals and fluids caused by dehydration. Abdominal cramps may be caused by low back problems or menstruation. Diseases such as Parkinson's, untreated thyroid problems, or diabetes can also lead to cramps.

Muscle cramps are rarely serious, but heat cramps can be a sign of heat exhaustion. With dizziness or confusion, they can signal the onset of heat stroke, which can be fatal. (See **heat stroke** and **heat exhaustion,** page 40.)

WHAT YOU CAN DO NOW

- ➤ Stretch. For leg muscles, face a wall and put your hands or forearms against it. Keep your feet flat on the floor and step backward until you are leaning against the wall from several feet away.
- ➤ Massage. Begin at the edges of the cramp and move in toward the center, squeezing the muscle gently.
- ➤ For a stubborn cramp, immerse the area in warm water while stretching and massaging the muscle.
- ➤ If you have heat cramps, get out of the sun and sip cool water or a sports drink.
- ➤ For menstrual cramps, take warm baths or put a hot-water bottle or heating pad on your abdomen. Try ibuprofen to ease pain.

WHEN TO CALL THE DOCTOR

Call 911 or go to an emergency room **right away:**

- If you get a severe, cramping pain in your chest, shoulders, or arms; this can signal a heart attack.
- If you have heat cramps with dizziness or confusion; you may have heat stroke.

Call for advice and an appointment:

- If cramps are long-lasting or frequent.

HOW TO PREVENT IT

- Drink 6 to 8 glasses of water every day.
- Stretch often, and above all before bed.
- Warm up and stretch before exercising.
- To prevent heat cramps in hot weather, drink a small glass (about 4 ounces) of cool water before and after exercise and every 15 minutes during exercise. (Drinking lots of cold water at once may cause stomach upset.) If you use a sports beverage, drink one low in sugar.

FOR MORE HELP

Web access: FYIowa, The Fitness Files. After logging on to the Internet, type: *http://www.tms.tribune.com/fyiowa_fitness/crampinj.htm.* Explains muscle cramps and shows simple stretching exercises.

Osteoporosis

SIGNS AND SYMPTOMS

- A broken bone (may be the first symptom), often in the spine, hip, ribs, or wrist.
- Stooped and round-shouldered posture; loss of height (usually after age 70).
- Severe backache.

Osteoporosis means "porous bones." When you're young, your skeleton acts as a calcium bank for the rest of your body, taking in new deposits that help replace old bone. By the time you reach your mid-30s, though, it's easier to lose bone than to gain it. From then on, bones tend to lose calcium, becoming less dense and more brittle (see color illustrations, page 164).

Osteoporosis is most common in people over 70 and in women after menopause, when levels of bone-protecting estrogen drop. If you're thin, if you smoke or drink, or if others in your family have osteoporosis, you may have a higher risk as well. It can get worse without symptoms until a bone breaks—often in the spine, causing severe backache and a stooped posture.

Major bone breaks may require surgery and bed rest, which can lead to further weakness and other ailments such as blood clots or pneumonia.

That's the bad news. The good news? You can prevent osteoporosis, and if you have it, you can slow its progress. Self-care, including gentle exercise and calcium supplements, is important. Hormone therapy for menopausal women can cut the risk of fractures in half, but it may also increase the risk of breast cancer (see **hormone replacement** box, page 241). Your doctor may prescribe physical therapy and drugs that prevent bone loss or build new bone. One new drug, alendronate, works well to strengthen bones in the spine and hips.

WHAT YOU CAN DO NOW

- Ask your doctor about a bone density test; it can show whether you have lost bone.
- Get plenty of exercise. It lowers your risk of thinning bones. And it can strengthen bones that have begun to thin. Weight-bearing exercise, such as walking and dancing, is best (see **get some exercise,** page 298).
- Make sure you get lots of calcium in your diet. If you are past menopause, get at least 1,500 milligrams of calcium per day; men, younger women, or women taking hormone replacement therapy should get 1,000 mg per day (see **the nutrition top ten,** page 304).
- If you're not sure your diet has enough calcium, take over-the-counter calcium supplements. Some common antacids are good sources. Check the label to see how much "elemental" (usable) calcium a supplement or antacid contains. (If you have a problem with kidney stones, talk with

your doctor about calcium supplements; they may not be for you.)

- If you have osteoporosis that causes pain, take over-the-counter painkillers (see **pain relief** box on page 317).
- To prevent falls: Install handrails on stairs and grab bars in the bathroom. Cover slippery floors with carpet, rubber mats, or nonskid wax. Use bright lamps and night-lights.

WHEN TO CALL THE DOCTOR

- If you fracture a bone.
- If you have stubborn pain in your back, ribs, spine, or feet.
- If you have a backache or are getting a curved back ("dowager's hump").

HOW TO PREVENT IT

- All of the steps outlined above in What You Can Do Now will help prevent osteoporosis. Also:
- Try to gain a little weight if you're underweight; being too thin may decrease bone density.
- If you smoke, quit, and if you drink alcohol, don't drink much. If you drink, have no more than 2 drinks a day if you're a man, 1 if you're a woman. A drink is a 12-ounce beer, a 5-ounce glass of wine, or a 1.5-ounce shot of hard liquor.

FOR MORE HELP

Information line: National Osteoporosis Foundation, 800-223-9994, 24-hour line. Sends a free fact packet. **Web site:** *http://www.nof.org.*

Organization: Arthritis Foundation, 1330 W. Peachtree St., Atlanta, GA 30309. 800-283-7800, 24-hour recording, or 404-872-7100, M–F 9–5 EST. Offers lists of local chapters and a free brochure about osteoporosis.

Organization: Osteoporosis and Related Bone Diseases–National Resource Center, 1150 17th St. N.W., Suite 500, Washington, DC 20036. 800-624-BONE, M–F 9–5 EST. Sends a packet on osteoporosis. **Web site:** *http://www.osteo.org.* Click on *Osteoporosis* for an overview. Click on *Bone Links* for a list of resources.

Book: *Eating Well, Living Well With Osteoporosis,* by Mark K. Drezner, M.D., Kimberly P. Hoben, R.D., M.P.H., L.D.N., and Duke University Medical Center. Explains diet as a way to prevent and treat osteoporosis. Viking, 1996, $12.95.

Video: *Osteoporosis at Time of Diagnosis.* Clear overview of causes and treatments, with 4 reports—Understanding the Diagnosis, What Happens Next?, Treatment and Management, and Issues and Answers. Time Life Medical, 1996, $19.95. Sold in many pharmacies; for one near you, call 800-588-9959.

Overuse Injuries

SIGNS AND SYMPTOMS

The tip-off to an overuse injury is pain that gets worse with activity. Often, it follows this pattern:

- At first, there is dull pain and general fatigue (the normal effects of exertion).
- Pain becomes sharper and more local (it's felt mostly in one place, such as the knee, hip, or arm).
- Pain lingers from one day to the next, often with swelling.
- Pain or swelling makes it hard to do the activity that caused it.
- Pain or swelling makes it hard to do normal activities of daily living, such as walking or standing.

Overuse injuries result from using bones, muscles, tendons, or joints in the same way, over and over again, without enough rest—often in the repeated motions of a sport. Runners more than others are likely to get overuse injuries of the knees and feet; throwing a ball or swinging a tennis racket can be hard on the shoulders and elbows. But these injuries can be caused by any repeated motion, such as typing, or by activities you do only now and then, such as trimming the

FIRST AID FOR INJURIES: R•I•C•E

RICE stands for **Rest, Ice, Compression,** and **Elevation.** This is the best treatment for either an overuse injury or a sudden injury such as a sprain. Start it as soon as you notice symptoms. If begun right away, it can save you days or weeks of pain.

Rest: Try not to use the injured part until the pain and swelling go away (often 1 to 3 days).

Ice: Apply ice as soon as you can to reduce swelling and pain. Place a damp towel over the injured spot and a plastic bag full of ice on top of it. A bag of frozen peas also works well. Hold the cold pack in place for 10 to 30 minutes, then leave it off for 30 to 45 minutes. Repeat as often as you can. Icing should go on for 3 days; for severe bruises, up to 7 days. For chronic pain, ice whenever you have symptoms.

Compression: Use an elastic bandage to apply gentle but firm pressure until the swelling goes down. Wrap the bandage in an upward spiral, starting a few inches below the injured area. Apply even pressure to start, then wrap more loosely after you've passed the injured area. (To use ice and pressure at the same time, wrap a bandage over an ice pack.)

Elevation: For the first 1 to 3 days, keep the injured area raised above heart level when you can to help drain excess fluid from the area.

Note: Also for the first 1 to 3 days after an injury:

- Do not apply heat (hot showers, compresses, or baths).
- Do not work the injured part.
- Do not massage the injury.
- Do not drink alcohol.

These can increase swelling.

hedge for the first time in the spring.

Overuse injuries can take longer to heal than other kinds. Without rest, therapy, and prevention, they may come back or cause more serious problems, such as **arthritis** (see page 184).

WHAT YOU CAN DO NOW

- Stop or change what causes pain.
- Use the **RICE** treatment (see box above) on the sore spot.
- Take over-the-counter painkillers (see **pain relief** box, page 317) for pain and swelling. But even if this helps, don't assume it's okay to return to whatever caused the pain in the first place. Allow plenty of time for the injury to heal.
- When pain and swelling have eased, slowly resume your normal activities. If this causes more pain, though, stop and rest some more. Find other things to do that don't hurt. For instance, if walking hurts your knee, try swimming until the pain in the knee is gone.

WHEN TO CALL THE DOCTOR

- If a week of home care doesn't help.

HOW TO PREVENT IT

- Allow at least 48 hours between hard workouts in sports such as running, tennis, or swimming.
- Don't increase the time or intensity of a sport too much at one time. For example, if you walk or run 10 miles a week, increase your distance no more than about 1 mile each week.
- Know your body. Change your activities if you know you have a problem. For instance, people with flat feet (over-pronation) are more likely to have knee or foot trouble from running; they might want to try swimming or tennis instead.
- Use the right gear. If you walk or run, your shoes should be sturdy enough for your weight to help absorb the shock. (If you have foot problems, ask your doctor about orthotics, shoe inserts that can help prevent knee and foot trouble.)

Foot and Ankle Pain

The feet take a beating, especially when we stuff them into shoes that don't fit. That's why it's important to catch foot problems early, when they can be treated most easily.

SYMPTOMS	WHAT IT MIGHT BE	WHAT YOU CAN DO
Pain in ankle or foot after injury; maybe swelling, bruising, or bleeding; can't support weight.	Broken bone (see fractures and dislocations, page 37).	Call doctor for prompt advice. If you can't get one, call 911 or go to emergency room.
Pain and fatigue in feet, thighs, calves, or hips when active; pain stops with rest; most common in older adults.	Peripheral vascular disease (see artery disease, page 106).	Call doctor for prompt appointment.
Pain, swelling, stiffness, and maybe redness in joints of ankles, feet, or toes.	Arthritis (see page 184).	Call doctor for advice and appointment.
Sharp pain or tender feeling under foot or heel; worse when walking or running, often worse in morning.	Plantar fasciitis—inflamed tissue that runs along heel and supports arch. Most often caused by stress on arch. Common among runners (see overuse injuries, page 199).	Stay off foot, take over-the-counter pain relievers to ease pain and swelling, and use RICE treatment (see box, page 200). Ask doctor or physical therapist about ways to stretch ligament.
Pain in Achilles tendon in back of ankle, or in other tendons in ankle or foot; may restrict foot movement.	Tendinitis (see page 204).	Call doctor for advice and appointment.
Hard, painful lump on side of foot, at base of big toe (bunion). Toe clenched and painful (hammertoe).	Bunion or hammertoe.	See bunions and hammertoes, page 187.
Patch of thickened skin on foot; may be painful.	Corn or callus.	See corns and calluses, page 150.
Wart on sole of foot, making walking painful. Tight shoes may make it worse.	Plantar wart.	See warts, page 182.

Knee Pain

The knee is a hinge meant to swing one way—forward and back—within limits. Twisting to the side or bending too far back can cause injury. Most knee trouble can be prevented. When things do go wrong, treatment often gets good results.

SYMPTOMS	WHAT IT MIGHT BE	WHAT YOU CAN DO
Pain and perhaps a "pop" at moment of injury; swelling, stiffness, a "wobbly" knee, trouble walking.	Ligament sprain or rupture, and/or cartilage damage (see sprains and strains, page 46, and illustration, next page).	Call doctor for prompt appointment. Use RICE treatment for pain and swelling (see box, page 200).
In teens: pain and swelling about 2 inches below kneecap; may cause limping or prevent running.	Osgood-Schlatter disease—inflamed tendon and bone.	Call doctor for advice and appointment. Use RICE treatment (see box, page 200).
Pain, swelling, and stiffness in knee joint.	Arthritis (see page 184).	Call doctor for advice and appointment.
Tender, stiff, and swollen knee; pain when bending knee; possibly fever or redness.	Bursitis (see page 189).	Call doctor for advice and appointment.
Pain just below kneecap, may be worse when sitting or straightening leg; may be felt after running or jumping; knee pain and tightness that worsen with movement.	Patellar tendinitis, or "jumper's knee" (see tendinitis, page 204, and overuse injuries, page 199).	Call doctor for advice and appointment. Use RICE treatment for pain and swelling (see box, page 200).

- If a certain motion causes you problems, change your technique. You may want to learn a new swimming stroke if you're prone to shoulder problems, for instance.
- Vary your routine so you don't work the same muscles and joints over and over. Jog one day, perhaps, and swim the next.
- Warm up before exercise. Stretch gently and walk briskly for a few minutes. Warm muscles, ligaments, and tendons are less likely to get hurt.
- Dress in layers for a workout. Layering clothing allows you to add and remove clothes as needed, keeping your muscles, ligaments, and tendons warm and loose.
- Make sure your work site is comfortable (see **carpal tunnel syndrome,** page 190).

FOR MORE HELP

Book: *Dr. Scott's Knee Book,* by W. Norman Scott, M.D. A guide to symptoms, treatment, and prevention of a number of knee problems. Fireside, 1996, $11.

Book: *The Sports Medicine Bible,* by Lyle J. Micheli, M.D. Guidelines for the casual athlete to help prevent and treat injuries. HarperPerennial, 1995, $20.

THE KNEE

Tendons (the ends of muscles attached to bone) and ligaments keep your knee bones in place; cartilage cushions the bones.

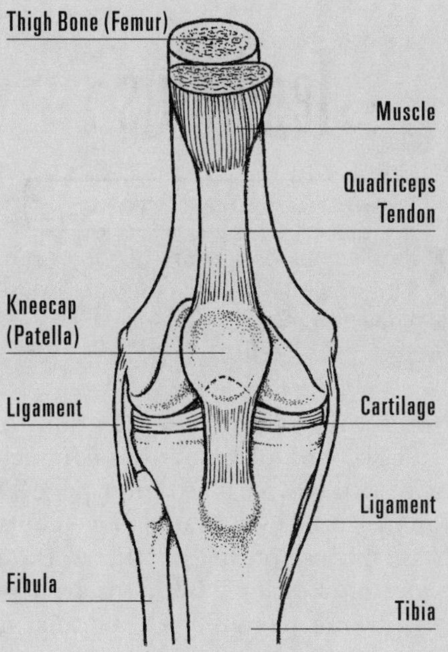

Temporomandibular Disorder

SIGNS AND SYMPTOMS

- Pain in the chewing muscles or jaw joint on either side of the head.
- Headaches or earaches.
- Clicking, popping, or grating sounds in the jaw joints when opening or closing the mouth.
- Pain that spreads to the face, neck, or shoulders.
- Jaw is locked shut or painful to open.

Because we talk, chew, and yawn every day, the jaw is always busy. The hinges called temporomandibular joints, which connect the lower jaw to a bone on each side of the head, help the jawbone move smoothly (see illustration, next page). Pain in or around these joints is known as temporomandibular disorder (TMD, also called TMJ). Perhaps two-thirds of Americans have bouts of such pain now and then.

Many things can cause TMD, including strain on the jaw muscles from clenching the teeth (see **tooth grinding,** page 85), arthritis, injury to the jaw, and even **stress** (see page 222). Poor posture (from thrusting the chin forward) may also cause the problem.

TMD often clears up in a few days with rest and painkillers such as ibuprofen. When it is severe or chronic, treatments include physical therapy, anti-inflammatory drugs, tranquilizers to relieve muscle tension, and a bite guard to ease the strain on the joint. Surgery and injections are last resorts; there is little agreement on whether they really help.

WHAT YOU CAN DO NOW

- Take an anti-inflammatory painkiller such as ibuprofen (see **pain relief** box, page 317).
- Massage the muscles above and in front of your temples, as well as the large muscles along your jawline. Use small motions in circles.
- Limit talking and chewing for a few days. Rest your jaw by eating soft or liquid foods.
- Apply a hot or cold pack, available in drugstores, or a damp warm or cool towel for pain relief. Hold in place for a few minutes at a time.
- Don't clench your teeth.

WHEN TO CALL THE DOCTOR

- If the pain of TMD interferes with eating or talking.
- If you grind or clench your teeth and think you may need a bite guard to protect them.

HOW TO PREVENT IT

- Whenever you find yourself clenching or grinding your teeth, stop.
- Reduce stress (see box, page 223, and

TEMPOROMANDIBULAR JOINT

Pain can spread far beyond the hinge that connects the jawbone and skull.

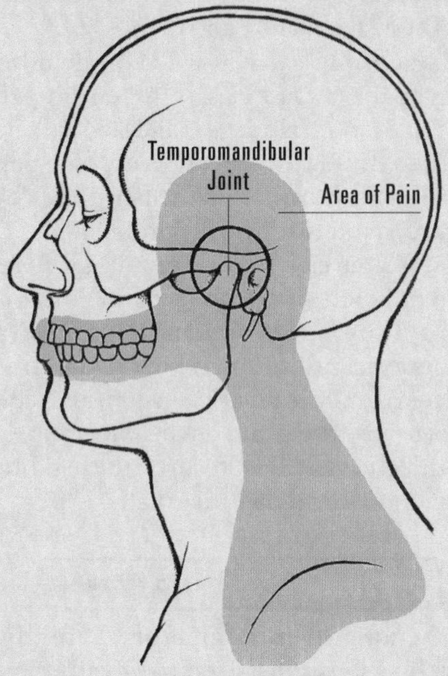

relax, page 309). This may be the best treatment.

➤ If you are prone to jaw pain, stay away from chewy foods such as steak and bagels, and hard foods such as carrots and apples. Don't chew gum, pencils, or other objects.

➤ To lessen the strain on the jaw, don't sleep on your stomach.

➤ Never cradle a telephone receiver between your shoulder and jaw.

FOR MORE HELP

Information line: National Oral Health Information Clearinghouse, 301-402-7364, M–F 9–5:30 EST. Provides free brochures, packets, and fact sheets on oral health, including TMD.

Organization: American Academy of Otolaryngology–Head and Neck Surgery, One Prince Street, Alexandria, VA 22314. 703-836-4444, M–F 8:30–5 EST. Send a stamped, self-addressed, business-size envelope with a request for "Pain and TMJ." **Web site:** *http://www.entnet.org.*

Web access: Healthtouch. After logging on to the Internet, type: *http://www.healthtouch.com.* Click on *Health Information,* then scroll to *TMJ & Jaw Joints.* Covers the symptoms and treatment of TMJ.

Tendinitis

SIGNS AND SYMPTOMS

- Pain around a joint, often worse with movement and in bed at night.
- Muscle spasms.

Tendinitis is an inflamed tendon—the tough band of tissue that connects a muscle to a bone (see illustration, page 203). It's often caused by repeated movements in sports or in assembly-line or office work. (See **overuse injuries,** page 199, and **carpal tunnel syndrome,** page 190.) Other causes are injury, not enough warm-up before exercise, calcium deposits in the tendon, and breakdown of the tendon because of aging.

Tendinitis is most common in shoulders ("golfer's shoulder"), the outside of elbows ("tennis elbow," see box on next page), the fingers ("trigger finger"), the wrist, and the back of the lower leg (Achilles tendinitis).

Most tendinitis heals with about 2 weeks of rest. More stubborn tendinitis can be treated with drugs to ease the pain and swelling, plus physical therapy, ice packs, ultrasound treatments, and gentle exercise.

WHAT YOU CAN DO NOW

➤ Rest the area until pain and swelling ease.

➤ Use a splint if the cause is overuse, and if you can't rest the painful joint.

➤ Take anti-inflammatories such as aspirin or ibuprofen to relieve the pain and swelling (see **pain relief** box, page 317).

➤ If it comes on quickly after an injury or heavy use, put an ice pack on the area for 10 to 30 minutes at a time to relieve the swelling. Wait 30 to 45 minutes, and repeat.

Repeat as often as you can. After 2 days, apply a towel soaked in hot water and wrung out or a heat pack (available in drugstores) to relieve the pain. (See **RICE** treatment box, page 200.)

- After a few days, start to gently exercise.

WHEN TO CALL THE DOCTOR

- If the area around the joint appears discolored or deformed.
- If pain and swelling continue for more than 2 weeks despite rest and over-the-counter pain relievers. These could be early signs of arthritis.

HOW TO PREVENT IT

- When you have symptoms, rest the joint to prevent the problem from getting worse.
- If you perform the same tasks over and over during work—for instance, a lot of typing—ask your doctor or employer about an ergonomic specialist who can suggest ways to change your workplace to ease the stress on tender tendons.
- Stretch before and after work. When you have to do the same movements over and over, take a 5- to 10-minute break every hour or so.
- Exercise often to maintain muscle and tendon strength. This will help prevent injuries.
- Always warm up before exercise or sports, and cool down after with gentle stretching.
- Wear shoes with flexible soles and good heel control when you exercise. If you have weak ankles, wear high-top sports shoes.
- Don't grip tools, pens, or sports gear too tightly. Wrap utensils in felt or rubber to create larger grips.
- Switch to low-impact exercise, such as swimming or low-impact aerobics, if you think higher-impact sports are to blame.

FOR MORE HELP

Organization: Arthritis Foundation, 1330 W. Peachtree St., Atlanta, GA 30309. 800-283-7800, 24-hour recording, or 404-872-7100, M–F 9–5 EST. Sends a brochure about tendinitis. Local chapters have arthritis support groups.

Book: *The Sports Medicine Bible,* by Lyle J. Micheli, M.D. Guidelines for casual athletes to help prevent and treat injuries. HarperPerennial, 1995, $20.

Web access: American College of Rheumatology. After logging on to the Internet, type: *http://www.rheumatology.org/patient/tendin.htm.* Covers tendinitis and offers lists of doctors near you.

TENNIS ELBOW

Anyone who uses the arms and elbows in sports or on the job can get tennis elbow. It results when the forearm is snapped, rolled, or twisted, or when people lift heavy objects with the elbow locked and the arm extended. In tennis, it can occur when the grip is wrong.

The remedies for tennis elbow and tendinitis are the same. But the symptoms of tennis elbow may last from 6 to 12 weeks. The best home care is rest and over-the-counter painkillers, then gentle exercise. You can also try wearing a Velcro tennis-elbow strap, sold in sporting goods stores, to support muscles and tendons. Don't wear the strap for long periods, though, because it can reduce blood flow.

Prevent tennis elbow the same way you prevent tendinitis. If tennis is the cause of your pain, try a more flexible racket or one with a slightly larger grip; ask a coach to help you change your grip to ease the stress on your elbow.

Behavior & Emotions

Alcohol Abuse and Alcoholism

SIGNS AND SYMPTOMS

Alcohol abuse:

- Blackouts or memory loss.
- Unusual bad temper and aggression (sometimes).
- Using alcohol more and more to relax, sleep, cheer up, deal with problems, or feel "normal."

Alcoholism (alcohol addiction):
Same symptoms as those above. Other symptoms can include:

- Withdrawal—headaches, insomnia, anxiety, or nausea—when you stop drinking.
- Depression and anxiety.
- Trouble with family relationships and holding a job.
- Often drinking alone.
- Drinking early in the day.
- Drinking in secret (hiding cans or bottles).
- Failed attempts to control drinking.
- Broken capillaries and flushed skin on the face.
- Shaky hands.
- Yellowish skin, which may mean cirrhosis—a disease of the liver.

Alcohol abuse causes more health problems in the United States than all illegal drugs combined. Some 18 million adults suffer drinking-related problems. Alcohol abuse can disrupt a person's work, family, and social life, and can damage organs in every system of the body—the kidneys, liver, brain, heart, and intestines. It may increase the risk of many forms of cancer as well. Drinking when pregnant can cause severe damage to the growing fetus. Alcohol also plays a role in about half of all car-accident deaths in the United States.

The line between abuse and alcoholism can be hard to see. But alcoholism is marked by a loss of control: The alcoholic keeps drinking even when it causes physical, psychological, or social harm. Most experts class alcoholism as a disease, not a character flaw. The causes still are not known, but they seem to be a mixture of many factors. Some research suggests that a person's risk of alcoholism is 3 to 4 times greater if a parent is an alcoholic.

Treatment can't begin until an alcoholic admits he or she has a problem and agrees to stop drinking and get help. Those who also have psychological problems, or don't have much social support or desire to quit, often start drinking again after treatment. But a person with basic good health plus support and desire has a good chance of kicking the habit. As one expert puts it, "Alcoholism is the most treatable untreated disease in America."

Confusion

Everyone gets confused once in a while, but severe, frequent, or long-term confusion may signal a problem. Confusion is the inability to think clearly or make decisions; in severe cases, people may not know where or who they are. Confusion can come on quickly or slowly. Depending on the cause—physical or mental illness, injury, poisoning, or drug side effects—it can require prompt medical care.

SYMPTOMS	WHAT IT MIGHT BE	WHAT YOU CAN DO
Confusion; severe headache or agitation; drowsiness, sluggishness, maybe coma.	Poisoning from carbon monoxide fumes. Causes include car running in garage, or old-fashioned gas or kerosene appliances in poorly vented room.	Get person into open air **right away.** Call 911 or go to emergency room **right away.** Check for pulse and breathing; if none, begin CPR (see page 16).
Head wound or bruise, confusion or loss of consciousness, slurred speech.	Head injury causing concussion or internal bleeding (see head, neck, and back injuries, page 38).	Call 911 or go to emergency room **right away.**
After being in cold air or water: shivering and numbness, confusion, slurred speech, stumbling.	Hypothermia (see page 41).	Call 911 or go to emergency room **right away.**
Confusion, anxiety, or loss of consciousness; weak or rapid pulse; cold, clammy, pale, or bluish skin; rapid, shallow breathing.	Shock—vital organs are deprived of blood due to sudden illness or injury, or severe allergic reaction (see page 24).	Call 911 or go to emergency room **right away.** Check for breathing and pulse; if none, begin CPR (see page 16).
Sudden, temporary confusion; dizziness; loss of coordination; light-headedness; tingling; weakness or numbness, usually on one side of body; double vision or temporary blindness; speech problems; hearing loss; headache.	Transient ischemic attack (TIA) or stroke—interrupted blood flow to brain from temporary artery blockage (see stroke, pages 46 and 115).	Call 911 or go to emergency room **right away.**
Confusion, fever over 100, chills, fatigue, and/or weakness; maybe nausea and vomiting, loss of appetite, headache.	Bacterial or viral infection, such as pneumonia (see page 98), meningitis (see page 57), toxic shock syndrome (see page 248), or kidney infection.	Call doctor for advice. If you can't get one, call 911 or go to emergency room.

(continued)

Confusion *(continued)*

SYMPTOMS	WHAT IT MIGHT BE	WHAT YOU CAN DO
Confusion, anxiety, dizziness, sweating, shakiness, hunger, headache, impaired vision, rapid heartbeat, numbness, lack of coordination.	Hypoglycemia—low blood sugar, especially in people who take insulin (see diabetes, page 282).	People with diabetes should eat or drink something with sugar; for others, sugarless foods. If symptoms persist, call doctor for advice. If seizures or loss of consciousness, call 911 or go to emergency room **right away.**
Confusion, sleepiness, loss of consciousness, muscle spasms, shortness of breath.	Chronic kidney disease.	Call doctor for prompt appointment.
Confusion, bruising or bleeding for no clear reason, jaundice.	Chronic liver disease.	Call doctor for prompt appointment.
Coming on over time: confusion; faulty judgment and thinking; inability to complete simple tasks; memory problems that get worse; tendency to lose things, and to wander and become lost.	Alzheimer's disease (see page 50).	Call doctor for advice and appointment.
Confusion, drowsiness, chronic breathing or sleep problems.	High levels of carbon dioxide in blood from chronic lung disease, blocked airway, or obesity.	Call doctor for advice.
Forgetfulness, poor concentration, bad temper, anxiety, depression, falling asleep at wrong times.	Sleep deprivation or sleep apnea (see sleep disorders, page 292).	Call doctor for advice.

WHAT YOU CAN DO NOW

Alcohol abuse:

- If you think you might have an alcohol problem, keep careful track of how much you drink over a given time (a week or more), and don't fudge. Experts say women—whose bodies use alcohol differently than men's do—should have no more than 1 drink a day, and men no more than 2. (A "drink" is one 12-ounce beer, one 5-ounce glass of wine, or 1.5 ounces of spirits.) New research suggests that if you drink at all, for best health you should limit yourself to 3 or 4 drinks a week.
- Never have more than 1 drink in an hour. The liver can't process more than an ounce of alcohol per hour.
- Don't drink on an empty stomach.
- If you notice yourself getting drunk despite your best intentions, hoarding alcohol, saying you drink less than you do, or

getting angry if someone confronts you about your drinking, get professional help.

- Don't drink any beer, wine, or other alcohol if you are pregnant, trying to get pregnant, or nursing.

Alcoholism:

- If you suspect that a partner or loved one depends on alcohol, talk to your doctor or contact an alcohol treatment program for advice on how to deal with him or her.
- If you often drink too much, admit the problem and resolve to stop drinking on your own. If you have no success, call your doctor or a treatment center for advice. In most cases, early treatment improves the chance of recovery.
- Join a self-help group or attend a meeting. Alcoholics Anonymous (AA) is the best-known; it has groups throughout the country. If you are not at ease with AA's spiritual approach, you might want to explore other programs such as Rational Recovery or Women for Sobriety. Family members may want to look into Al-Anon Family Groups, a support program for the parents, children, and spouses of alcoholics.
- Exercise regularly. Exercise can provide a sense of well-being.
- Eat well. Alcohol robs your body of nutrients.

WHEN TO CALL THE DOCTOR

- If you have symptoms of alcohol abuse or alcoholism.
- If you regularly get drunk and often feel depressed.
- If you tried to stop drinking and had symptoms of withdrawal such as headache, anxiety, insomnia, nausea, or, in rare cases, shaking limbs and strange visions.
- If you can't give up alcohol and are pregnant or think you may be.

HOW TO PREVENT IT

Alcohol abuse:

- Don't drink to try to escape anxiety or depression (see **depression,** page 213).
- Try other, more healthful activities in place of social drinking if, during the day, you find yourself eagerly waiting for a drink.

Alcoholism:

Most experts believe that staying away from alcohol completely is the key for alcoholics. That might not be easy. These steps can help prevent a relapse:

- Avoid places and events that you connect with alcohol, and don't spend time with friends when they are drinking.
- Ask your family and friends to help. Tell them you are trying not to drink, and let them know how they can support you.
- Replace your need for alcohol with other activities. Take a class or volunteer.
- Get a checkup, and ask your doctor for advice about foods and vitamins that can aid your recovery.
- If you have a relapse, don't use it as an excuse to give up all your gains. Think about what led to the relapse and how to do things differently next time.

FOR MORE HELP

Hotline: Adcare Hospital Helpline. 800-252-6465, 24-hour line. Staff answers questions, provides support, and suggests places to find help.

Organization: National Council on Alcoholism and Drug Dependence. 800-622-2255, 24-hour recording. Sends information on alcoholism and lists local chapters. **Web site:** *http://www.niaaa.nih.gov.*

Organization: National Clearinghouse for Alchohol & Drug Information, Box 2345, Rockville, MD 20847-2345. 800-729-6686, M–F 8–7 EST. Sends fact sheets on alcohol and drug abuse prevention and treatment.

Organization: Alcoholics Anonymous, Box 459, Grand Central Station, New York, NY 10163. 212-870-3400, M–F 8:30–4:45 EST. Call for the number of a local AA group, or look in your phone book under "Alcoholics Anonymous."

Organization: Al-Anon/Alateen Family Groups, Box 862, Midtown Station, New York, NY 10018-0862. 800-356-9996, M–F 9–6 EST. Al-Anon is a mutual support program for families and friends of alcoholics. Alateen is a support program for teenagers and young people whose lives are affected by alcoholism.

Organization: Rational Recovery, Box 800, Lotus, CA 95651-0800. 916-621-4374, M–F 8–4 PST. A self-help program for people with alcohol or drug problems. Groups are available in 700 U.S. cities.

Organization: Women for Sobriety, Box 618, Quakertown, PA 18951. 215-536-8026, M–F 8:30–3 EST. Operates mutual-help groups that address the special needs of women with alcohol problems. **Web site:** *http://www.mediapulse.com/wfs*.

Book: *Educating Yourself About Alcohol and Drugs: A People's Primer,* by Marc Alan Schuckit, M.D. A guide to recovery by an expert. Plenum Publishing, 1995, $28.95.

Web access: Web of Addictions. After logging on to the Internet, type: *http://www.well.com/user/woa*. Offers news, fact sheets, resources, and other links.

Video: *Alcoholism at Time of Diagnosis*. Clear overview of causes and treatments, with 4 reports—Understanding the Diagnosis, What Happens Next?, Treatment and Management, and Issues and Answers. Time Life Medical, 1996, $19.95. Sold in many pharmacies; for one near you, call 800-588-9959.

Anxiety and Phobias

SIGNS AND SYMPTOMS

Generalized anxiety disorder:
Severe long-term worry, tension, bad temper, or depression, for no clear reason. Plus some of the following:

- Inability to relax, sleep, or concentrate.
- Fatigue.
- Headaches.
- Sweating or hot flashes.
- Tension, trembling, or twitching.
- Being easily startled.

Phobias:

- Constant, irrational fear of certain things, such as heights, blood, insects, flying, or snakes.
- Fear of social settings in which you think you will be shamed or criticized.

Panic disorder:
Feelings of terror—"panic attacks"—that strike suddenly, sometimes in times of stress but often for no clear reason, and typically last a couple of minutes. They are marked by:

- Racing or pounding heart, sometimes with chest pain.
- Shortness of breath.
- Dizziness, weakness, or faintness.
- Nausea.
- Flushes or chills.
- Feelings of unreality or a sense of losing control.
- Fear of doom or dying.

Panic disorder often comes with fear of situations that might bring on a panic attack and would be hard to escape.

Obsessive-compulsive disorder:

- Constant unwelcome thoughts, such as images of germs or dirt; violent urges; or fear of harming people.
- Repeated actions and rituals performed in an effort to prevent or cast out unwelcome thoughts. Examples include washing the hands over and over, counting things, and rearranging objects.

Post-traumatic stress disorder:

- Inability to escape thoughts about past ordeals such as war, disasters, rape, or abuse.
- Flashbacks and nightmares.
- Trouble sleeping.
- Frequent bad temper.
- Aggressive or violent feelings and actions.
- Withdrawal, numbness, or loss of interest in things that used to be enjoyable (see **depression,** page 213).

Feeling anxious sometimes is normal and healthy: It rouses you to action when you face a real threat. But too much worry disrupts daily life.

Anxiety can be mild or immobilizing. Experts believe that heredity, along with life events, may incline a person to it. Some believe it is a learned response that comes from childhood trauma or other trauma and conflict. Recent research suggests it also has a physical basis: Studies show that chemical changes in the body can set off panic attacks and anxiety in some people.

There is most likely more than one cause. Treatment can involve drugs, psychotherapy, stress reduction, biofeedback, or a mix of all of these. Most people improve with treatment. If you are troubled by anxiety, ask your doctor for advice. You may want to be treated by someone who specializes in this disorder.

WHAT YOU CAN DO NOW

- Be honest about how your anxiety affects you: Is it keeping you from doing things you want to do?
- Learn about the problem from up-to-date books, tapes, and studies and by getting news from mental health groups.
- Talk to a friend about your fears and feelings. Telling others can release stress.
- Find a good therapist. Ask your friends or doctor to refer you to someone experienced in treating anxiety. Go to a session to see if you like the therapist's approach.
- Get some daily exercise, such as a brisk walk or a sport you enjoy. Research shows that people who get frequent exercise feel less anxious than those who don't.
- Cut down on alcohol and caffeine. Too much caffeine often causes anxiety and may trigger panic attacks. Don't use street drugs such as cocaine.
- Simplify your life by making your schedule less hectic (see **stress**, page 222).
- Spend less time on stressful projects. Do something you enjoy.
- Get enough rest. If you have trouble sleeping, see **sleep disorders**, page 292.
- Do volunteer work.
- Join a support group.
- Do deep breathing and relaxation exercises, especially when your anxiety level starts to rise. Learn yoga or meditation (see **relax,** page 309).

WHEN TO CALL THE DOCTOR

- If you feel troubled, anxious, or out of control, and can't function.
- If, along with being anxious, you have lost weight and your eyes seem to bulge; you may have a **thyroid problem** (see page 294) or other ailment.

FOR MORE HELP

Information line: National Institute of Mental Health. 800-647-2642, M–F 8AM–9PM EST. Sends fact sheets and lists of resources on panic disorder.

Information line: National Mental Health Association, 800-969-6642, 24-hour recording, or 703-684-7722, M–F 9–5 EST (messages taken 24 hours a day). Sends free pamphlets on anxiety and other mental health problems, provides counseling, and refers to services and support groups.

Organization: Anxiety Disorders Association of America, Box 96505, Washington, DC 20077-7140. For $3, sends a fact pack about anxiety disorders and a list of places to find help.

Organization: "Vet Centers" of the Department of Veterans Affairs. Counseling centers for Vietnam veterans and other vets with post-traumatic stress disorder are in many cities. Check your phone book or call local information for the number of the one nearest you.

Book: *Triumph Over Fear: A Book of Help for People with Anxiety, Panic Attacks, and Phobias,* by Jerilyn Ross and Rosalynn Carter. Bantam, 1995, $12.95.

Book: *The Sky is Falling: Understanding and Coping with Phobias, Panic and Obsessive Compulsive Disorders,* by Raenn Dumont. Stories and advice from people with anxiety disorders. W.W. Norton, 1995, $25.

Web access: Veritas Programming. After logging on to the Internet, type: *http: //www.sover.net/~schwcof/books.html.* Full text of 4 "Attacking Anxiety" booklets.

Video: *Stress & Anxiety at Time of Diagnosis.* Clear overview of causes and treatments, with 4 reports—Understanding the Diagnosis, What Happens Next?, Treatment and Management, and Issues and Answers. Time Life Medical, 1996, $19.95. Sold in many pharmacies; for one near you, call 800-588-9959.

Attention Deficit Disorder

SIGNS AND SYMPTOMS

- Frequent inability to pay attention.
- Trouble focusing on work.
- Strong pattern of making careless mistakes or trouble following instructions.
- Impulsive actions.
- Talking too much and interrupting others frequently.
- Sometimes, hyperactivity—squirming and running around in quiet situations.

Attention deficit disorder (ADD) is one of the most often diagnosed behavioral problems. Because some experts believe it is widely overdiagnosed, it is also one of the most controversial. Genuine ADD may run in families, although other factors also play a role in causing it. If a woman smokes, uses drugs or alcohol, or is exposed to lead during pregnancy, her fetus may be harmed so that symptoms of ADD appear later in childhood. Children exposed to lead can also get ADD.

The symptoms should be seen as a problem only if they affect a person's ability to function in more than one setting—at school *and* at home, or at work *and* at play. Many children are labeled with ADD when their behavior is really quite normal for their age and their situation.

Also, symptoms of ADD can be triggered by problems other than ADD: Learning disabilities, physical or sexual abuse, tension, **depression** (see page 213), **stress** (see page 222), and family violence can all cause children to act in ways that look like ADD.

ADD is most common in children (mostly boys), though adults can also have it. When people with symptoms of ADD are also hyperactive, they are said to have attention deficit hyperactivity disorder (ADHD).

People with ADD do not lack intelligence; rather, they have trouble focusing, and as a result they don't perform at their best. Life can be baffling for children with ADD: They have problems at school, they become known as troublemakers or slow learners, they often get angry, they see themselves as bad or stupid.

Since there is no known cure for ADD, the normal treatment is to try to manage it with drugs, chiefly the stimulant methylphenidate (brand name Ritalin). This drug and other stimulants help some children, but many experts think doctors prescribe them too often. Doctors may also prescribe antidepressants for some children.

Many doctors now believe that most children with ADD will have some symptoms as adults, in other forms. Adults may be highly disorganized, given to wild temper outbursts, and feel unable to cope with the stresses of life. They may have trouble getting along with other people and problems with drug or alcohol abuse.

WHAT YOU CAN DO NOW

- If you suspect that your child has ADD, take him or her to an expert you trust. Child psychiatrists, pediatricians, neurologists, and psychologists are among those who work with ADD. Your family doctor may be able to refer you.

After diagnosis:

- Think about getting a second opinion if a doctor says you have ADD or your child does—above all if the doctor prescribes Ritalin or another drug or does not specialize in childhood psychological problems.
- Know your child's patterns and habits, strengths and weaknesses. Some children with ADD do best with lots of planned time and few distractions, while others need lots of variety and do poorly if they are too controlled.
- Learn about ADD.
- Don't punish your child for acting in ways he or she can't control.
- Join an ADD support group .
- An adult with ADD should follow the same advice.

WHEN TO CALL A MENTAL HEALTH PROFESSIONAL

➤ If you or your child show symptoms of ADD that disrupt daily life and work or school.

FOR MORE HELP

Organization: Children and Adults with Attention Deficit Disorder (CHADD), 800-233-4050, 24-hour recording. Leave your name and address to receive reports about ADD and a list of local support groups.

Organization: National ADD Association, 800-487-2282, 24-hour recording, or 313-769-6690 M–F 9–4:30 CST if you have questions. Leave your name and address to receive a list of local ADD support groups. **Web site:** *http://www.add.org*

Brochure: National Institute of Mental Health, Public Inquiries, 5600 Fishers Lane, Room 7C-02, Rockville, MD 20857. 301-443-4513, M–F 8:30–4:30 EST. Ask for the "Attention Deficit" brochure or look it up on the Web at: *http://www.nimh.nih.gov/publicat/adhd.htm*.

Book: *The Misunderstood Child,* by Larry Silver, M.D. A guide for parents of children with learning disabilities and ADD. McGraw Hill, 1995, $9.95.

Book: *Driven to Distraction: Recognizing and Coping With Attention Deficit Disorder From Childhood Through Adulthood,* by Edward M. Hallowell, M.D., and John J. Ratey, M.D. Touchstone, 1994, $12.

Depression

SIGNS AND SYMPTOMS

- Constant feelings of pessimism or sadness.
- Feelings of worthlessness, hopelessness, guilt, or despair.
- Lack of interest or pleasure in life: in work, relationships, food, and sex.
- Lack of energy.
- Sleep problems: insomnia, oversleeping, or often waking too early.
- Trouble focusing, remembering, making decisions, and doing simple tasks; a feeling of moving in slow motion.
- Unusual weight loss or gain.
- Frequent thoughts of death.
- Nagging ailments—such as headaches or stomach pain—that don't get better with treatment.

Feeling blue is normal—up to a point. When people are so unhappy that they can't work, enjoy life, or simply function, they have the distinct ailment called depression.

The causes—and treatments—of depression are hotly debated, but clearly your genes, surroundings, brain chemistry, and life experiences each play a part. Depression can strike at any age, even in childhood, though its severe forms most often affect adults. Women are twice as likely as men to be diagnosed as depressed.

Depression can take many forms. Feelings such as sadness, pessimism, or self-pity in response to painful events are sometimes called **depressive reactions.** These feelings, which are normal, can be quite severe but most often go away in a short time without treatment.

There's also a form of chronic, low-level depression called **dysthymia**. People who have it aren't severely depressed or suicidal, but they have little joy in life and feel downcast about the future. Some suffer from fatigue, sleep problems, and low self-esteem. They tend to heap blame on themselves. They have a hard time making choices or shaking their gloomy mood, and they sometimes fall into major depression.

A woman may feel blue after childbirth. But **postpartum depression** that is severe and lasts more than a few weeks may need treatment.

People who suffer from **major depression** feel so miserable that they have trouble living day to day. They are often in despair and are troubled by guilt, sleep problems, fatigue, crushing sadness, and feelings of emptiness and worthlessness. They may be suicidal or obsessed with death.

In rare cases, they may lose touch with the real world and have delusions and hallucinations. Their depression—which may have started with a major loss and can last for months—may lift, only to return later. Research suggests this may sometimes run in a family or have links to the brain chemicals that affect mood and behavior.

When depression comes in fall or winter and then fades in the spring or summer, it is called **seasonal affective disorder** (SAD). People with SAD are affected by the lack of sunlight and often go through major mood shifts between the seasons.

Mood swings are even more extreme for people with **manic depression,** also known as **bipolar affective disorder.** They go back and forth from being very active or high (though they may also be moody, unfocused, and paranoid) to feeling sluggish and beaten down by despair.

WHAT YOU CAN DO NOW

- Get help. See your family doctor to rule out illness. Sometimes depression is a symptom of disease.
- Ask your doctor or pharmacist if any medicine you are taking could be causing it.
- Ask your doctor about counselors who work with depressed people, and about medication for depression.
- Get some physical exercise every day—join a class or group. Research shows people who exercise regularly are less likely to be depressed or stressed.
- Try a support group. Many are peer-led groups such as those geared for people who had traumas in childhood (for instance, alcoholic parents or abuse) or who have had major losses (see **grief,** page 219). It's important to get support from people who will treat you with respect and understanding.
- Learn about depression. Self-help and professional organizations give out information, and you can find many on-line.
- Don't use alcohol or street drugs to feel better: Alcohol is a depressant.
- If you have SAD, ask an expert about indoor lighting that mimics sunlight. Get out in the sun when you can, or take a trip to a sunny place.

WHEN TO CALL A MENTAL HEALTH PROFESSIONAL

- If you, your child, or someone close to you has suicidal thoughts or depression that doesn't seem to lift. (Check your phone book: Many cities have suicide hotlines.)
- If depression seriously disrupts your work, school, or relationships. Psychologists, psychiatrists, social workers, and peer counselors all work with people who are depressed. They take varied approaches to treatment, from psychotherapy ("talk therapy") to medication.

HOW TO PREVENT IT

- Don't isolate yourself.
- When you're feeling blue, find a friend or someone to talk with about your troubles.
- Stay active. Research shows that regular exercise can improve your mood.
- Be sure to get enough sleep (see **sleep disorders,** page 292).
- Eat balanced meals.

FOR MORE HELP

Information line: National Mental Health Association, 800-969-6642, 24-hour recording, or 703-684-7722, M–F 9–5 EST. Sends free pamphlets on depression and other mental health issues; provides counseling, and suggests services and support groups.

Organization: National Empowerment Center, 800-POWER-2U (769-3728), M–F 8–4 EST. Mental health consumers' group suggests support groups and drop-in centers as well as print and audio items.

Organization: National Institute of Mental Health, Public Inquiries, 5600 Fishers Lane, Room 7C-02, Rockville, MD 20857. 301-443-4513, M–F 8:30–4:30 EST. Offers brochures on depression. **Web site:** *http://www.nimh.nih.gov.* Click on *Publications,* then scroll to the topic you want.

Book: *Depression: The Mood Disease,* by Francis Mark Mondimore, M.D. Offers advice on dealing with depression. Johns Hopkins University Press, 1995, $15.95.

Video: *Depression at Time of Diagnosis.* Clear

overview of causes and treatments, with 4 reports—Understanding the Diagnosis, What Happens Next?, Treatment and Management, and Issues and Answers. Time Life Medical, 1996, $19.95. Sold in many pharmacies; for one near you, call 800-588-9959.

Drug Abuse

SIGNS AND SYMPTOMS

- Changes in looks, dress, and/or attitude.
- Behavior changes that affect work and relationships.
- Bad temper or abrupt changes in mood.
- Restlessness, or sometimes extreme lethargy.
- Puzzling absences.
- Odd money problems.
- Blackouts and memory lapses.
- Drug cravings, inability to stop using, lying about drug use, constant thoughts about getting a drug and using it.

The use of drugs to obtain pleasure, relieve pain, or alter reality has been common in most cultures throughout history. But drug use can lead to abuse and sometimes to addiction.

Drug abuse is the use of a substance—legal or illegal—often enough or in large enough doses to result in physical, mental, emotional, or social harm. Addiction is loss of control over drug use.

Experts still don't know why some people can use drugs now and then while others get hooked almost right away. Many experts agree that drug addiction is a disease, not simply a sign of weak character, and should be treated as such.

Abuse of illegal drugs can be risky and even fatal (see **street drugs** chart, page 216). But abuse of *legal* drugs is also a major problem. In the United States some 21 million people have abused prescription drugs, such as painkillers, sleeping pills, and tranquilizers, at least once. Alcohol and tobacco alone claim more lives than all illegal drugs combined. Death from car and other accidents as a result of drinking is a major risk.

Like alcoholics, drug abusers can be hard to treat because they often deny their problem—even when it threatens to destroy their lives. Successful treatment programs aim to create social support, enhance self-esteem, and teach ways to avoid situations that can trigger relapse.

WHAT YOU CAN DO NOW

- If you believe you have a drug problem and have tried to stop using but could not, call a drug treatment program or professional right away. It's hard to stop drug abuse on your own.
- If you see 2 or more of the listed symptoms in a family member or friend (above all a child or teenager) and suspect drug abuse, call your doctor. Or contact one of the organizations listed here for names of drug treatment specialists or clinics.

WHEN TO CALL THE DOCTOR

Call for a prompt appointment:

- If you are pregnant (or think you might be) and have been abusing drugs.
- If someone (above all a child or teenager) shows symptoms of drug abuse.

HOW TO PREVENT IT

Staying drug-free often requires major changes in habits and lifestyle. Depending on the depth of the drug problem, recovery (the stage that follows withdrawal) can be difficult. Still, you can take steps to help yourself stay clean:

- Seek the support of family members, friends, and colleagues.
- Join a support group such as Narcotics Anonymous or Cocaine Anonymous.
- Avoid places and situations that you connect with drug use. Make new friends who don't use drugs, and try to stay away from friends when they are using drugs.
- Be careful not to substitute some other

Some Street Drugs: Symptoms and Risks

Abuse of any drug can cause major personal and social problems. But street drugs, because they are illegal, carry special risks, the least of which is jail. The drugs themselves are dangerous and are often mixed with deadly fillers. Users have no way of knowing what they are really getting, how strong it is, or how it will affect them. New street drugs keep appearing. Here are some that are widely used.

TYPE OF DRUG	SYMPTOMS OF USE	RISKS
Amphetamines (speed, uppers); methamphetamine (ice).	Restlessness; talkativeness; decreased appetite with weight loss; dilated pupils; insomnia; trembling; dry mouth; angry, paranoid, or violent behavior.	Stroke or heart failure; violence.
Opiates, including heroin (smack) and opium.	Fatigue, euphoria, weight loss, sweating, poor appetite, needle marks on arms (sometimes), sniffling and runny nose (if snorted).	Overdose can lead to coma and death. If injected, risk of HIV infection and hepatitis from contaminated needles.
Cocaine (coke); called crack or rock when smoked.	Decreased appetite; mood swings; talkativeness; dilated pupils; apparent intoxication; sniffling, runny nose, and nosebleeds (if snorted); weight loss; paranoia; disconnected speech.	Holes in cartilage separating nostrils (if snorted); seizures and coma; death by cardiac arrest or respiratory failure; suicidal behavior after prolonged use.
Inhalants, including nitrous oxide (laughing gas), amyl nitrite (poppers), butyl nitrite (rush), chlorohydrocarbons (aerosol sprays), and hydrocarbons (glue, paint thinner).	Agitation, nausea, coughing, nosebleeds, fatigue, lack of coordination, violent behavior.	Suffocation; with glue or paint thinner, permanent damage to brain and nervous system; violence.
Designer drugs, including synthetic heroin (China white), MPTP, MDMA (ecstasy); and ephedrine, pseudoephedrine, or the herb ephedra, mixed with caffeine (herbal ecstasy).	Euphoria, tremors, impaired speech, nausea, sweating, fainting.	Synthetic heroin can lead to Parkinson's-like symptoms, including tremors, paralysis, and impaired speech or permanent brain damage. Ecstasy may cause paranoia and depression.

Street Drugs: Symptoms and Risks

TYPE OF DRUG	SYMPTOMS OF USE	RISKS
Sedatives (downers), including tranquilizers and barbiturates; Rohypnol (roofies) ; ketamine.	Lethargy, confused speech, lack of balance, impaired judgment and motor ability, memory loss.	Overdose; combined with alcohol, can lead to coma and death.
Hallucinogens, including LSD (acid), mescaline, and PCP (angel dust).	Seeing things that aren't there, nausea, sweating and trembling, mood disorders, increased heart rate, paranoia, violent behavior (PCP).	PCP in large doses can lead to seizures, coma, and violence. LSD can cause panic or loss of control.
Cannabis, including marijuana (pot, grass) and hashish (hash).	Mood swings, increased appetite, red eyes, slowed time sense and reflexes, anxiety, lethargy, alienation (sometimes).	Not physically addictive, but may cause psychological dependence and damage to lungs from smoking.

kind of addictive act—such as gambling, smoking, or overeating—for the one you're quitting.

- Make sure your diet is healthy and that you exercise. Workouts help your body release chemicals that make you feel good.
- Remember, recovery doesn't happen in a day. If you have a relapse, don't use it as an excuse to go back to your old habits. Think about what led to the relapse, and plan how to avoid it next time.

FOR MORE HELP

Hotline: National Drug Information Treatment and Referral Hotline of the Center for Substance Abuse Treatment, 800-662-4357, M–F 24-hour line. Refers callers to treatment programs for drug and/or alcohol problems.

Hotline: Phoenix House, 800-COCAINE (262-2463), 24-hour line. Gives names and numbers of local treatment programs.

Information line: Cocaine Anonymous National Hotline, 800-347-8998, 24-hour line. A mutual support program patterned on the Alcoholics Anonymous 12-step approach. Call for meetings near you.

Information line: National Council on Alcoholism and Drug Dependence Hope Line, 800-622-2255, 24-hour line. Provides fact sheets and other items. State and local affiliates give names of drug treatment specialists and programs.

Organization: Narcotics Anonymous, Box 9999, Van Nuys, CA 91409. 818-773-9999, M–F 8–5 PST. A self-help/mutual support program patterned on the Alcoholics Anonymous 12-step approach. Call about local meetings.

Organization: National Clearinghouse for Alcohol and Drug Information, Box 2345, Rockville, MD 20847-2345. 800-729-6686 in Maryland, 301-468-2600 elsewhere, M–F 8–7 EST. Provides facts about alcohol and drug abuse.

Book: *Educating Yourself About Alcohol and Drugs: A People's Primer,* by Marc Alan Schuckit, M.D. A guide to recovery by an expert. Plenum Publishing, 1995, $28.95.

Web access: Web of Addictions. After logging on to the Internet, type: *http://www.well.com/user/woa.* Offers news, fact sheets, resources, and other links.

Eating Disorders

SIGNS AND SYMPTOMS

Anorexia:

- Eating very little food and dieting even while losing large amounts of weight.
- Feeling fat even when far below normal weight.
- Compulsive exercising.
- Irregular menstrual periods, or none.
- In women, increase in facial and body hair.
- Dry, yellow, or sallow skin.
- Depression, moodiness, impatience, social withdrawal.
- Constant use of over-the-counter diet pills or laxatives.

Bulimia:

- Frequent periods of overeating, followed by vomiting in secret.
- Spending long times in the bathroom, especially after meals, and signs of frequent vomiting (such as bloodshot eyes) or laxative or diuretic use (dizziness).
- Damage to tooth enamel, cavities, and gum disease caused by stomach acids from frequent vomiting.
- Compulsive exercising.

As many as 8 million people in the United States are thought to have eating disorders: mental illnesses in which the person becomes obsessed with food and body image. Anorexia nervosa (self-starvation) and bulimia nervosa (binge eating and/or purging) are the most common. Both can be fatal if untreated, and they require prompt professional care.

Anorexia is most common in young women, but it can affect anyone. It often looks at first like a normal concern about weight. But it grows out of control as the person becomes locked into a vicious cycle of frantic dieting and overexercise. The person with anorexia views himself or herself as fat even when emaciated. A person with bulimia, in contrast, goes on eating binges—sometimes eating up to 20,000 calories at one sitting.

Anorexia and bulimia are closely linked: About one-fourth of those with bulimia have also had anorexia. The cause is still not known, but it seems to involve low self-esteem, troubled family life, worries about body changes during adolescence, and social pressure to look thin.

Treatment may include nutrition counseling, individual or family therapy, and support groups. Antidepressant drugs can help with bulimia, even in those who aren't depressed. Hospitalization is sometimes needed in serious cases or for people with severe **depression** (see page 213).

WHAT YOU CAN DO NOW

- Get help from a doctor specializing in eating disorders as soon as you can. The longer an eating disorder goes untreated, the harder it is to reverse. Your family doctor may be able to refer you.
- Treat yourself or someone who has the problem with love and understanding—be aware that this is a mental illness.
- Avoid diet pills, laxatives, and diuretics. Overuse of diet pills can result in stroke; overuse of laxatives and diuretics can cause heart failure.

WHEN TO CALL THE DOCTOR

- If you see symptoms of anorexia or bulimia, most of all with depression and/or talk of suicide.
- If you find yourself or a family member worrying all the time about weight and looks.

HOW TO PREVENT IT

- Provide your children with healthy views of food and body image. Handle issues of eating and weight with sensitivity. Don't criticize or joke about your child's looks.
- As a parent, be willing to admit your own mistakes and to accept those of your children. Anorexia and bulimia are more common in families that value high

achievement and perfection. Be careful to keep the pressure down.

FOR MORE HELP

Information line: National Association of Anorexia Nervosa and Associated Disorders, Box 7, Highland Park, IL 60035. 847-831-3438, M–F 9–5 CST. Staff answers questions, sends information, and refers callers to lists of experts and support groups.

Organization: National Eating Disorders Organization, Laureate Eating Disorders Program, 6655 S. Yale Ave., Tulsa, OK 74136-3329. 918-481-4044, 8–5 M–F CST. Provides materials and refers to therapists and programs.

Organization: Overeaters Anonymous. A 12-step program with chapters around the world. Check the white pages for the chapter nearest you. If you don't find one, write OA's Worldwide Service Office, Box 44020, Rio Rancho, NM 87174-4020, or call 505-891-2664 (24-hour recording) for a list of chapters.

Book: *Fat Is a Feminist Issue: A Program to Conquer Compulsive Eating,* by Susie Orbach. Latest edition of a classic antidiet book. Berkeley Books, 1995, $4.95.

Book: *Overcoming Binge Eating,* by Christopher Fairburn, D.M. Offers facts and a self-help program for binge eating. The Guilford Press, 1995, $14.95.

Web access: Alliance to Fight Eating Disorders. After logging on to the Internet, type: *http://www.fsci.umn.edu/~AFED.* Offers basic facts on eating disorders and lists more resources.

Video: *Anorexia & Bulimia at Time of Diagnosis.* Clear overview of causes and treatments, with 4 reports—Understanding the Diagnosis, What Happens Next?, Treatment and Management, and Issues and Answers. Time Life Medical, 1996, $19.95. Sold in many pharmacies; for one near you, call 800-588-9959.

Grief

SIGNS AND SYMPTOMS

Grief is normal after any deep loss. Symptoms vary, but may include:

- Extreme depression and fatigue.
- Sudden shifts in emotions—being numb and cool one minute and sobbing out of control the next.
- Feeling helpless, confused, and lost.
- Major changes in sleep patterns, such as trouble getting to sleep, waking up often at night, or wanting to sleep all the time.
- Physical pain or discomfort.
- Loss of appetite or overeating.
- Lack of focus; trouble making choices or concentrating.
- Self-destructive behavior, including reckless driving or abuse of drugs or alcohol.

Few things can be as wrenching and as hard to get over as the death of a loved one. But other losses can also leave people stunned with grief. These include divorce, miscarriage, the end of a friendship or serious relationship, a disabling illness or accident, and even the loss of a pet.

Grieving often happens in stages. The first stage is often marked by a mixture of numbness, shock, and denial. You may feel you're in a trance and unable to make decisions. Many people feel so drained, or so badly neglect their own needs (such as eating or sleeping), that they get sick. Others try to pretend the shock is not so bad: "Don't worry about me. I'm fine."

After a while, you may go through phases of intense feeling. When someone close to you has died, feelings may include anger (at the unfairness of the death), fear (that you or other loved ones will also die), guilt (for having survived or for something you think you failed to do for the person who died), depression, and aimlessness.

Don't block your grief. Experts advise letting yourself (and others) feel numb, sad, angry, or depressed. Then, at your own pace, move on with your life. "Grief is not a sign of weakness," is a saying of the Theos Foundation, which sets up support groups for widowed people. "Allow grief to have its way for a while; then, gradually and gently, you can release yourself from its grip."

WHAT YOU CAN DO NOW

- Don't hide your grief from friends. If you express your needs, they will be more able to help.
- Find a support group. Being with others who are going through the same process can help. (Many groups also work with people who have a loved one who is dying.)
- Find help for your children. If there is a death or other hurtful event in your family, your children need to grieve too, and may need your support. Grief groups for children exist but may be hard to find. For young children, counseling may be better.
- Put off making major decisions—whether to move from your home, what to do with your loved one's possessions—while you're in the midst of grieving.
- Don't leave important things unsaid or undone before someone dies. Seek the person out and make sure you resolve as much as you can; you'll spare yourself much grief and guilt later.
- If you know someone who is grieving, don't be afraid to make contact and talk with him or her.

WHEN TO CALL THE DOCTOR

- If you feel ill and think you need help. Ailments caused by grief are real.
- If symptoms of **depression** (see page 213) last longer than 2 months, or if you feel you might kill yourself.

FOR MORE HELP

Information line: Theos Foundation, 412-471-7779, M–Th 9–4 EST. For widows and widowers; connects callers with local support groups and sends information on the grieving process.

Information line: Compassionate Friends, 708-990-0010, M–F 9–4 CST. Refers bereaved parents and siblings to local support groups, and sends brochures related to death.

Information line: Kara, 415-321-5859, M–F 9–5 PST. Connects children and teens who have lost a parent or sibling with support groups, and sends brochures. Adults have their own support line at 415-321-5272.

Information line: Pregnancy and Infant Loss Center, 612-473-9372, M–F 9–4 CST. Provides names of experts who can help parents coping with miscarriage, stillbirth, and infant death. **Web site:** *http://sids-network.org/pil.htm.*

Book: *Doors Close, Doors Open: Widows, Grieving and Growing,* by Morton Lieberman, Ph.D. Offers advice and support for widows and widowers. Putnam Publishing, 1996, $23.95.

Book: *The Mourning Handbook,* by Helen Fitzgerald. Offers advice on coping with every kind of loss. Fireside, 1994, $11.

Web access: Hygeia... An Online Journal for Pregnancy and Neonatal Loss. After logging on to the Internet, type: *http://www.connix.com/~hygeia.* Offers support and further resources.

Smoking and Illness

SIGNS AND SYMPTOMS

- Shortness of breath, wheezing.
- Fatigue.
- Lasting or hacking cough.
- Poor sense of smell and taste.
- Bad breath.
- Poor blood flow (cold hands and feet are a sign).
- Frequent bouts of throat and lung illnesses such as bronchitis.
- Early wrinkling of the skin.

Cigarette smoking is the leading cause of preventable illness and death in the United States. It kills more Americans every year than do alcohol, cocaine, heroin, murder, airplane and automobile accidents, and

AIDS combined—more than 120,000 a year from lung cancer and about 180,000 from heart disease. (See **lung cancer,** page 97, **congestive heart failure,** page 111, **chronic bronchitis and emphysema,** page 92 , and **high blood pressure,** page 112.)

Smoking harms more than just the person who lights up: Secondhand smoke (other people's tobacco smoke) may kill as many as 50,000 Americans a year. Smoking by parents can make asthma worse in children and increase their risk of colds, ear infections, and sudden infant death syndrome. Smoking during pregnancy increases the risk of miscarriage, premature birth, and fetal death.

Nicotine is a strongly addictive drug; that's why so many people keep smoking despite the known risks. Still, if you're a smoker, there are things you can do to quit—and to help yourself stay away from tobacco.

WHAT YOU CAN DO NOW

The best advice is to quit smoking. The benefits of quitting kick in right away. Within 20 minutes after your last puff, your blood pressure—which rises when you smoke—returns to normal. Within 8 to 48 hours, excess carbon monoxide (a deadly gas) in your blood drops to normal. One year after that, your risk of heart disease will be half that of a smoker's. Fifteen years after giving up cigarettes, your risk of heart disease will be the same as that of someone who never smoked. You'll also reduce your risk of getting many types of cancer.

Tips for making quitting easier:

- Get support. Some people find that it helps to quit with a friend or relative, or to join a "quitting support group." Your doctor may be able to refer you.
- Pick a day to quit ahead of time, to give yourself time to prepare, and to get your support system ready.
- If you are a heavy smoker, ask your doctor about using nicotine gum or skin patches. They're now sold over the counter, without a prescription. These aids are meant to reduce the physical urge for a cigarette. Never smoke while using the gum or patches, though, or you'll risk a bad nicotine overdose.
- Exercise daily. Walks, bike rides, or any workouts that make you breathe hard help your body overcome its need for nicotine.
- Know your "triggers"—situations and places that make you want to smoke—and avoid them. Find other things to do when you're tempted to light up.
- Explore acupuncture, meditation, guided imagery, hypnotherapy, and biofeedback. All of these can be useful.
- Drink lots of water and have low-calorie snacks on hand during the first weeks when you have an urge to put something in your mouth.

What to expect when you quit:

The good news is you plan to quit smoking. The bad news? You may have at least one of these withdrawal symptoms: headache, nausea, constipation or diarrhea, fatigue, drowsiness, loss of concentration, and trouble sleeping. You may also feel more crabby, anxious, or depressed than usual, or want to eat more. Some people start craving sweets.

That's because your body is scrambling to adjust to the sudden absence of nicotine. But don't be alarmed—and don't rush out to buy a pack of cigarettes. Withdrawal symptoms don't last, and once they pass, you'll feel better than you have in years.

WHEN TO CALL THE DOCTOR

Call for a prompt appointment:

- If you are wheezing and have a lasting cough, trouble breathing, and chest pains.

Call for advice:

- If you are a tobacco user and become concerned about your health for any reason. Smokers are more likely to get many major illnesses than nonsmokers.

FOR MORE HELP

Information line: Smoking, Tobacco, and Health Information Line, Centers for Disease Control and Prevention, 800-232-1311, 24-hour recording. Free information about smoking. **Web site:** *http://www.cdc.gov/nccdphp/osh/tobacco.htm.*

Organization: American Lung Association, 1740 Broadway, New York, NY 10019. 800-586-4872, M–F 9–5 your time. Has many local offices; some run support groups. Offers programs and information. **Web site:** *http://www.lungusa.org.*

Organization: American Cancer Society, 1599 Clifton Rd., Atlanta, GA 30329-4251. 800-227-2345, M–F 9–5 your time. Provides facts about smoking and refers callers to local chapters. **Web site:** *http://www.cancer.org.*

Organization: Smokenders, 4455 E. Camelback Rd., #D-150, Phoenix, AZ 85018. 800-828-4357, M–F 8–4:30 MST. A private group with a quit-smoking program.

Brochure: Agency for Health Care Policy and Research. 800-358-9295 M–F 9–5 EST. Ask for "You Can Quit Smoking."

Stress

SIGNS AND SYMPTOMS

Physical:

- Frequent headaches.
- Trouble sleeping.
- Fatigue.
- Digestive illness.
- Skin problems.
- Back or neck pain.
- Poor appetite or overeating, or heavy drinking.

Psychological:

- Anxiety, tension, or anger.
- Withdrawal from social life.
- Pessimism or cynicism.
- Boredom.
- Bad temper or resentment.
- Loss of ability to concentrate or perform as usual.

Stress is our reaction to anything—good or bad—that upsets our balance. Stressful events trigger the release of hormones—including adrenaline—that provide a quick supply of oxygen and energy.

But these hormone surges, if sparked again and again, can deplete the body's ability to bounce back and can cause problems such as ulcers, high blood pressure, and loss of appetite. Constant stress also puts you at risk of migraine **headaches** (see page 54), **depression** (see page 213), **chronic fatigue syndrome** (see page 281), adult-onset **diabetes** (see page 282), and digestive ailments. Constant stress can also upset your body's immune system and lower your resistance to disease.

Stress often comes from painful situations you feel you can't control: job burnout, money problems, grief, or divorce. Minor stresses range from arguments to traffic jams. Even a good event, such as marriage, a job promotion, or a new baby, can trigger stress. Other causes include illness, loneliness, pain, and the drive to be perfect.

WHAT YOU CAN DO NOW

- Do things that calm you. Take walks or long, hot baths. Talk with friends, or rent movies that make you laugh.
- Exercise 30 minutes a day at least 3 times a week. You'll reduce your level of stress hormones and gain a sense of well-being.
- Spend time outdoors. Some research shows contact with nature can help reduce stress.
- Enroll in a stress reduction course. Ask your doctor to refer you, or check with your local hospital. Also, some employers offer courses or will send you to one.
- Learn relaxation techniques such as deep breathing, stretching exercises, yoga, visualization, or meditation (see **relaxation exercises** box, next page).

WHEN TO CALL THE DOCTOR

- If you believe you are anxious, depressed, or troubled beyond routine stress (see **depression,** page 213, and **anxiety and phobias,** page 210).
- If you have symptoms of stress with any of these: new sleep patterns, mood swings, loss of sex drive, crying jags, exhaustion, great difficulty with minor tasks, agitated or slow movement, or a change in menstrual cycles (in women). You may have a form of clinical depression.
- If your symptoms of stress are long-lasting and trouble you.

THREE EASY RELAXATION EXERCISES

Relax your body and your mind will follow. These easy exercises start to banish stress right away. For best results, do one or more each day.

- Loosen up: 4 minutes. Find a quiet place to lie down. Begin by tensing your body: Tighten your fists, scrunch up your face, and tense your hands, arms, feet, legs, neck, and head. Hold for 5 or 10 seconds. Now let everything go all at once. Feel the tension drain away. Relax for 1 minute. Repeat 3 times.
- Watch your breath: 10 minutes. Sit or lie down in a quiet place where you won't be disturbed. Breathe normally through your nose. Focus on each breath as it flows in and out. Don't try to control it—just watch. When your attention wanders, bring it gently back to your breathing. Repeat as often as you like.
- Meditate: 20 minutes. Find a quiet place. Sit in a chair with your feet on the floor and your hands in your lap. Close your eyes and in your mind say a simple word or phrase. Try the word *one*.

  When thoughts come to mind, ignore them and return to the word. Make it the focus of your attention, but don't force it or work at it—let it come as though you are hearing it, not thinking it. As you relax, your mouth may fall open, and you may slump over or even drift briefly into sleep. Don't worry, just allow yourself to let go. Practice this once a day (twice is better) for lasting results. If you don't have 20 minutes, try 10.

HOW TO PREVENT IT

- Figure out what causes your stress and where you can make changes. Set reachable goals for yourself and be forthright with other people about what you can and can't do, and will and won't do.
- Don't try to be perfect. If you are juggling too many things, let a ball or two drop. Your house doesn't have to be spotless, and you don't always have to be the last one to leave the office. Practice giving yourself a break.
- Take a true slow-paced, pressure-free vacation, leaving your work behind.

FOR MORE HELP

Information line: National Mental Health Association. 800-969-6642, 24-hour recording, or 703-684-7722, M–F 9–5 EST. Sends free pamphlets on stress and other mental health issues, provides counseling, and lists services and support groups.

Organization: American Institute of Stress, 124 Park Ave., Yonkers, NY 10703. 800-24-RELAX, M–F 9–5 EST. Offers a monthly newsletter and a $35 fact packet.

Organization: The Stress Reduction Clinic, University of Massachusetts Medical Center, 55 Lake Ave. N, Worcester, MA 01655. 508-856-2656 M–F 8–4 EST. Offers meditation workshops around the country.

Organization: Re-evaluation Counseling. 719 Second Ave. N, Seattle, WA 98109. 206-284-0311 M–F 9–5:30 PST. Offers nationwide peer support network and counseling classes, and publications. **Web site:** *http://www.rc.org*.

Book: *Why Zebras Don't Get Ulcers: A Guide to Stress, Stress-Related Diseases, and Coping*, by Robert M. Sapolsky. Freeman, 1994, $14.95.

Book: *Full Catastrophe Living: Using the Wisdom of Your Body and Mind to Face Stress, Pain, and Illness*, by Jon Kabat-Zinn. Delta, 1991, $13.95.

Web access: "How to Avoid Burning Out," from the Medical Reporter. After logging on to the Internet, type: *http://www.ihr.com/medreprt/articles/burnout.html*.

Video: *Stress & Anxiety at Time of Diagnosis*. Clear overview of causes and treatments, with 4 reports—Understanding the Diagnosis, What Happens Next?, Treatment and Management, and Issues and Answers. Time Life Medical, 1996, $19.95. Sold in many pharmacies; for one near you, call 800-588-9959.

Sexual Health

AIDS

SIGNS AND SYMPTOMS

As HIV progresses to AIDS:

- Sore throat, fever, swollen glands, rash.
- Constant swollen glands in the neck, underarms, and groin.
- Fatigue, overall sick feeling.
- Fevers, chills, and night sweats.
- Frequent colds, cold sores, fungal or yeast infections in the mouth.
- Sudden weight loss, chronic diarrhea.
- Dry cough, breathing problems.
- Skin sores, mostly the purple lesions of Kaposi's sarcoma.
- Rapid vision loss.
- Finally, confusion, memory loss, and personality changes; dementia.

AIDS, or acquired immune deficiency syndrome, was first reported in 1981. Now it is a worldwide epidemic.

AIDS is caused by HIV (the human immunodeficiency virus), found in blood, semen, and vaginal fluids, and sometimes in saliva and breast milk. HIV is spread mostly through sexual contact or by sharing intravenous needles, and can infect men, women, and children of any age. An infected woman can pass it to her child during childbirth or breast-feeding. Blood transfusions before 1986 also spread HIV—but now, research suggests the current risk of getting HIV from a transfusion is only 1 in 500,000. HIV can't be spread by contact as casual as hugging, or sharing a towel or a drinking glass.

HIV destroys the blood cells (T cells) that fight off disease. The first symptoms of HIV infection are similar to those of mononucleosis—fatigue and swollen glands. Years may pass before more symptoms appear. Symptoms may progress slowly. A person is said to have full-blown AIDS when his or her T cell count falls to one-fifth of a healthy person's, and he or she has many infections (see **tuberculosis,** page 105) or a cancer such as Kaposi's sarcoma. Death comes when the immune system is too weak to fight off cancer, **pneumonia** (see page 98), or some other infection.

So far, AIDS has no cure and no vaccine. But new treatments—some combine 3 or more drugs—seem to attack the virus, slow its growth, and help infected people live longer, healthier lives. A new class of drugs, protease inhibitors, also looks promising. It's easy to prevent the spread of AIDS: Don't share body fluids with others unless you know they—and you—are HIV-free.

WHAT YOU CAN DO NOW

➤ If your sexual partner has the virus or if you have symptoms, get an HIV test right away. In most cities, you can get the test without giving your name. If you are infected, the sooner you know it the better, so you can start treatments to slow the onset of AIDS.

➤ Get tested again in 3 to 6 months. HIV

Sexually Transmitted Diseases

Every sexually transmitted disease (STD) listed here may produce no symptoms at first. When symptoms do show up, they may be confused with those of other diseases. If you are infected but don't have any symptoms, you can still pass an STD on to your partner. Note, too, that any STD with open sores or irritated skin, either on the inside or outside of the genitals, puts you at greater risk of catching HIV. That's why, if you have sex with more than one person, testing and checkups are vital, as is safe sex.

SYMPTOMS	WHAT IT MIGHT BE	WHAT YOU CAN DO
Watery mucus from penis or vagina, burning with urination, mild lower abdominal pain 1–3 weeks after infection. Some (mostly women) may have no symptoms.	Chlamydia—bacterial disease. Can result in pelvic inflammatory disease in women (see page 242) or sterility. In newborns exposed during childbirth, can cause pneumonia and eye infections.	Call doctor for prompt appointment. You and your partner(s) should be treated with antibiotics.
Itching or burning pain in genital area, then red bumps in or on genitals that may turn into blisters or open sores 2–10 days after infection. These go away within 3 weeks. Later attacks (with same symptoms) heal faster.	Genital herpes—viral infection spread through sex, from cold sores (see page 81), or, rarely, by hands that have herpes blisters or sores. Most catching when symptoms are present. Can be transferred from mother to baby during childbirth.	Call doctor for prompt appointment. Medications shorten outbreaks and make them less severe. Don't have sex until sores heal. **For more help:** ASHA Resource Center, 800-230-6039, M–F 9–7 EST. National Herpes Hotline: 919-361-8488, M–F 9–7 EST.
Small, round, red, flat, itchy bumps on genitals, around anus, or inside vagina; can also appear in mouth of someone who has had oral contact with genitals of infected person.	Genital warts—viral infection. Some strains may increase risk of cervical or penile cancer. After warts are removed, virus remains and can cause future outbreaks.	Call doctor for prompt appointment. Treatment can include drugs or laser surgery. Don't use over-the-counter wart treatments, which are too harsh. Women who've had warts should get Pap smear every 6 months.
Thick yellowish discharge from vagina or penis, burning and itching with urination, maybe discharge from rectum 2–10 days after infection. In later stages in women: abdominal pain, bleeding between periods.	Gonorrhea—bacterial infection. Left untreated, may spread to joints, tendons, or heart. May also cause pelvic inflammatory disease in women (see page 242). Infants exposed during birth can become blind.	Call doctor for prompt appointment. Treatment consists of antibiotics and painkillers. Don't have sex until doctor says it's safe. Your partner(s) should be tested and treated even if they have no symptoms.

(continued)

Sexual Health

Sexually Transmitted Diseases *(continued)*

SYMPTOMS	WHAT IT MIGHT BE	WHAT YOU CAN DO
Painless sores on or in genitals, rectal area, or mouth, and enlarged lymph nodes near sores 10 days to 3 months after infection. If untreated, in second stage (3 weeks to several months later): mild fever, rash, patchy hair loss, sore throat. In third stage (5–30 years later): loss of balance, paralysis, dementia, numbness in legs, and blindness (rarely).	Syphilis—bacterial infection. Can damage brain, nervous system, and heart; can be fatal. Highly catching in first 2 stages but not in third stage. Infected mothers may pass infection to infants during childbirth.	Call doctor for prompt appointment. Antibiotics can cure syphilis, although in later stages some damage cannot be reversed. Don't have sex during treatment. Your partner(s) should be tested and treated.
In women, heavy greenish-yellow or gray discharge from vagina, pain during intercourse, vaginal odor, painful urination 4–20 days after infection. Men may have no symptoms.	Trichomoniasis—infection caused by parasite. May increase risk that baby born to infected mother will be premature or underweight.	Call doctor for prompt appointment. You and your partner(s) will be treated with antibiotics. A man may have no symptoms but can infect others if not treated. Don't have sex until treatment is finished.

FOR MORE HELP

Hotline: National STD Hotline of the Centers for Disease Control and Prevention, 800-227-8922, M–F 8AM–11PM EST. Staff answers questions and gives lists of doctors and testing sites.

Organization: American Social Health Association, 800-972-8500, 24-hour recording. Provides pamphlets on sexual health.

Organization: National Institute of Allergy and Infectious Diseases, Office of Communications, Bldg. 31, Room 7A-50, 9000 Rockville Pike, Bethesda, MD 20892. Write for free STD packet.

Pamphlet: American Foundation for the Prevention of Venereal Disease, 799 Broadway, Suite 638, New York, NY 10003. Send a self-addressed, stamped envelope and $1 for a copy of "STD Prevention for Everyone."

Book: *Choices: Sex in the Age of STDs*, by Jeffrey S. Nevid, Ph.D. A guide to STDs and how to prevent them. Allyn and Bacon, 1995, $15.

Web access: The Safer Sex Page. After logging on to the Internet, type: *http://www.safersex.org*. Offers tips on safe sex, facts about STDs (treatment and prevention), counseling resources, and other links on the Web.

Web access: Go Ask Alice. After logging on to the Internet, type: *http://www.cc.columbia.edu/cu/healthwise/alice.html*. Columbia University's health question & answer service. Covers a wide range of topics, including sexual health.

can take that long to show up on a test.

- If you are pregnant (or trying to conceive), get an HIV test. Treatment can greatly reduce the chances that a woman with HIV will pass it on to her baby.

After diagnosis:

- Practice **safe sex** (see box, this page). You can catch other HIV strains, or spread HIV even if you have no symptoms.

WHEN TO CALL THE DOCTOR

- If you have symptoms of HIV or AIDS.
- If you have HIV or AIDS, and your symptoms get worse or you get a new symptom.
- If you have had a high-risk exposure—a needle-stick from an HIV-infected person, or sex with a person who might be HIV-positive. Early treatment can help you fight off the disease.

HOW TO PREVENT IT

- Practice **safe sex** (see box, this page).
- Don't inject drugs. If you do use intravenous drugs, don't share needles.
- Avoid contact with other people's blood, including menstrual blood.
- If you engage in high-risk sex acts, you and your partner(s) should be tested every 6 to 12 months.

FOR MORE HELP

Hotline: National HIV/AIDS Hotline, Centers for Disease Control and Prevention. English: 800-342-AIDS, 7 days a week, 24-hour line. Spanish: 800-344-7432, 7 days a week, 8AM–2AM EST. Staff answers questions and refers callers to experts on health, legal, and financial issues. Calls are confidential.

Hotline: Project Inform. 800-822-7422, M–SAT 10–4 PST. Staff answers questions about drug treatments. You can also request a free drug fact packet.

Organization: National AIDS Clearinghouse, Centers for Disease Control and Prevention, Box 6003, Rockville, MD 20849-6003. 800-458-5231 (English and Spanish), M–F 9–7 EST. Provides free publications and referrals. **Web site:** *http://www.cdcnac.org*.

Organization: National Association of People With AIDS. 202-898-0414, M–F 9–6 EST. Staff answers questions, sends pamphlets, and refers to support groups. **Web site:** *http://www.thecure.org*.

Organization: American Foundation for AIDS Research (AmFAR), 733 3rd Ave., 12th Floor, New York, NY 10017-3204. 800-392-6327, M–F 9–5 EST. Offers a twice-yearly treatment directory for $50.

Book: *The Essential AIDS Fact Book,* by Paul Harding Douglas and Laura Pinsky. Clear guide to prevention, treatments, and other resources. Pocket Books, 1996, $7.

Book: *What You Can Do to Avoid AIDS,* by Earvin "Magic" Johnson. Easy-to-read book about AIDS prevention. Times Books, 1996, $4.99.

Book: *Take These Broken Wings and Learn to Fly,* by Steven D. Dietz and M. Jane Parker Hicks, M.D. Support for anyone touched by AIDS. Harbinger, 1992, $10.95.

Web access: The Body: A Multimedia AIDS and HIV Information Resource. After logging on to the Internet, type: *http://www.thebody.com*. Covers causes of AIDS, prevention, treatment, and quality-of-life issues.

HOW TO HAVE SAFE SEX

- Have sex only with a person you know to be free of diseases.
- If you have more than one sex partner, use latex condoms (even during oral sex). Never reuse a condom. A water-based lubricant will help prevent the condom from tearing.
- Use condoms with anyone whose sexual history you don't know or who isn't willing to be tested for HIV.
- Don't have anal sex; it increases your risk of HIV because of the chance of bleeding.
- It is safe to hug, kiss, massage, and touch others.

Birth Control Health Risks

Choosing a birth control method takes careful thought. How well does each method prevent pregnancy? How well does it protect against HIV and other sexually transmitted diseases (STDs)? How easy is the method to use, and how willing is each partner to use it? How much does it cost? How does it affect each person's health?

The health risk is one of the most important things to think about.

Birth control pills: With today's lower-estrogen birth control pills, severe side effects are rare in women under 30. The Pill does pose real risks, though. Among them are blood clots in the veins, heart attack, and stroke, as well as higher rates of breast cancer and cervical cancer. Discuss the risks with your doctor. You are at higher risk:

- If you have high blood pressure, blood clots, or diabetes, or any close relative does.
- If you have a history of breast cancer, uterine cancer, or uterine fibroids, or any close relative does.
- If you smoke, especially if you're over 35.

If you are at high risk, ask your doctor about the mini-Pill, which doesn't contain estrogen and has fewer side effects. Although it does not prevent pregnancy as well as the standard pill, and may cause bleeding between periods, it is believed to be safer.

If you take either type of birth control pill, be sure to get a Pap smear each year to check for cervical cancer.

Implanted or injected hormones: The hormones found in the Pill can also be injected or implanted under the skin on a woman's arm. Side effects can include:

- Bleeding or spotting between periods, heavy or prolonged bleeding, or no bleeding at all for months.
- Headache, dizziness, or nausea.
- Weight gain or change in appetite.

There is also a slight risk of skin infection where hormones are implanted.

You should not use implants or shots if

CHOOSING THE RIGHT BIRTH CONTROL METHOD FOR YOU

Nearly half of all women who use birth control become pregnant anyway. Birth control—no matter how respected or well known the method—is not foolproof. Even if used perfectly, it only reduces the risk of pregnancy. In fact, studies show that unplanned pregnancy often results not from a flaw in a method but from using it wrong.

To reduce your chances of getting pregnant (as well as your risk of a sexually transmitted disease), don't depend on just one type of birth control. Combine 2 or more—and make sure you know how to use them.

Here are success rates, pros and cons, and costs of birth control methods, listed in the order of their numbers of users. (Success rates are for the first year of use.)

Sterilization

The most effective, most common—and most lasting—form of birth control.

Success rate: More than 99 percent—although in rare cases sterilization has failed to prevent pregnancy.

Pro: Very effective; no loss of sexual mood.

Con: General anesthesia for tubal ligation has some risk; hard to undo; no defense against STDs.

Cost: Tubal ligation (for women): $1,000–2,500; vasectomy (for men): $240–520.

The Pill

The most popular form of birth control after sterilization. Early research questioned the Pill's long-term safety. Now researchers believe that today's low-hormone Pill is safe for most women who don't smoke. Ask your doctor whether it's right for you.

Success rate: 94 percent; higher if used "perfectly," without skipping days.

Pro: Effective; no loss of sexual mood.

Con: Side effects (see this page); risk of breast and cervical cancers; must be taken daily (mini-Pills must be taken at the same time every day); no defense against STDs.

Cost: $35–125 for exam; $15–25 monthly.

Condoms

The only method that also protects against most STDs—as long as the condom is latex. The condom is the cheapest, and the simplest to use, of all contraceptives.

Success rate: 84 percent for the male condom, 79 percent for the female condom (vaginal pouch). The success rate for condoms is much higher when they are used every time you have sex, used only with water-based lubricants (oil-based jellies and creams eat away at the latex), and handled carefully—watch the fingernails.

Pro: Best defense against STDs; low cost; easy to buy at drugstores and supermarkets, and from restroom dispensers.

Con: Can tear, slip, or come off during sex; may disrupt sexual mood.

Cost: 25–35 cents each for male condoms; up to $2.50 for the vaginal pouch.

Cervical Cap and Diaphragm

Less medical risk than most other women's contraceptives. Not as effective as most other forms of birth control; must be used with a spermicide.

Success rate: 82 percent.

Pro: Low cost; few serious side effects; some defense against STDs.

Con: Some loss of sexual mood; hard to use.

Cost: $50–125 for the exam; $13–25 for the device; $3–10 per tube for the spermicide.

Implanted and Injected Hormones

Next to sterilization, the most effective form of birth control. Norplant, a contraceptive implant, and Depo-Provera, an injectable contraceptive, are the newest and most effective forms of birth control on the market. Although both are FDA approved, long-term studies have not yet been done.

Success rate: 99 percent.

Pro: Highly effective; no loss of sexual mood; fewer side effects than the Pill.

Con: Expensive; no defense against STDs; harder to reverse than the Pill.

Cost: Norplant: $500–750 for the exam, 5-year implant, and insertion; $100–200 for removal. Depo-Provera: $35–125 for exam and $22–30 for the 90-day injection.

Spermicides

Most effective when used with another form of birth control such as a diaphragm, cervical cap, or condom.

Success rate: 70 percent.

Pro: No medical side effects; easy to buy at most drugstores; easily combined with other birth control methods.

Con: Used alone, less effective than other methods; no defense against STDs.

Costs: $3–10 (spermicide is found in foams, creams, jellies, films, and suppositories).

Intrauterine Device (IUD)

A hotly debated, but very effective, form of birth control. Although many doctors feel the IUD is safe, it has been linked to a slightly higher risk of pelvic inflammatory disease and may not be a good choice for women who want to have children later.

Success rate: 96 percent.

Pro: Effective; no loss of sexual mood.

Con: May decrease chance of future fertility; no defense against STDs.

Cost: $150–300 for exam and insertion.

Natural Method

The withdrawal and rhythm methods of birth control result in pregnancy about 25 percent of the time. If you use no birth control, you and your partner have an 85 percent chance of a pregnancy over time.

Pro: Low cost; natural.

Con: Not an effective form of birth control (unless you are very careful with the rhythm method); no defense against STDs.

Cost: None for the method; $3,225 or more for unintended pregnancy.

Emergency Birth Control

Because birth control methods don't always work and because a woman may have been raped, women sometimes need to take action after intercourse to avoid pregnancy. Your doctor can write a prescription for Emergency Mini-Pills or Emergency Contraceptive Pills within 48–72 hours after unprotected sex. For advice, call the Emergency Contraception Hotline at 800-584-9911, 24-hour recording.

you might be pregnant or if you have ever had vaginal bleeding for no clear reason, breast cancer, liver disease, or blood clots in your legs, lungs, or eyes.

Also, certain illnesses may worsen the side effects or raise your risk of other trouble. Talk to your doctor if you have had, or anyone in your family has ever had:

- Breast nodules or fibrocystic breasts (see **breast pain or lumps** chart, page 243), bleeding from the nipples, or an abnormal mammogram.
- High blood pressure, high cholesterol levels, or diabetes.
- Kidney, heart, or gallbladder disease.
- Irregular or very light menstrual periods.
- Migraines or frequent headaches.
- Asthma or epilepsy.
- Depression.

Condoms: This method of birth control—including the female condom, which fits inside the vagina—has few health risks or side effects. It is also the only form of birth control that can protect against HIV, the virus that causes AIDS.

On the other hand, some people are allergic to latex. You can use lambskin or other nonlatex condoms, but be aware that they may not protect you against HIV, because the virus may pass through a nonlatex condom.

Diaphragm, cervical cap, and spermicide: When used in the correct way, diaphragms and cervical caps pose few health risks. Some women who use diaphragms get urinary tract infections; being fitted with a smaller diaphragm can sometimes help.

Very rarely, a person is allergic to the spermicide used with a diaphragm or cervical cap (or used by itself); the result is genital itching and redness. Try switching to another brand or type (cream, jelly, or foam).

Careless use of a diaphragm or cervical cap may increase your risk of **toxic shock syndrome** (see page 248). Never leave a diaphragm in your body for more than 24 hours (or for more than 6 to 8 hours during your period), and never leave a cervical cap in place for more than 48 hours.

Intrauterine device (IUD): A doctor or other trained health worker places a T-shaped copper or plastic device in the uterus. It can cause cramping pain and heavy menstrual bleeding. Women who have heavy or painful periods should not use IUDs. They are also risky for women who have an STD or who have more than one sex partner, which increases the risk of getting STDs.

The worst problems with IUDs are pelvic infections (see **pelvic inflammatory disease,** page 242) and ectopic pregnancy (pregnancy outside the uterus).

Call your doctor for a prompt appointment if you are using an IUD and:

- You think you might be pregnant.
- You have pain in the pelvic area.
- You have fever with no cause.
- You have foul-smelling vaginal discharge.

Tubal sterilization: Surgery to close off the fallopian tubes (see color illustration, page 175) is a common type of permanent birth control for women. Although it's a simple operation, it poses some risk, such as infection or a reaction to the anesthesia.

Vasectomy: Men who want permanent birth control can have minor surgery to tie the tubes through which the sperm travel from the testicles into the penis (see color illustration, page 175). It doesn't affect sexual performance. Doctors often advise vasectomy for couples because it's simpler, cheaper, and safer than tubal sterilization. Problems may include heavy bleeding and infection.

FOR MORE HELP

Information line: Office of Population Affairs Clearinghouse, Box 30686, Bethesda, MD 20824-0686. 301-654-6190, M–F 9–5 EST. Ask for facts about birth control.

Organization: Planned Parenthood, 800-230-PLAN, 24-hour recording. Connects you to a local chapter, which offers information on birth control. **Web site:** *http://www.ppfa.org/ppfa*.

Book: *The Birth Control Book,* by Samuel A. Pasquale, M.D., and Jennifer Cadoff. A woman's guide to choosing the safest and most effective method of birth control. Ballantine, 1996, $10.

Web access: Ann Rose's Ultimate Birth Control Links. After logging on to the Internet, type: *http://gynpages.com/ultimate/index.html.* Offers facts on birth control and a range of other links on the Web.

Loss of Sexual Desire

SIGNS AND SYMPTOMS

- Lack of interest in sex for more than 2 months.
- In couples, sex less often than every other week, or anxiety about sex.
- Sometimes, erection problems, premature ejaculation, painful intercourse, or trouble reaching orgasm.

A short-term loss of sexual desire is quite normal; people of all ages go through peaks and declines. A lack of desire is the most common complaint at sex therapy clinics. The problem is often caused by psychological factors: **depression** (see page 213), anger, boredom, conflict in a relationship, stress, fear of pregnancy, or memories of sexual abuse. It may also result from fatigue, **alcohol abuse** (see page 206), or the use of antidepressants, tranquilizers, or antihistamines. Less often, the cause is a hormonal imbalance or a disease such as **diabetes** (see page 282).

A marriage counselor or sex therapist can often help if the problem is an emotional or psychological issue. Easing stress or treating any health problems may also help. Testosterone shots have helped some men as well as some women who are past menopause.

WHAT YOU CAN DO NOW

- See whether a drug you are taking might be the cause. Many drugs have side effects that can cause lack of desire. Ask your doctor.
- Cut back on alcohol or stop drinking (see **alcohol abuse and alcoholism,** page 206).
- Check your stress level (see **is stress putting your health at risk?** page 308). Worry and conflict chill interest in sex.
- Wait before you worry: If you have had a recent crisis—a loss, an illness, a major change—your sex drive may just be taking a rest (see **grief,** page 219, and **erection problems,** page 232).
- Try something new. Have sex at a different time or place, or try varied positions.
- Relax when making love. Take your time and try more foreplay. Tell your partner what arouses you.
- Share your feelings and worries about your sexual performance—but not while making love.
- Try reading or using erotic materials, watching videos, or playing out sexual fantasies, if this appeals to you.

WHEN TO CALL THE DOCTOR

- If you have erection problems or pain during intercourse.
- If loss of sexual desire is causing problems in your relationship.
- If you don't respond to self-help measures; you may have an illness.
- If you think a drug is the cause.
- If you are depressed.

HOW TO PREVENT IT

- Take steps to reduce **stress** (see page 222, and **relax,** page 309).
- Exercise regularly and eat good food (see **eat well,** page 302). Get plenty of sleep.
- Devote time to your relationship. Set aside time to go out on "dates," or create romantic evenings at home.
- Try to solve problems in your relationship before they build up.

FOR MORE HELP

Information line: Sexuality Information and Education Council of the United States, 212-819-9770, M–F 12–5 EST. Suggests clinics and hospitals dealing with sexual problems; sends facts for a fee.

Organization: American Association of Marriage and Family Therapists, 1133 15th St. NW, Suite 300, Washington, DC 20005. Send a self-addressed, stamped envelope for a list of counselors near you.

Organization: American Association of Sex Educators, Counselors, and Therapists, Box 238, Mount Vernon, IA 52314. Sends lists of sex therapists near you.

Men's Health

Erection Problems

SIGNS AND SYMPTOMS

- Frequent trouble getting and keeping an erection for intercourse.

Erection problems are more common than people think—though people differ about what's a "problem." Many men have trouble getting an erection now and then, maybe more often as they age. If you are often unable to get erections and this bothers you, talk to your doctor.

An erection is a complex process, and many things can interfere with it. The most common are physical problems, including **diabetes** (see page 282); reduced blood flow to the penis (see **artery disease,** page 106); a sports injury; and too much alcohol (see **alcohol abuse and alcoholism,** page 206). Drugs prescribed for high blood pressure and depression, and psychological stresses such as **depression** (see page 213), worry, guilt, or "performance anxiety" can also cause trouble.

Although erection problems may embarrass or upset you, they can almost always be treated.

WHAT YOU CAN DO NOW

- See if a drug you are taking might be the cause. Many blood pressure drugs, among others, can affect sexual function. Ask your doctor or pharmacist.
- Don't drink alcohol or smoke (see **alcohol abuse and alcoholism,** page 206, and **smoking and illness,** page 220). Both make the problem worse.
- Check your stress level (see **is stress putting your health at risk?** page 308). Tension, worry, and conflict can chill interest in sex.
- Wait before you worry: If you have had a recent crisis—a loss, a breakup, a major change—your sex drive may just be taking a rest (see **loss of sexual desire,** page 231, and **grief,** page 219).
- Relax when making love. Take your time and try more foreplay. Tell your partner what arouses you.
- Share your feelings and worries about your performance—but not while making love. Set aside some time to talk with your partner about it.
- Try reading or using erotic materials, watching videos, or playing out sexual fantasies, if this appeals to you and your partner.
- See if you can get an erection while masturbating, when just waking up, or at other times when you aren't making love. If you can, the problem is most likely not physical.

WHEN TO CALL THE DOCTOR

- If erection problems often keep you from having intercourse or cause tension with your partner.

Testicle Problems

Pain, swelling, and tenderness in the testicles can have any number of causes, from sports injuries to illness (including mumps, when you get it as an adult). A lump can signal testicular cancer, the leading cancer for men between the ages of 20 and 35. Most doctors advise a monthly testicular self-exam (see self-exams, page 320).

SYMPTOMS	WHAT IT MIGHT BE	WHAT YOU CAN DO
Extreme pain and tenderness in either testicle; may spread to lower abdomen. Scrotum may be swollen, firm, and red. Sometimes faintness and nausea.	Testicular torsion—twisting of testicle and the tube that carries sperm to the prostate, cutting off blood supply to testicle.	Call doctor for prompt appointment. Can cause permanent damage if not treated promptly.
Firm, most often painless lump or swelling on one testicle. Testicle may feel heavy or hard, sometimes painful.	Testicular cancer. Most common in men between 15 and 34. Rarely fatal.	If you notice symptoms, call doctor for prompt appointment. Do a self-exam once a month after warm bath or shower. (See self-exams, page 320.)
Swelling and pain around testicle; comes on slowly, then becomes severe. Swollen area is hot and tender; swelling may spread to scrotum.	Epididymitis—inflamed sperm-storage tube (epididymis) behind each testicle. Causes include prostate infections and sexually transmitted diseases.	Call doctor for prompt appointment. Bed rest and ice packs may help. Antibiotics most often cure it; sex partners may also need treatment.
Soft, painless swelling in scrotum.	Hydrocele—excess fluid that builds up in membrane around each testicle. It's harmless.	Treatment of small hydroceles is most often not needed. If very large or painful, call doctor for advice and appointment.
Swollen veins in scrotum, almost always on left side. Most often no pain. Swelling lessens when you lie down.	Varicocele—varicose or enlarged veins in scrotum. Very common and most often harmless. In 20% of cases, can cause infertility.	Call doctor for advice.
Tenderness and pain in testicles or scrotum; not severe, may come and go.	Orchialgia—pain in testicles; no known cause, may be viral.	Take over-the-counter painkillers and warm baths. Call doctor for advice if pain lasts more than a week.

- If one of your medicines might be causing the problem.
- If physical causes have been ruled out, ask to be referred to a counselor or therapist.

HOW TO PREVENT IT

- Exercise regularly and eat well (see **staying healthy,** page 297).
- Reduce your stress: Try deep breathing, meditation, or yoga (see **relax,** page 309).
- Sometimes, daily pelvic muscle exercises help men with artery disease or other circulation problems. Called Kegel exercises, they also tone the muscles that control urination. Begin by sensing which muscles you use to start and stop urination. Later, contract and release them in 15 to 20 squeezes, 3 times a day. Work up to holding the squeeze for at least 10 seconds each time.

FOR MORE HELP

Information line: Impotence Institute of America, 8201 Corporate Dr., Suite 320, Landover, MD 20785. 800-669-1603, M–F 9–5 EST. Staff answers questions and sends brochures.

Organization: American Foundation for Urologic Disease, 300 W. Pratt St., Suite 401, Baltimore, MD 21201. 410-727-2908, M–F 8:30–5 EST. Ask for the brochure on erection problems.

Organization: National Kidney and Urologic Diseases Information Clearinghouse, Box NKUDIC, 3 Information Way, Bethesda, MD 20892-3580. Write for facts about erection problems.

Web access: National Institute of Diabetes and Digestive and Kidney Diseases. After logging on to the Internet, type: *http://www.niddk.nih.gov.* Scroll to *Information on Disorders,* then click on *Urologic Diseases* under that heading.

Prostate Problems

SIGNS AND SYMPTOMS

General symptoms:

- Frequent, urgent, sometimes painful need to urinate; urine may be bloody.
- Weak or dribbling stream of urine.
- Incontinence (sometimes).

Enlarged prostate:

- Sometimes a feeling the bladder is not emptied.

Prostate cancer:

Often no symptoms in early stages, sometimes followed by the symptoms above. In later stages:

- Pain in the lower back or pelvis, or sometimes in other places.
- Weight loss.

Prostatitis:

- Pain between the anus and scrotum.
- Painful ejaculation; blood in the semen or urine.
- Fever and chills (acute prostatitis).
- Lower back pain.

The prostate is a chestnut-size gland that wraps around the urethra (the tube that runs between a man's bladder and the end of his penis; see color illustration, page 175). It makes most of the fluid in semen that carries sperm.

Enlarged prostate: In most men, the prostate gland grows larger with age—75 percent of men over 50 have somewhat larger prostates. As it grows, it can squeeze the urethra and obstruct urine flow. This benign enlarged prostate isn't cancer. It doesn't lead to cancer. Nor does it need to be treated unless difficult or frequent urination becomes a problem. Then surgery or drugs can help.

Prostate cancer: A tumor in the prostate is the most common cancer in American men. It can exist for many years without symptoms, until the tumor grows large enough to affect urination and produce other symptoms.

Prostate cancer grows slowly and can be treated best when caught early. If untreated, it may spread to other organs or bone. Treat-

DO YOU HAVE A PROSTATE PROBLEM?

Urinary problems are key signs of an enlarged prostate gland. The American Urological Association's Symptom Score Index, aimed at spotting such problems, can help a man check his prostate health. It does not detect prostate cancer.

Circle your response to each question. A total score of 7 or below means no problem or no more than a mild problem; 8 to 19 is mild; 20 to 35 is severe. Note: The AUA advises that your doctor explain the results of this test.

In the last month, how often have you:	**Never**	**Less than one time in five**	**Less than half the time**	**About half the time**	**More than half the time**	**Almost always**
Had a feeling of not having emptied your bladder completely after you finished urinating?	0	1	2	3	4	5
Had to urinate again less than 2 hours after you last urinated?	0	1	2	3	4	5
Found your flow stopped and started again several times when you urinated?	0	1	2	3	4	5
Found it difficult to postpone urination?	0	1	2	3	4	5
Had a weak urinary stream?	0	1	2	3	4	5
Had to push or strain to begin urination?	0	1	2	3	4	5
In the last month, about how many times a night did you:	**Never**	**One**	**Two**	**Three**	**Four**	**Five or more**
Get up to urinate from the time you went to bed until the time you got up in the morning?	0	1	2	3	4	5

Adapted with permission of the *Journal of Urology*

ment can include surgery, radiation, or hormone therapy.

Prostatitis: This is an inflamed prostate. One form is caused by bacteria, which can move to the prostate from the urinary system. In acute cases, an abscess may form that has to be drained. In chronic cases, the infection causes lasting discomfort but rarely a fever. Sometimes its only symptom is repeated bladder infections. Another, more common form of prostatitis is not caused by bacteria—it has no known cause—and does not respond to antibiotics.

PENIS PROBLEMS

Most problems with the penis are rare.

An erection that won't go away (priapism): This painful problem occurs when blood cannot drain from the penis. It may result from penile injections (including those intended to produce erections), diseases such as leukemia or sickle-cell anemia, side effects of some drugs, or injury. Priapism has nothing to do with arousal. If an erection does not subside after 4 hours, call your doctor for emergency advice. If you can't get him or her, call 911 or go to an emergency room.

A small, pimplelike sore: Most often on the head of the penis, a sore that lasts more than 1 or 2 weeks can be a sign of penis cancer or of a **sexually transmitted disease** (see chart on page 225). In later stages, cancer symptoms may include bleeding or discharge, pain with urination, and enlarged lymph nodes in the groin. Penis cancer is most common in uncircumcised men. Call your doctor for prompt appointment if you detect any lasting sore or growth.

Blisters: One or more, on or around the penis, can mean a herpes infection. An outbreak can be itchy, painful, or both, and needs a doctor's care.

A bend in the penis (Peyronie's disease): This occurs during an erection and can be painful. It may be caused by scar tissue in the penis—mainly from an injury—that does not stretch enough. The problem most often goes away without treatment. In rare cases, it may require surgery.

Soreness and inflammation of the tip of the penis (balanitis): This can be caused by infection or by irritation from clothing, condoms, or spermicides. It's most common in men who are uncircumcised. Call your doctor for advice and an appointment.

Tight foreskin (phimosis): Sometimes the foreskin in uncircumcised boys or men is too tight to retract easily; this may make erections painful. Phimosis can also be caused by an infection under the foreskin. Uncircumcised men and men with diabetes have a higher chance of getting such infections. Call your doctor for advice and an appointment.

WHAT YOU CAN DO NOW

- Drink water all day, as much as you can.
- If you are getting up often to urinate at night, avoid caffeine and alcohol.
- Warm baths may help relieve pain.
- Take the prostate quiz (see box on page 235). Go over the results with your doctor.
- Try an over-the-counter painkiller for painful urination.

WHEN TO CALL THE DOCTOR

- If you have the symptoms listed.

HOW TO PREVENT IT

Enlarged prostate:

- There is no known way to prevent this.

Prostate cancer:

- Know your genes (see **a family tree,** page 319): If your father or brother had prostate cancer, your risk is much higher than if they didn't. This makes the next steps even more vital.
- Cut down on animal fat in your diet; men who eat a lot of fat may increase their risk.
- Get a rectal exam each year after age 50 to check for lumps on the gland. African Americans and men with a family history of prostate cancer should begin their yearly tests at age 40.
- Some doctors also advise a blood test for prostate-specific antigen, or PSA, that can detect prostate cancer.

Prostatitis:

- Treat any urinary tract infection before it can spread.

FOR MORE HELP

Information line: American Prostate Society, 1340 Charwood Rd., Hanover, MD 21076, 800-308-1106, M–F 9–5 EST. Volunteers answer questions and send out brochures.

Organization: American Foundation for Urologic Disease, 300 W. Pratt St., Suite 401, Baltimore, MD 21201. 410-727-2908, M–F 8:30–5 EST. Staff sends facts about prostate problems.

Book: *The Prostate Book: Sound Advice on Symptoms and Treatment,* by Stephen N. Rous, M.D. A fine guide to the male genital and urinary anatomy and prostate conditions. W. W. Norton, 1995, $12 paperback.

Book: *The Prostate: A Guide for Men and the Women Who Love Them,* by Patrick Walsh, M.D., and Janet Farrar Worthington. Covers prostate problems and treatment. Johns Hopkins University Press, 1995, $15.95.

Web access: American Cancer Society. After logging on to the Internet, type: *http://www.cancer.org.* Click on *Prostate Cancer.*

Videos: *Prostate Cancer at Time of Diagnosis* and *Prostate Disorders at Time of Diagnosis.* Clear overviews of causes and treatments, with 4 reports—Understanding the Diagnosis, What Happens Next?, Treatment and Management, and Issues and Answers. Time Life Medical, 1996, $19.95 each. Sold in many pharmacies; for one near you, call 800-588-9959.

Women's Health

Menopause

SIGNS AND SYMPTOMS

Many women have few or no signs that they are entering menopause. If you do feel some changes, they may include:

- Hot flashes or flushes—a sudden feeling of heat, mostly on the face, neck, and chest. May include profuse sweating during the day and night sweats that disrupt sleep.
- Irregular periods. Menstrual flow may be very heavy or very light and then periods cease.
- Irritability and mood swings.
- Sleep disorders.
- Vaginal dryness.
- Pain during intercourse.

Sometime between her late 30s and late 50s, a woman's body begins to prepare for menopause. The levels of hormones needed for pregnancy—estrogen and progesterone—decline. As a result, her periods become irregular. Her ovaries stop releasing eggs and, finally, she stops menstruating.

Menopause can come earlier or later. The average age is about 51. Illness or surgery that removes the ovaries can also bring it on quickly, but it is most often a gradual process, taking 2 to 5 years.

Some women don't notice any major changes in their bodies except the end of their periods. Many have some or all of the signs listed above, but don't find the process very uncomfortable. About 1 in 4 will have a stronger response to the shift in hormone levels and may feel emotional or physical distress.

The decline in hormone levels can lead to health problems for some women. Low estrogen levels can cause bone loss (see **osteoporosis,** page 198), which can result in broken bones and spinal problems. It can also raise cholesterol levels, leading to a higher risk of heart disease. For these reasons, many doctors prescribe **hormone replacement** therapy (see box, page 241), but the treatment has some risks. Discuss it with your doctor.

For many women, menopause is a positive life change that means freedom from menstrual periods and from concerns about birth control and pregnancy. It can also be a time of sadness and loss, as a woman's parents enter old age or die, and she and her partner face signs of their own aging. If a woman has children, they may be leaving home at about the same time her fertility ends.

And all change—even good change—can lead to **stress** (see page 222). Exercise, diet, support systems, and lifestyle adjustments can help lower stress levels as you move through this "change of life."

WHAT YOU CAN DO NOW

➤ Ask if your local hospital has a menopause support group. Talk to your family and friends about the changes you are going through and how they affect your feelings.

Menstrual Irregularities

All women should have pelvic exams as often as once a year if they are sexually active, so that any problems can be found and treated early. Be sure to tell your doctor about any changes in your menstrual cycle.

SYMPTOMS	WHAT IT MIGHT BE	WHAT YOU CAN DO
Missed menstrual periods or very heavy, painful periods; cramps, pain, or sense of pressure in lower abdomen; vaginal spotting or bleeding.	Ectopic pregnancy—pregnancy outside uterus, usually in fallopian tube (see color illustration, page 175).	Call doctor for prompt appointment. If bleeding or abdominal pain is severe, call 911 or go to emergency room **right away.**
Bleeding or spotting during pregnancy.	Common, but may signal a problem.	Call a doctor for prompt advice. If you can't get one, call 911 or go to emergency room **right away.**
Very heavy or painful periods, chiefly toward the end; pain in lower abdomen, vagina, or lower back that may begin just before period and worsen just after; pain during intercourse; blood in urine or stool while menstruating; nausea and vomiting just before period begins.	Endometriosis—disorder in which tissue that lines uterus grows outside uterus and becomes attached to other organs.	If you have symptoms for the first time or if pain is severe, call doctor for prompt appointment.
Very heavy, irregular, or missed menstrual periods; pain in lower abdomen or back; foul-smelling vaginal discharge; pain during intercourse; fever and sometimes chills.	Pelvic inflammatory disease (see page 242)—infection of reproductive organs, often caused by sexually transmitted diseases (see chart on page 225).	Call doctor for prompt appointment.
Changes in heaviness of flow, length of periods, or time between periods; aches or pain in abdomen; feeling of fullness, swelling, or pressure in abdomen; frequent urination.	Noncancerous ovarian cyst. • Noncancerous ovarian tumor. • Ovarian cancer.	Call doctor for prompt appointment. It's vital to diagnose cancer right away.

(continued)

Menstrual Irregularities *(continued)*

SYMPTOMS	WHAT IT MIGHT BE	WHAT YOU CAN DO
Very heavy or painful menstrual period that begins a week or more late.	Early pregnancy and miscarriage.	If you think you may be pregnant and you are bleeding, call doctor for advice and appointment.
No menstrual period for several months.	Amenorrhea (absence of menstruation), which can be caused by emotional distress, hormone imbalance, dieting or eating disorders (see eating disorders, page 218), or strenuous athletic training. • Pregnancy (see page 244). • Breast-feeding. • Menopause (see page 238). • Abnormality of reproductive organs. • Use of certain drugs. • Stopping use of birth control pills.	Call doctor for advice. **Note:** If a young woman is over 16 and has never had a menstrual period, schedule appointment with doctor.
Very heavy periods; bleeding between periods; pain or discomfort in lower back or abdomen; frequent urination; constipation; possibly sudden, sharp pain in lower abdomen.	Uterine fibroid tumors—common, noncancerous masses in uterus. Sometimes tumor becomes twisted, cutting off its blood supply and causing severe pain.	Call doctor for advice and appointment. Write down dates you are bleeding and how many pads or tampons you use each day.
Very heavy or painful menstrual periods while using IUD or after you stop taking birth control pills.	Common side effect of IUDs. • Hormonal changes caused by going off the Pill (see birth control health risks, page 228).	Call doctor for advice about your birth control method.
Very heavy menstrual period soon after childbirth.	Normal.	If you have more than 2 heavy periods after giving birth, call doctor for advice.
Menstrual flow that is always heavy; periods that last more than 7 days; large clots of blood.	Probably no problem, but heavy bleeding can result in anemia (see page 278).	If bleeding is very heavy (you use more than 1 pad or tampon in an hour), call doctor for advice.

- Don't stop using birth control when your periods get irregular—keep using it for a year or two even after they stop, since you may still be releasing eggs and could get pregnant.
- If you are on birth control pills, you may have periods even after menopause. If you are near 50 and taking the Pill, ask your doctor about a blood check, called an FSH test, that can tell if it's safe to stop.
- Wear cotton clothes if you are having night sweats or hot flashes. Take naps during the day if night sweats are costing you sleep.
- Dress in layers so you can cool down. Use a fan.
- Drink at least 8 glasses of water a day.
- For vaginal dryness, use a lubricant. If you and your partner use condoms, use a water-soluble lubricant rather than petroleum jelly, which breaks down latex.
- Reduce stress (see **relax,** page 309).
- Reduce your risk of heart disease by making efforts to lose weight if you are overweight, by quitting smoking (see **smoking and illness,** page 220), and by switching to a low-fat diet.
- Try to get 1,200 to 1,500 mg of calcium a day in your diet or from supplements.
- Get regular weight-bearing exercise (such as walking, dancing, or lifting light weights) to guard against osteoporosis.
- Cut back on caffeine and alcohol.

WHEN TO CALL THE DOCTOR

- If you have heavy bleeding for a long time, or any bleeding a year after your period stops. This could be a sign of uterine cancer.
- If you have any symptoms that bother you.

FOR MORE HELP

Organization: National Institute on Aging, Information Center, Box 8057, Gaithersburg, MD 20898. 800-222-2225, M–F 8:30–5 EST. Sends fact sheets on menopause and estrogen therapy.

Organization: National Women's Health Resource Center, 202-293-6045, M–F 9–5 EST. Ask for a copy of the *National Women's Health Report;* it covers menopause ($5). Staff also refers callers to women's centers and support groups.

Book: *What Every Woman Needs to Know About Menopause,* by Mary Jane Minkin, M.D., and Carol V. Wright. Yale University Press, 1996, $22.50.

IS HORMONE REPLACEMENT RIGHT FOR YOU?

As a woman enters menopause, she'll face a decision about hormone replacement therapy. Studies have shown that estrogen—the major ingredient in hormone therapy—can prevent bone loss and fractures, and can reduce the risk of heart disease. Hormone replacement therapy also helps ease the short-term effects of menopause.

Doctors often prescribe a mixture of estrogen and progestin for women who have not had a hysterectomy. This protects women against endometrial cancer, which taking estrogen alone does not. Combined hormone therapy has also been shown to raise levels of HDL ("good") cholesterol and lower levels of LDL ("bad") cholesterol, and to help prevent bone fractures in women who already have osteoporosis.

After menopause, women may take these hormones for the rest of their lives to protect against osteoporosis and heart disease. Questions remain about this therapy. Some studies have shown that it may increase the risk of breast cancer if taken for more than 5 years. Others suggest that the increased risk is due to aging. If you are thinking about hormone replacement therapy, be sure to discuss all the risks with your doctor.

Estrogen creams can help women with vaginal dryness or discomfort. Women who use these regularly must take progestin to reduce their risk of endometrial cancer.

Book: *The Complete Book of Menopause,* by Carol Landau, Ph.D., Michele G. Cyr, M.D., and Anne W. Moulton, M.D. Pedigree, 1994, $15.

Web access: Doctor's Guide to Menopause Information & Resources. After logging on to the Internet, type *http://www.pslgroup.com/Menopause.htm.* Offers medical news, drug therapies, discussion groups, and links to other sites.

Video: *Menopause at Time of Diagnosis.* Clear overview of causes and treatments, with 4 reports—Understanding the Diagnosis, What Happens Next?, Treatment and Management, and Issues and Answers. Time Life Medical, 1996, $19.95. Sold in many pharmacies; for one near you, call 800-588-9959.

Pelvic Inflammatory Disease

SIGNS AND SYMPTOMS

Often PID has no symptoms. Sometimes it can cause:

- Mild to severe aching in the lower abdomen, sometimes with backache.
- Pain during intercourse.
- Fever, sometimes with chills.
- Absent or irregular periods, or very heavy bleeding.
- Heavy or foul-smelling discharge from the vagina.
- Frequent urination with burning pain.
- Nausea and vomiting.
- Trouble getting pregnant (chronic or prior PID).

Pelvic inflammatory disease (PID) is an infection of the female reproductive organs, including the ovaries, the fallopian tubes, the cervix, and the uterus. (See color illustration, page 175.) Untreated, it can result in fatal illnesses, such as blood poisoning or infection of the abdominal cavity. It can also cause infertility or ectopic pregnancy (in which a fertilized egg settles outside the uterus).

PID is often caused by the bacteria that produce gonorrhea and chlamydia (see **sexually transmitted diseases** chart, page 225). It may also be brought on by other bacteria that get into the upper genital region through sexual intercourse, abortion, miscarriage, childbirth, or hysterectomy.

Sexually active teens, women with more than one sexual partner, and those with a partner who has sex with others are most likely to get PID. Some experts believe that frequent douching may also increase the risk by pushing bacteria farther up into the reproductive system. Intrauterine devices (IUDs) increase the risk. Birth control pills, however, hinder the passage of bacteria and may slightly lower the chance of getting PID or may keep it from getting more severe.

PID can be treated with antibiotics, but it often comes back and may become chronic. (You may have it for a long time, with symptoms that come and go.) When antibiotics don't help, a doctor may have to remove or repair infected tissue.

WHAT YOU CAN DO NOW

After diagnosis:

- Take all of your drugs, even if symptoms are gone.
- If gonorrhea or chlamydia caused your PID, make sure your partner is treated. Otherwise, he may reinfect you or infect others.
- Don't have sex until all symptoms are gone.
- Get plenty of bed rest.
- If needed, take an over-the-counter painkiller such as ibuprofen.

WHEN TO CALL THE DOCTOR

- If you have symptoms of PID.

HOW TO PREVENT IT

- Practice **safe sex** (see box on page 227) to protect yourself from STDs.
- Have regular medical checkups if you are sexually active.

Breast Pain or Lumps

Breasts change with puberty, with your menstrual cycle, and with pregnancy, and they change with age. Starting at puberty, women should examine their breasts every month, so that they know their structure and can detect any masses or lumps (see **breast self-exam** box, page 245). Most changes in breasts are normal and no cause for concern. Some, however, require medical care.

SYMPTOMS	WHAT IT MIGHT BE	WHAT YOU CAN DO
Lump (usually painless) in breast or underarm area; flat area or indentation on breast; change in contour, texture, size, or symmetry of breast; change in nipple (such as indrawn or dimpled look, itching or burning feeling, or discharge that may be dark or bloody).	Noncancerous cyst. • Noncancerous tumor. • Breast cancer (if breast is painful, could signal advanced stage).	Call doctor for prompt appointment. Most lumps are not cancerous, but it is very important to have an exam. Biopsy may be needed to diagnose or rule out breast cancer.
After having just given birth: pain and tenderness in breast, hard or swollen breast, fever, area with redness and pain.	Infection of breast (mastitis), caused by bacteria. Redness and pain can mean an abscess.	Call doctor for advice and appointment. Keep on breast-feeding. If you get an abscess, use a breast pump on infected side and feed on uninfected side. If you have a fever, rest in bed and drink plenty of fluids.
Pain, tenderness, or swelling in breasts; missed period; fatigue; nausea.	Pregnancy (see page 244).	Call doctor for advice and make appointment for pregnancy test. Wear support bra.
Less than 5 days after having given birth: tenderness, hardness, or swelling in breast. Also, when breast-feeding mother cannot keep to feeding schedule.	Swelling with milk.	Nurse more often, or try using warm compresses to reduce discomfort. Call doctor for advice if symptoms persist.
In women who are breast-feeding: sore nipple or sharp pain in nipple while nursing.	Sore or cracked nipples, common during first few weeks of breast-feeding.	Gently wash nipples after nursing and apply pure vitamin E oil. With fever, call doctor for advice.
Breast pain while taking estrogen.	Drug side effect.	Call doctor for advice.

(continued)

Breast Pain or Lumps *(continued)*

SYMPTOMS	WHAT IT MIGHT BE	WHAT YOU CAN DO
Lumpy or swollen breasts; pain or discomfort, chiefly in the week before menstrual period.	Fibrocystic breasts. More than half of all women develop this harmless condition, most often between ages of 25 and 50.	Call doctor for advice if you notice lumps for first time; if you notice a new lump; or if a lump becomes larger, harder, or more painful. Limit intake of caffeine. Wear support bra.
Pain or tenderness in breasts before menstrual period.	Premenstrual syndrome. • Irregular periods.	See premenstrual syndrome, page 247, and menstrual irregularities chart, page 239.

For more help: You can buy the videos *Breast Lumps at Time of Diagnosis* and *Breast Cancer at Time of Diagnosis.* Each provides a clear overview of causes and treatments, with 4 reports—Understanding the Diagnosis, What Happens Next?, Treatment and Management, and Issues and Answers. Time Life Medical, 1996, $19.95. Sold in many pharmacies; for one near you, call 800-588-9959.

➤ To prevent infection after pelvic surgery or a minor gynecologic procedure, don't douche or have intercourse for a week.

FOR MORE HELP

Hotline: National STD Hotline, Centers for Disease Control and Prevention, 800-227-8922, M–F 8AM–11PM EST. Staff answers questions about STDs and refers callers for testing.

Organization: American College of Obstetricians and Gynecologists, Resource Center, 409 12th St. NW, Box 96920, Washington, DC 20024-6920. Send a business-size, self-addressed, stamped envelope; ask for the brochure on PID.

Web access: Duke University. After logging on to the Internet, type: *http://h-devil-www.mc.duke.edu/h-devil/women/women.htm.* Covers PID and pelvic exams.

Pregnancy

The best time to start taking better care of your health is before you become pregnant. The first few weeks of your pregnancy can be crucial for the rapidly growing fetus. If you eat poorly, drink, smoke, or take drugs, you can harm your baby.

Good health habits and good prenatal care help assure a healthy baby. They also help you cope with the stress that comes with pregnancy, childbirth, and parenthood. If you are planning a pregnancy, you may want to visit your health care provider to discuss your diet, lifestyle, past pregnancies, medical history, and any medicines you are taking.

WHAT YOU CAN DO NOW

Diet, Rest, and Exercise

During your pregnancy, get plenty of rest and exercise, maintain a well-balanced diet, and avoid anything that can harm the fetus. Follow your health care provider's advice as well as these guidelines:

➤ Get enough calories, protein, iron, calcium,

HOW TO DO A BREAST SELF-EXAM

A regular breast self-exam is one of the best ways to find a cancerous tumor when it is small, before the cancer has a chance to spread. Check yourself at the same time every month, 2 to 3 days after your period. (Remember, self-examination is not a substitute for regular exams by a doctor.)

❶ Stand facing a mirror with your arms at your sides. Look for anything unusual on your breasts: dimples, scaly patches, puckers, or discharge coming from a nipple.

❷ Check for changes in the contours of your breasts. Watch in the mirror as you lift your hands behind your head, clasp your hands, and press them against the back of your head.

❸ Check again with your hands on your hips and your elbows pulled forward.

❹ Squeeze your nipples gently to check for discharge.

❺ With one arm raised, use the fingertips of your other hand to feel your breast for any lumps under the skin. Start in your armpit and move toward your breast, pressing in small areas about the size of a quarter. (Try this in the shower; your fingers will slide more easily over soapy skin.)

Use a definite pattern—a spiral, line, or wedge. Cover the entire breast, as well as the upper chest and underarm. Repeat on other side.

Spiral: Start at the outer edges of the breast and slowly work your way around the breast in smaller and smaller circles.

Line: Start under your arm and slowly move toward and across the breast.

Wedge: Start at the outer edge of the breast and move slowly toward the middle, then back to the edge. Repeat until you have covered the whole breast.

❻ Repeat step 5 lying on your back, with one arm over your head and a pillow under your shoulder. Use one of the patterns above to check each breast.

If you find a lump, unusual firmness, a change in shape, or any discharge from a nipple, call your doctor for a prompt appointment.

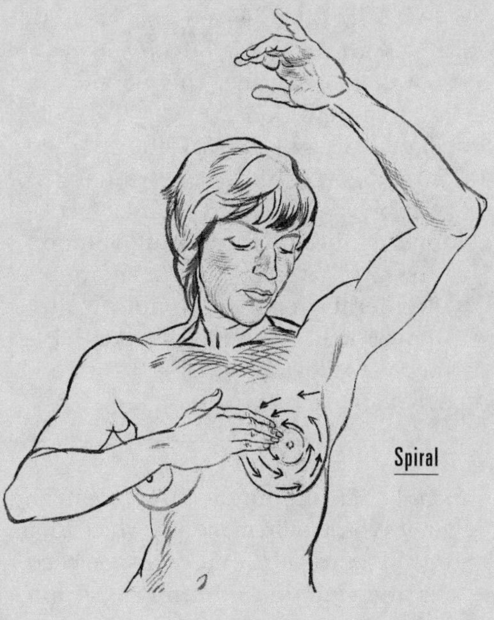

Spiral

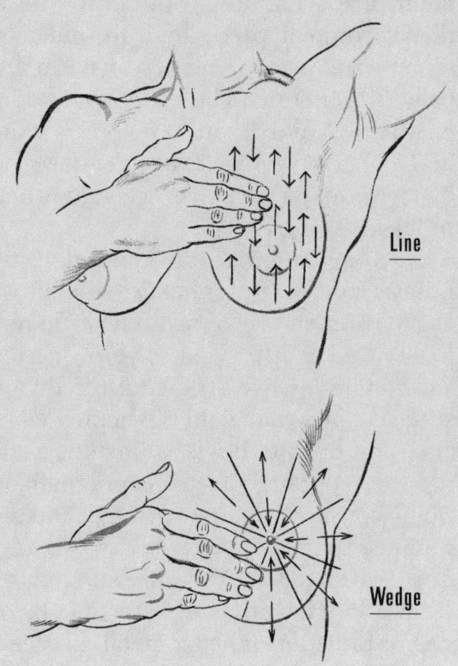

Line

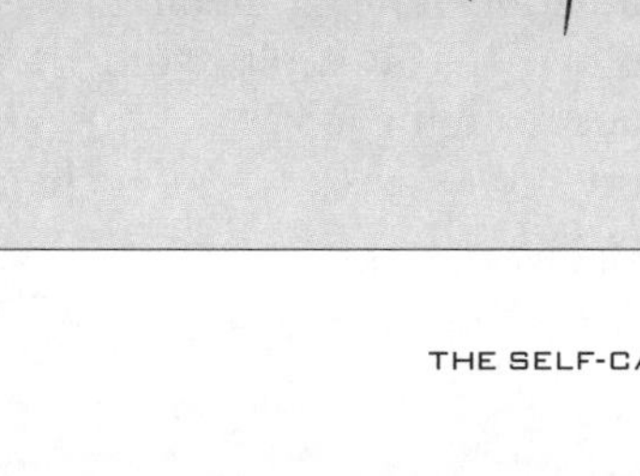

Wedge

DANGER SIGNS IN PREGNANCY

Call your doctor for a prompt appointment if you have:

- Vaginal bleeding or spotting. This is common, but it sometimes signals a miscarriage or other problem.
- Fever over 100 degrees; backache; chills; and frequent, burning urination or bloody urine. This may mean a kidney infection.
- Sudden weight gain, swelling of the hands and face, severe headache with blurred vision. These are signs of preeclampsia, a form of high blood pressure that can be very dangerous.
- Less fetal movement or none at all for more than a day (if the fetus has begun to move). The fetus may be in trouble.

and folic acid in your diet. (Ask about any changes you should make and which foods are good sources of the nutrients you need.)

- Take any vitamin and mineral supplements prescribed for you, but no more than the amount prescribed. Too much of some vitamins and minerals can harm the baby. (Recent research showed that women who took more than 10,000 IU of vitamin A per day were more likely to have babies with major heart defects and other problems.)
- Avoid things known to cause birth defects, miscarriages, or other harm to the fetus: Don't drink, smoke, or take any drugs not prescribed or approved by your doctor. That includes over-the-counter drugs such as aspirin and cold medicines. (You also should avoid those that include alcohol when you are trying to get pregnant or when you are breast-feeding. Consult your health care provider.)
- Cut down on caffeine (in coffee and sodas).
- Be aware of hazards in your workplace, such as radiation or heavy metals like lead and mercury. If you can't avoid them, think about changing jobs.
- Avoid paint fumes, gas, and other chemical vapors.
- Don't touch cat feces or litter boxes, and cook meat well-done. Cat feces and raw meat can spread toxoplasmosis, a disease that may cause miscarriage or birth defects.
- Exercise at least 3 times a week. Brisk walking, jogging, swimming, yoga, and low-impact aerobics are all good during pregnancy. Avoid heavy exercise, though, especially in hot weather. Wear a support bra to protect your breasts.
- Get enough rest. Go to bed early, and take breaks throughout the day to relax and put your feet up. Share more of the housework or child care with your partner, family, or friends.

Staying Comfortable

Try the following for some of the common discomforts of pregnancy:

Abdominal pain:

- Use a hot-water bottle or heating pad to relieve pain or cramps from stretched abdominal muscles.
- Don't change positions quickly, above all when turning at the waist.
- Call your doctor for advice if your pain persists or gets worse.

Backache:

- Don't take any over-the-counter drugs. Instead, use a hot-water bottle or a heating pad to relieve pain.
- Don't stand for a long time.
- Sit in chairs that have good support for your back, or use a small pillow behind your lower back. Keep your back straight and put your feet up.
- Sleep on a firm mattress, on your side, and put a pillow between your knees for support.
- Wear low-heeled shoes with good support, or shoe inserts made for pregnant women. Don't wear high heels.
- Try pregnancy underwear, or an elastic sling for abdominal support.

Breast discomfort:

- Wear a support bra.

Constipation: See page 121.

Headache: See page 54.

- Get enough rest.
- Eat small meals often, and drink at least 8 glasses of water a day.
- Learn yoga or meditation to relieve stress.

➤ Call your doctor if your headache lasts or is severe, or if it comes with nausea or blurred vision.

Heartburn: See page 127.

Hemorrhoids: See page 128.

➤ Don't use over-the-counter hemorrhoid treatments without asking your health care provider.

Nausea and vomiting (morning sickness): See page 133.

➤ Eat crackers or plain toast as soon as you wake up. Sit on your bed for a few minutes before getting up.

➤ Try to eat often so you never have an empty stomach. Snack all day rather than eating 3 full meals. (The best snacks are high-protein foods such as nuts, yogurt, granola, and peanut butter on apple slices or celery.) Have a snack at bedtime and when you get up during the night.

➤ Drink plenty of water and other liquids, but avoid milk, citrus juices, coffee, tea, and sodas with caffeine.

➤ Try papaya juice or almonds to ease nausea. Also try fresh ginger—put a small piece on your tongue or make a tea by grating and steeping ginger in hot water.

➤ Call your doctor if you have severe nausea and vomiting; rapid heartbeat; pale, dry skin; or signs of dehydration (dry mouth, sticky saliva, dizziness, decreased urination, sometimes thirst).

Urinary tract infections:

➤ Call your doctor if you have pain when you urinate, or if you think you have a bladder or other urinary tract infection (see **painful urination,** page 140).

➤ Use a hot-water bottle or heating pad on your lower abdomen for pain.

➤ Drink at least 8 to 10 glasses of water a day.

➤ Drink cranberry juice daily to help prevent urinary tract infections.

Varicose veins and swelling in the legs: See page 116.

➤ Exercise daily.

➤ Don't stand or sit for long periods.

➤ Put your legs up when you can.

FOR MORE HELP

Organization: Healthy Mothers, Healthy Babies Coalition, 800-673-8444, ext. 2458, M–F 9–5 EST. Offers facts about prenatal and baby health education programs.

Book: *What to Expect When You're Expecting*, by Arlene Eisenberg, Heidi E. Murkoff, and Sandee E. Hathaway, B.S.N. The classic guide to pregnancy. Workman Publishing, 1991, $10.95.

Web access: Childbirth.org. After logging on to the Internet, type *http://www.childbirth.org*. Offers pregnancy and childbirth information, personal stories, and links to other sites.

Video: *Pregnancy at Time of Diagnosis.* Clear overview with 4 reports—Understanding the Diagnosis, What Happens Next?, Treatment and Management, and Issues and Answers. Time Life Medical, 1996, $19.95. Sold in many pharmacies; for one near you, call 800-588-9959.

Premenstrual Syndrome

SIGNS AND SYMPTOMS

- Bloating and weight gain.
- Breast swelling or tenderness.
- Headaches.
- Dizziness.
- Fatigue.
- Decrease or increase in sex drive.
- Outbreaks of acne.
- Mood swings, bad temper, nervousness, or depression.
- Food cravings.
- Diarrhea or constipation.

PMS, or premenstrual syndrome, affects many women some of the time, and some women nearly every month. It is marked by a range of physical and emotional changes that begin 1 to 2 weeks before a woman's period and stop when her period starts. The symptoms can be mild or severe. Some women feel just a little low on energy, while a small number get so depressed or tense that they can barely function.

No one knows for sure what causes PMS. It may result from changes in hormone levels, monthly changes in brain chemicals, or poor diet.

WHAT YOU CAN DO NOW

- Change your diet. For the week before your period, don't use salt, sugar, or caffeine (in coffee, tea, sodas, and chocolate). Limit fats, and add grains, fruit, and vegetables (see **eat well,** page 302).
- Cut out alcohol in the week before your period—it can worsen headaches, fatigue, and depression.
- Eat small meals often—6 times a day—and snack to maintain a steady level of blood sugar.
- Exercise daily. Raising your body temperature can help your body balance hormones.
- Reduce stress (see **relax,** page 309). Practice yoga or meditation. Take a stress reduction course.
- Take good care of yourself. Get more sleep. Take long, warm baths. Get a massage.
- PMS medication or an over-the-counter painkiller may help with bloating, cramps, and aches.
- Join a PMS support or self-help group.

WHEN TO CALL THE DOCTOR

- If you've tried the advice above, but your symptoms still bother you.

HOW TO PREVENT IT

There are no ways to prevent PMS, but the advice above about diet, rest, and exercise can help soften the impact.

FOR MORE HELP

Organization: PMS Research Foundation, Box 14574, Las Vegas, NV 89114. Send a letter describing your symptoms along with $5 postage for advice and names of doctors near you.

Book: *All About Eve: The Complete Guide to Women's Health and Well-Being*, by Tracy Chutorian Semler. Contains a chapter on PMS. HarperCollins, 1995, $16.

Book: *PMS: Solving the Puzzle,* by Linaya Hahn. Offers theories on causes and treatment of PMS. Chicago Spectrum Press, 1996, $16.95.

Web access: Duke University. After logging on to the Internet, type: *http://h-devil-www.mc.duke.edu/h-devil/women/women.htm.* Covers PMS and cramps.

Toxic Shock Syndrome

SIGNS AND SYMPTOMS

Call 911 or go to an emergency room **right away** if you have:

- Sudden fever (over 102 degrees).
- Diarrhea.
- Vomiting.
- A deep red, sunburnlike rash, most often on the palms of the hands or soles of the feet.
- Headache, confusion, or dizziness.
- Weakness or fainting.

Toxic shock syndrome comes on suddenly and can cause severe illness. It is caused by common bacteria (*Staphylococcus aureus*) that release toxins into the bloodstream.

Toxic shock occurs chiefly among menstruating women who use tampons—most of all superabsorbent tampons. When a tampon is left in place for a long time, it can trap the bacteria and give them an ideal place to grow. Toxic shock has also been linked to the use of birth control sponges and—very rarely—to diaphragms and cervical caps.

The disease can also affect children, men, and women of all ages who are exposed to the bacteria through surgery, a burn, or an open wound.

Toxic shock syndrome requires emergency care. In most cases, people are hospitalized and given intravenous antibiotics to kill the bacteria. If untreated, it can cause liver or kidney failure, severe shock, and—in rare cases—death. Most patients recover though, if they are treated quickly.

WHAT YOU CAN DO NOW

- If you have symptoms of toxic shock, call 911 or go to an emergency room **right away.** If you have a tampon, a menstrual sponge, a birth control sponge, a diaphragm, or a cervical cap inside you, remove it right away.

WHEN TO CALL THE DOCTOR

Call 911 or go to an emergency room **right away:**

- If you have symptoms of toxic shock syndrome—above all if you are menstruating and have been using tampons.

Call for a prompt appointment:

- If you are being treated for toxic shock syndrome and you get new symptoms. Drugs used to treat the illness may produce side effects.

HOW TO PREVENT IT

- Use tampons less often. If you don't want to stop using them, wear tampons made of cotton, which pose the least risk. Switch between tampons and sanitary pads. If you've ever had toxic shock syndrome, don't use tampons at all.
- Don't use superabsorbent tampons.
- Change tampons at least every 4 to 6 hours.
- Don't use tampons or menstrual sponges overnight.
- If you use a diaphragm or cervical cap, never leave the diaphragm in for more than 24 hours (8 hours during your period) or the cervical cap in for more than 48 hours.
- Wash your diaphragm or cervical cap after each use in warm, soapy water. Rinse and dry it well with a clean towel.
- Wash your hands well before you insert a tampon or any other device.
- Always clean and disinfect cuts or scrapes anywhere on your body. If a wound appears to be infected, get medical help.

FOR MORE HELP

Organization: National Women's Health Network, 202-628-7814, M–F 9–5 EST. Staff answers questions on toxic shock syndrome and sends a fact packet for a small fee.

Vaginal Problems

SIGNS AND SYMPTOMS

Yeast infection:

- Redness, itching, and sometimes burning during urination.
- Pain during intercourse.
- White, cheesy, odorless discharge (sometimes).

Bacterial vaginosis:

- Watery, grayish white or yellow discharge with a fishy odor.
- Mild burning or irritation.

Contact dermatitis:

- Redness and itching of the vulva (the outer genital area).

The term *vaginitis* refers to many irritations of a woman's genital area.

A **yeast infection** is the most common. It's caused by overgrowth of a fungus normally found in the vagina. It can be brought on by pregnancy, diabetes, use of antibiotics, and sometimes use of the Pill. Hot weather and clothing made of synthetic materials such as polyester (which doesn't allow air to reach your skin) can cause it. Some experts believe that feminine hygiene products also cause it. If you get frequent yeast infections, your doctor can prescribe antifungal pills.

Bacterial vaginosis occurs when bacteria normally found in the vagina grow out of control or when bacteria normally found in the rectum spread to the vagina. Poor health, poor hygiene, or clothing made of material that does not allow air to reach the skin can make it more likely.

Contact dermatitis may be caused by chemicals in latex condoms, spermicides, or diaphragms; feminine hygiene sprays; colored or scented toilet tissue; soaps, detergents, or fabric softeners; and deodorant tampons or sanitary pads (see **dermatitis,** page 151). Your doctor can prescribe an ointment for contact dermatitis that won't go away.

WOMEN'S HEALTH RESOURCES

Organization: National Women's Health Resource Center, 202-293-6045, M–F 9–5 EST. Offers fact sheets and brochures on a range of women's issues and publishes the *National Women's Health Report* newsletter (6 issues for $25). Staff members will perform a search on a specific topic and supply lists of women's centers near you.

Organization: American College of Obstetricians and Gynecologists, Resource Center, 409 12th St. SW, Washington, DC 20024-6920. Offers pamphlets on a range of topics, from birth control and pregnancy to menopause, PMS, and cancer. Send a business-size, self-addressed, stamped envelope and request the topic you need.

Book: *The New Our Bodies, Ourselves,* by the Boston Women's Health Book Collective. The bible of women's self-help medical books. Touchstone, 1992, $20.

Book: *American Medical Association Complete Guide to Women's Health* with medical editor Ramona Slupik, M.D. Covers health issues for every age group, from safe sex and weight control to depression and hormone replacement therapy. Random House, 1996, $39.95.

Book: *Dr. Susan Love's Breast Book,* by Susan M. Love, M.D. Latest edition of the classic breast care guide. Addison-Wesley, 1995, $17.

Web access: Breast Cancer Information Clearinghouse. After logging on to the Internet, type: *http://nysernet.org/bcic.* Covers most issues related to breast cancer prevention and treatment and lists other resources.

Web access: Women's Medical Health Page. After logging on to the Internet, type: *http://www.best.com/~sirlou/wmhp.html.* Offers the latest news on a range of women's health issues.

WHAT YOU CAN DO NOW

For all vaginitis:

- Don't have intercourse for 2 weeks, or until all soreness is gone.
- Don't scratch. Use cool compresses or sitz baths to ease itching.
- Use plain yogurt with live acidophilus cultures (check the label) to make a compress or to put in the vagina. You can apply it as a douche, or with a spoon or applicator made for vaginal treatments.
- Keep your vulva clean, and dry it well after urinating or showering. You can use a hair dryer set on low to blow warm, dry air on the sore area—just be careful of the heat.
- If urinating causes pain, urinate through a plastic or paper cup with the bottom cut out. Press it against your vulva to keep urine from touching sore skin. Or use a spray bottle to squirt warm water over the vulva while urinating.
- Wash all underwear in mild, fragrance-free soap or detergent (soap made for baby laundry is good) and rinse twice. Don't use fabric softener or bleach.

Yeast infection:

- If you are sure it is a yeast infection, use an over-the-counter antifungal cream made for yeast infections. Be sure to use all of the cream as directed, even after your symptoms are gone.
- The infection can spread, so stop having sex until you finish treatment. Your sexual partner may need treatment also to keep from reinfecting you.

WHEN TO CALL THE DOCTOR

Call for a prompt appointment:

- If you have bleeding between menstrual periods or after menopause; a firm, raised lesion or bump on the vulva or inside the vagina; or vaginal pain and itching that doesn't go away. These may be signs of cancer of the vagina or vulva.
- If you notice a vaginal discharge that is yellow or green and foul-smelling. This may be a symptom of a **sexually trans-**

mitted disease (see chart on page 225).

Call for advice and an appointment:

- If you have symptoms of bacterial vaginosis. Your doctor can treat the infection with an oral antibiotic. It can spread, so be sure your partner is also treated.
- If you have any vaginal symptoms for the first time, or if they recur more than twice a year.
- If symptoms don't go away after treatment, or are severe.

HOW TO PREVENT IT

- Wipe from front to back after a bowel movement to avoid spreading bacteria from the rectum to the vagina.
- Don't use scented toilet paper or perfumed soaps, feminine hygiene sprays, douches, or scented or deodorant tampons or sanitary pads.
- Change tampons and sanitary pads at least 4 times a day.
- Clean diaphragms, cervical caps, and spermicidal applicators well after each use.
- Don't wear tight pants, fabrics and clothing that can trap moisture, or underwear or panty hose with a crotch that's not cotton.
- If you are taking antibiotics, ask your doctor if you should use an antifungal cream in your vagina to prevent a yeast infection.
- Eat a cup of yogurt with live cultures every day (check the label).
- Check your vulva monthly for changes.

FOR MORE HELP

Organization: National Women's Health Network, 202-628-7814, M–F 9–5 EST. Staff answers questions and sends facts about vaginitis and yeast infections ($6 members, $8 nonmembers).

Organization: American College of Obstetricians and Gynecologists, Resource Center, 409 12th St. SW, Washington, DC 20024-6920. Send a business-size, self-addressed, stamped envelope, and request the pamphlet on vaginitis.

Book: *Every Woman's Body: Everything You Need to Know to Make Informed Choices About Your Health,* by Diana Korte. Fawcett Columbine, 1994, $15.

Web access: Duke University. After logging on to the Internet, type: *http://h-devil-www.mc.duke.edu/h-devil/women/women.htm.* Covers vaginal and urinary tract infections.

Children's Health

Bed-Wetting

SIGNS AND SYMPTOMS

Bed-wetting now and then is normal. It may be a problem:

- If your child is 6 or older and seldom stays dry overnight.
- If you are concerned about it, or your child is.

Bed-wetting is common, even well beyond the time of toilet training. About 1 child in 10 will wet the bed past the age of 5. Boys are more prone to bed-wetting than girls, and it tends to run in families. Some children who wet the bed simply have small bladders, or their nerves and muscles have not matured enough to control their bladders all night. Less often, a child doesn't have enough of a hormone that helps the kidneys hold urine. Most children outgrow these problems by their teens.

If your child has been dry during the night for a while and then starts wetting the bed, this could be a warning sign of something such as diabetes or a bladder infection. Or it may be a reaction to a stressful recent event, such as the birth of a brother or sister.

WHAT YOU CAN DO NOW

- Remind your child to use the bathroom just before bed each night.
- Limit the amount your child drinks before bedtime.
- Don't give your child drinks with caffeine, such as colas and teas. Caffeine increases the flow of urine.
- If your child has been sleeping for more than an hour, wake him or her to use the toilet again before you go to bed.
- Praise your child for staying dry. (Never scold a child for bed-wetting; you may make the problem worse.)

WHEN TO CALL THE DOCTOR

Call for a prompt appointment:

- If it is painful for your child to urinate, or your child has bloody or very cloudy urine, abdominal pain, or a very narrow urine stream. Any of these could signal a bladder infection.

Call for advice:

- If your child feels frustrated, or you do.

HOW TO PREVENT IT

- Try bladder training: Once a day, tell your child to hold his or her urine for a few minutes past the first feeling of a full bladder. Be patient: Practice for 3 months to give the child a chance to master it.

FOR MORE HELP

Information line: National Kidney Foundation Information Center, 800-622-9010, M–F 8:30–5 EST. Staff answers questions and sends reports on bed-wetting.

Children's Rashes

It's hard to tell if a childhood rash is a sign of a serious disease or a minor ailment. Also, babies and young children have delicate skin that may become inflamed and then clear up on its own. Look for other symptoms with the rash, and any changes in it—they are major clues to its cause.

SYMPTOMS	WHAT IT MIGHT BE	WHAT YOU CAN DO
Itchy red welts with pale centers, anywhere on body.	Hives (see page 157).	If child begins wheezing or has trouble swallowing, call 911 or go to emergency room **right away.** Otherwise, call doctor for advice .
Purple rash, pale skin, overall fatigue, headache, aching limbs, swollen glands, many infections, mouth sores.	Childhood leukemia.	Call doctor for prompt appointment.
First symptoms: sore throat, slight fever; 2 weeks later: painless, purple, spotted rash on ankles, elbows, shins, or buttocks.	Allergic purpura—a reaction that causes bleeding under the skin, forming a rash.	Call doctor for prompt appointment.
First symptoms: low fever, swollen glands; 2–3 days later: slightly raised red rash on face that spreads to rest of body.	German measles (rubella) (see page 263).	Call doctor for prompt appointment. Keep child away from pregnant women (this virus can damage a fetus).
First symptoms: fever as high as 105, cough, runny nose, pinkeye, overall sick feeling; 1–2 days later: rash of small red bumps starts on face and neck, then spreads to rest of body.	Measles (see page 267).	Call doctor for prompt appointment.
First symptoms: sore throat, fever of 101–104, headache; 1–2 days later: red, sandpaperlike rash begins on face and groin, spreads to torso, arms, and legs; may itch.	Scarlet fever (see page 271).	Call doctor for prompt appointment.

(continued)

Children's Health

Children's Rashes *(continued)*

SYMPTOMS	WHAT IT MIGHT BE	WHAT YOU CAN DO
Whitish patches in mouth and throat, or red patches in genital area.	Thrush (in mouth) or yeast infection (see fungal infections, page 155).	Call doctor for prompt appointment.
Blisters in mouth; blistering rash on hands, feet, and sometimes buttocks; fever up to 102; sore throat; loss of appetite.	Hand, foot, and mouth disease (see page 264).	Call doctor for prompt appointment if child has extreme trouble swallowing.
Small red itchy spots that turn into clear fluid–filled blisters; slight fever. Rash starts on face and torso.	Chicken pox (see facing page).	Call doctor for appointment. Ease itching with oatmeal baths or calamine lotion.
Bright red rash that looks like slapped cheeks starts on cheeks, then spreads, may itch; fever as high as 102; sometimes sore throat, headache, or fatigue.	Fifth disease (see page 262).	Call doctor for advice. Keep child away from pregnant women (this virus can damage a fetus).
First symptoms: fever as high as 105; mild cough, runny nose; 3–6 days later: red, spreading rash that disappears in a few hours to a few days.	Roseola (see page 270).	Call doctor for advice. If child's fever reaches 102 or higher, call doctor right away.
Round, scaly, itchy rash that appears mainly on scalp, feet, or around nails; creates bald patches on scalp.	Ringworm—a contagious fungal infection.	Call doctor for advice.
Dry, scaly skin; itchy red bumps; rash may cover small area or most of body; common on knees and elbows.	Eczema (see page 154).	If spreading, call doctor for advice. Soothe mild cases with cream; avoid lotions with preservatives, oils, or perfume.
Rash of small blisters, mostly on face, legs, or arms; blisters break and weep, forming golden crust.	Impetigo (see page 265).	Very contagious; keep rash and places around it clean with soap and water. If rash persists or gets worse, call doctor for advice.

Children's Rashes

SYMPTOMS	WHAT IT MIGHT BE	WHAT YOU CAN DO
Light red rash in spots or large blotches; occurs in hot weather.	Heat rash.	Remove clothing. Call doctor for prompt appointment if rash lasts 24 hours or if other symptoms appear.
Dry scales that turn into yellow, greasy patches; may be itchy. On scalp (in cradle cap); or in creases of neck, behind ears, in armpits, on face, or in diaper area (in seborrheic dermatitis).	Cradle cap. ● Seborrheic dermatitis (see dermatitis, page 151).	For cradle cap, loosen scales by rubbing with baby oil and combing with a fine-tooth comb. If it persists, call doctor for advice.
Bright red, tight, and/or sore skin in diaper area; rash that may consist of small bumps.	Diaper rash (see page 259).	Change wet diapers often, and right away after bowel movement. If doesn't improve in 3 days, call doctor for appointment.

Chicken Pox

SIGNS AND SYMPTOMS

- An itchy rash that most often appears on the face and torso. It starts out as small red spots; these turn into clear fluid–filled blisters. In the final stage of the rash, the blisters burst and scab over. The rash most often lasts 7 to 10 days.

Sometimes:

- Painful blisters in the mouth or vagina, or around the eyes.
- A low fever.

Chicken pox is a highly contagious childhood disease that affects about three-fourths of children before the age of 15. The rash and other symptoms appear 1 to 3 weeks after a person gets the virus. Infected people can give the disease to others for a day or two before the spots appear and 5 to 6 days after.

Most of the time, chicken pox is not serious. But it can lead to eye and lung problems in newborns and other people with weak immune systems, and it tends to make adults feel worse than it does children. A vaccine can now help prevent it.

You can do many simple things to help your child feel better. Above all, try to relieve the itching, since scratching can cause infections and scars.

WHAT YOU CAN DO NOW

- Give acetaminophen for pain. (Never give aspirin to a child under 12 who has chicken pox, a cold, the flu, or any other illness you suspect of being caused by a virus; see box on **Reye's syndrome,** page 96.) Don't give ibuprofen to a child with chicken pox. Some studies suggest it can increase the risk of strep infections.
- If your child wears diapers, leave them off as much as you can to let the blisters dry.
- Make sure your child gets plenty of rest and lots to drink.

To relieve itching:

- Apply calamine lotion to the rash, and try

RECOMMENDED CHILDREN'S IMMUNIZATIONS

During your child's early years, doctor checkups include immunizations. They protect against a range of major diseases, from polio to diphtheria. At one point, these diseases were widespread and deadly. Most states require children to get their shots before starting school. If a child is sick or has had a severe reaction to a previous vaccination, to neomycin, or to eggs, tell your doctor before any new vaccination.

Serious reactions are rare, but ask about symptoms to watch for.

CHILD'S AGE	VACCINE(S)	CHILD'S RECORD
Birth–2 months	Hep B (hepatitis B)—dose 1 of 3	
1–4 months	Hep B—dose 2	
2 months	DTP (diphtheria, tetanus/lockjaw, pertussis/whooping cough)	
	OPV (oral polio vaccine)	
	Hib (Haemophilus B conjugate). Immunizes children against *Haemophilus influenzae* type b, which can cause meningitis.	
4 months	DTP	
	Hib	
	OPV	
6 months	Hep B—dose 3 (given from 6–18 months)	
	DTP	
	Hib (may not need, depending on vaccines at 2 and 4 months)	
	OPV	
12–18 months	DTP or DTaP (diphtheria, tetanus, and acellular pertussis)	
	Hib	
	MMR (measles, mumps, rubella/German measles)	
	Var (varicella zoster virus). Immunizes against chicken pox.	
4–6 years	DTP or DTaP	
	MMR (recommended; may be given at 11–12 years instead if state law allows)	
	OPV	
11–12 years	Hep B (if not given before)	
	Td (tetanus and diphtheria). If at least 5 years since last dose, then every 10 years for rest of life.	
	MMR (if not given at 4–6 years)	
	Var (if not given before and child hasn't had chicken pox)	

This chart is based on recommendations by the American Academy of Pediatrics. These recommendations are subject to change, so be sure to ask your pediatrician for the most current schedule.

adding a handful of oatmeal, baking soda, or an over-the-counter anti-itch bath powder to your child's bathwater.

- Try an over-the-counter antihistamine—in a small dose for a child—to help control itching.
- For sores inside the mouth, see **canker sores,** page 80.
- Make a mouthwash of ½ teaspoon salt in an 8-ounce glass of warm water.
- For mouth sores, give ice chips and Popsicles to suck—they ease pain and add fluids.

To help prevent skin infections:

- Keep your child's skin, clothes, and bed linens clean.
- To keep your child from scratching, trim the fingernails and/or cover his or her hands with socks or mittens.

WHEN TO CALL THE DOCTOR

Call 911 or go to an emergency room **right away:**

- If your child is drowsy, and also has extreme sensitivity to light, eye pain, speech problems, loss of hearing, a stiff neck or back, or a severe cough. These may be symptoms of acute encephalitis, an inflammation of the brain (see **meningitis and encephalitis,** page 57).
- If it's hard for your child to breathe; this may be a symptom of **pneumonia** (see page 98), a rare complication of chicken pox (adults get it more than children).

Call for advice and an appointment:

- Whenever your child gets a rash. Most rashes are not serious, but they can be a sign of illness (see **children's rashes** chart, page 253).
- If areas of your child's rash get redder or more swollen or tender, or produce a yellow discharge.
- If your child still has a fever over 102 after 3 to 4 days; it may be a symptom of strep.

HOW TO PREVENT IT

- Children over 13 months can get a chicken pox vaccine. It can be combined with other routine immunizations. Children under 13 need only a single shot. Anyone over 12 needs 2 shots, 4 to 8 weeks apart.

FOR MORE HELP

Organization: American Academy of Pediatrics, Box 927, Elk Grove Village, IL 60009-0927. Include a business-size, self-addressed, stamped envelope with your request for reports on chicken pox.

Further resources: See box on page 275.

Colic

SIGNS AND SYMPTOMS

In a healthy infant under 3 months:

- Crying that goes on for 3 hours or more at a time, despite efforts to comfort the baby. Crying is often worse in the evening and at night.

When gas pain is the cause:

- Baby extends legs or pulls them up to the abdomen.
- Baby passes gas.

If your baby is acting colicky, don't despair. About 1 infant in 5 has colic. Often it seems to have no cause. But sometimes it can be the result of gas pains from certain foods in the nursing mother's diet or the type of milk in the baby's formula.

Although colic is harmless, it can be very tiring for parents. This phase of your baby's life may seem endless, but most colicky babies grow out of it by about the time they are 3 months of age. Sometimes, though, colicky crying may signal an illness, such as a **hernia** (see page 129) or an **ear infection** (see page 73).

WHAT YOU CAN DO NOW

- Stay calm. Never shake a baby—you can cause brain damage.
- Make sure a wet diaper or hunger is not the problem. See if the baby is too hot or cold—or bored.
- If gas pain seems to be the problem, place your baby stomach-down on your lap and gently massage the baby's back.
- Rhythmic motion often soothes babies. Walk with your baby in your arms or in a

body carrier. Rock him or her in a rocking chair or swing. Take him or her for a ride in a car.

- Try putting the baby near the sound of a clothes dryer or a vacuum cleaner. Some babies are calmed by "white noise" or rhythmic sounds.
- Wrap your baby snugly in a blanket for security and warmth.
- Spend 10 minutes alone, relaxing, while someone else holds the baby. When you feel yourself getting near the breaking point, ask a friend or neighbor for help.
- Don't give up. What doesn't work one time may work the next. And it's a short-term problem.

WHEN TO CALL THE DOCTOR

- If this is the first time your baby has had colic. Your doctor will want to rule out any illness.
- If the colic keeps getting worse.
- If your baby is more than 3 months old and is still colicky.
- If your colicky baby is not hungry and is not gaining weight.

HOW TO PREVENT IT

- If you're nursing, notice whether your baby is colicky after you eat certain foods, so that you can avoid them. Frequent problem foods include cabbage, onions, garlic, broccoli, and turnips, and the caffeine in coffee, tea, chocolate, and cocoa.
- For a colicky bottle-fed baby, switch to formula without cow's milk. Use nipples with a larger hole so your baby doesn't swallow air.
- Always burp your baby after a feeding.
- Try feeding your infant smaller amounts more often.

FOR MORE HELP

For a list of resources on children's health, see box on page 275.

Croup

SIGNS AND SYMPTOMS

- Loud, barking, seal-like cough.
- Trouble breathing.
- Shrill wheezing or grunting noise while breathing.
- Hoarseness.
- Sometimes fever (up to 104 degrees).

Children who have croup find it hard to breathe because their airways have become swollen and narrow. Croup most often starts as a respiratory infection caused by a virus. Some children are prone to croup and may get it every time they have a cold or other illness, most often between October and March.

Children between the ages of 6 months and 3 years are most likely to get croup. Those over 5 tend not to get it because their airways have grown larger, so swelling is less likely to affect breathing. Boys are more prone to croup than girls.

Croup most often clears up in about 6 days. Meanwhile, you can help your child feel better with simple at-home measures. But in rare cases, your child's airways may swell so much that he or she can barely breathe. If so, you may need to take him or her to the hospital.

WHAT YOU CAN DO NOW

- Have your child breathe moist air, either from a bowl filled with steaming water, a humidifier, or a hot shower (see **hints on humidifiers and vaporizers,** page 93). Your child's breathing should ease after 15 to 20 minutes.
- Take your child outside for a few minutes—dressed warmly if it's cold out. Cold, moist air may make breathing easier. A drive with the car windows open may also help.
- Sit your child up straight to ease breathing. For a baby, use an infant seat.
- Stay calm, and try to keep your child calm.

WHEN TO CALL THE DOCTOR

Call for advice right away (if you can't get it, call 911 or go to an emergency room):

- If your child starts to make loud, high-pitched wheezing noises while inhaling.
- If your child struggles to get a breath or can't speak for lack of breath.
- If your child has trouble swallowing.

Call for a prompt appointment:

- If your child breathes quickly and noisily.
- If your child has a fever of 102 or higher.

HOW TO PREVENT IT

- Get prompt treatment for any child with a respiratory illness.
- Make sure your children wash their hands often to reduce the chance of spreading illness.

FOR MORE HELP

For a list of resources on children's health, see box on page 275.

Diaper Rash

SIGNS AND SYMPTOMS

- Red skin or small bumps on a baby's buttocks, genitals, lower abdomen, thigh folds, or any place in contact with wet or soiled diapers.
- In the same areas, shiny, bright red skin or tight, paperlike skin.
- Strong ammonia odor (sometimes).

Most babies will get diaper rash at least once. Babies between 8 and 10 months old, or those just starting to eat solid foods, are most likely to get it. Formula-fed babies tend to get diaper rash more than breast-fed babies.

Most diaper rash is caused by too much contact with moisture, urine, or feces. Lotions or soaps used on the baby's skin, and detergents used to wash cloth diapers, can also cause rashes.

If home care doesn't get rid of diaper rash in 2 or 3 days, your baby may have a fungal or bacterial infection. Babies on antibiotics are very prone to fungal rashes (see **fungal infections,** page 155).

WHAT YOU CAN DO NOW

- Keep your baby's bottom as clean and dry as you can.
- Use a hair-dryer set on low to blow warm, dry air on your baby's bottom.
- After washing and drying your baby, apply an over-the-counter zinc oxide ointment to the sore area. Baby powder doesn't work well and can harm the lungs if inhaled.

WHEN TO CALL THE DOCTOR

- If it doesn't improve after 3 days of home treatment.
- If your baby's rash covers more than the diaper area.
- If the diaper area has red or pus-filled blisters that crust over. This may be **impetigo** (see page 265, and **children's rashes** chart, page 253).
- If a baby boy's foreskin becomes very red and inflamed.

HOW TO PREVENT IT

- Change soiled or wet diapers as soon as you can.
- Expose your baby's bottom to the air as much as you can.
- Make sure air can get inside your baby's diaper. You might want to stop using plastic pants or disposable diapers with tight gathers around the tummy or legs.
- If you wash cloth diapers yourself, use a mild laundry soap, and don't use fabric softeners, which can irritate skin. Put the diapers through at least 2 rinse cycles to remove all traces of soap. Add 2 tablespoons of vinegar to the rinse water. This helps fight bacteria.

FOR MORE HELP

Organization: American Academy of Pediatrics, Box 927, Elk Grove Village, IL

60009-0927. Include a business-size, self-addressed, stamped envelope with your request for reports on diaper rash.

Further resources: See box on page 275.

Diarrhea in Children

See **diarrhea,** page 122.

Ear Infections in Children

See **ear infections,** page 73.

Fever in Children

SIGNS AND SYMPTOMS

- A temperature of 100 degrees or higher (taken orally).
- Hot forehead.
- Flushed face.
- Sweating.
- Crying, irritability, or little appetite.

A fever of 100 degrees or higher is often the first sign that your child may be sick. Although 98.6 degrees is considered normal, body temperature varies with age, activity, and the time of day (it's most often lower in the morning and higher in the late afternoon). A temperature of 97 to 99 is no reason to worry.

A fever can be a sign of a childhood ailment, including viral or bacterial illnesses. In a baby or young child, fever can lead to a **seizure** (see box, this page).

Childhood illnesses marked by fever include chicken pox; croup; ear infection; German measles; hand, foot, and mouth disease; measles; mumps; rheumatic fever; strep throat; and whooping cough. (See the entry for each illness, and **fever** chart, page 279.)

FEVER SEIZURES

Watching a feverish child have a convulsion (febrile seizure) can be terrifying. These seizures are common in children from 6 months to age 5 whose temperatures have risen quickly. Despite the violence of a seizure, it is rarely harmful.

The signs of seizure include shaking or jerking of the arms and legs, a fixed stare or the eyes rolling back, drooling, heavy breathing, and the skin turning blue, mainly on the face. A seizure can last for less than a minute, more than 5 minutes, or, rarely, up to 20 minutes.

Take prompt action to prevent injury. Lay your child on a flat surface on his or her side, away from any sharp or hard objects. Turn your child's head to the side so that vomit or saliva can drain. If your child does vomit, clean out the mouth with your finger. Make sure the airway is clear, but don't force anything into your child's mouth. To reduce fever, take off his or her clothing and sponge the body with lukewarm water.

If the seizure lasts for more than a few minutes or is severe, call 911 or go to an emergency room **right away.** Always call your doctor for a prompt appointment to rule out a serious illness, such as **meningitis** (see page 57).

WHAT YOU CAN DO NOW

- Check your child's temperature with a thermometer (see **how to take a temperature,** next page).
- Make sure your child is not overdressed or in a place that's too hot. Remove extra clothing, and cool the room if you can.
- If a child is eating and sleeping well and is playful, there most likely is no serious problem. But complaints of feeling sick or tired, lack of appetite, and crying for no clear reason are likely signs of illness.
- Have your child drink plenty of cool fluids to help lower body temperature and prevent dehydration.

- Give your child acetaminophen to help lower the fever. (Never give aspirin to a child under 12 who has a fever, cold, chicken pox, flu, or any other illness you suspect of being caused by a virus; see box on **Reye's syndrome,** page 96.) Ask your doctor before giving medication to an infant under 3 months old.
- To lower body temperature, sponge your child with lukewarm water, especially if he or she has had seizures before or is vomiting. Don't use cold water or alcohol.

WHEN TO CALL THE DOCTOR

Take your child's temperature before you call the doctor (see **how to take a temperature,** this page).

Call for a prompt appointment:

- If your baby (3 months or younger) has a fever of 100.4 or higher, or if a child older than 3 months has a fever of 102 or higher.
- If your child has other symptoms, such as vomiting, diarrhea, trouble breathing, or a stiff neck; or if he or she cries all the time and is confused or delirious.

HOW TO TAKE A TEMPERATURE

Taking a sick child's or baby's temperature is no fun for anyone. Some new products make it easier (see below). The best places to measure your child's body heat are the mouth or the rectum and sometimes under the arm. A recent study shows underarm temperature can be as accurate as rectal temperature.

Some tips:

- Never leave a child or baby alone with a thermometer in place.
- For accurate oral readings: Don't take a temperature right after your child eats, drinks, or has a hot bath. You'll get a false reading.
- For oral readings with a mercury type (over age 5 only): Shake it down below 95 degrees. Put it under the tongue toward one side of the mouth. Have the child hold it for 3 minutes with lips and tongue—not teeth—and breathe through his or her nose.
- For rectal readings (under age 5): Use only a rectal thermometer. Lubricate the end with petroleum jelly. Hold the child (over your lap is good) with one hand. Gently insert the thermometer three-fourths of an inch. Hold it in place with the other hand for 2 minutes. It will read 1 degree higher than the oral temperature.
- For underarm reading: Put the thermometer in the deepest part of the armpit. Hold it in place by gently pressing the baby's elbow against his or her side for 4 to 5 minutes. Add 1.8 degrees to the reading.

Choosing a thermometer. Here's what experts say about accuracy, speed, and ease of use of some new choices.

- **Mercury** (cost: $1 to $3) comes as an oral type, and a thicker rectal type for babies and small children. Very accurate, but hard to read, bothersome to small children, and breakable. It has to be shaken down, and has to be held in the mouth 2 to 3 minutes, the rectum 2 minutes, or the underarm 4 to 5 minutes.
- **Digital** (cost: $4 to $10) works in the mouth, rectum, or underarm in about the same time as the mercury type. Very accurate, easy to read and use. Cons: Battery could wear out when you need it most.
- **Digital ear** (cost: $55 to $70) is the fastest and least trouble to use (even on a sleeping baby): Put the tip in the ear, then hold the button for 2 seconds. Cons: It's costly, and it may not be accurate unless you make a tight seal with the ear.
- **Contact strips** (you hold them on the child's forehead for 2 minutes) or pacifier styles ($2 to $3 each) are easy to use, but not always accurate. The pacifier shows only whether the temperature is higher than normal.

- ➤ If your child has a temperature of 105 degrees after spending time on a hot beach or in a closed car or other hot place. This is not really a fever; it is a **heat stroke** (see page 40). It needs emergency treatment.

Call for advice :

- ➤ If your child has a fever that lasts more than 3 days.
- ➤ Whenever your child gets a rash. Most rashes are not serious, but they can be a sign of illness (see **children's rashes** chart, page 253).

HOW TO PREVENT IT

There is no way to prevent most fevers. To avoid fevers caused by overheating:

- ➤ Don't overdress your child, and never leave your child alone in a closed car.
- ➤ Have your child drink lots of water, rest in the shade, and wear a hat when playing in hot sun.
- ➤ Keep your child's room at a safe temperature. Use a fan if the room is hot or stuffy, and never put a crib next to a radiator, heater, or heating vent.

FOR MORE HELP

For a list of resources on children's health, see box on page 275.

Fifth Disease

SIGNS AND SYMPTOMS

- ■ Fever as high as 102 degrees.
- ■ Later, a bright red rash on the cheeks; they may look as if they've been slapped. Over the next few days, rash becomes pink, slightly raised, and lacy-looking, and spreads to the buttocks, torso, arms, and thighs. Activity or hot baths may make the rash worse.
- ■ Coldlike symptoms, including sore throat, headache, reddish eyes, and fatigue (sometimes).
- ■ Itchiness (sometimes).

Fifth disease, a viral childhood illness, is so named because it is among the 5 common infections—along with measles, German measles (rubella), roseola, and scarlet fever—that cause a rash and fever, and that are catching (see entry for each illness). It is also called "slapped cheek." Children between the ages of 5 and 14 are most likely to get fifth disease, and outbreaks occur most often in the spring and early summer.

Once the virus has taken hold, the rash may take up to 14 days to appear. Meanwhile, your child, who may have the symptoms of a cold, can spread the disease to other children through the air. Your child is contagious before the rash shows up, but not while he or she has the rash or after it's gone.

Fifth disease is mild. Most children feel fine even while they have the rash, and the illness often clears up in about 10 days. But the virus (named parvovirus) can cause arthritis in older children and adults, miscarriages in pregnant women, and lead to other illnesses in children and teens who have sickle-cell anemia.

WHAT YOU CAN DO NOW

- ➤ If your child feels sick, have him or her rest in bed and drink plenty of water and other fluids.
- ➤ If the rash is itchy, apply an over-the-counter cream such as calamine lotion.
- ➤ For minor aches or pains, or for fever, you can give your child acetaminophen. (Never give aspirin to a child under 12 who has fifth disease, a cold, chicken pox, flu, or any other illness you suspect of being caused by a virus; see box on **Reye's syndrome,** page 96.)
- ➤ Keep your child away from pregnant women: Fifth disease can harm a fetus.

WHEN TO CALL THE DOCTOR

Call for advice:

- ➤ If your child gets any kind of rash. Most rashes are not serious, but they can be a sign of illness (see **children's rashes** chart, page 253).
- ➤ If your child has new symptoms or a fever of 102 degrees or higher.

HOW TO PREVENT IT

- Make sure your children wash their hands often to reduce the chance of spreading disease.

FOR MORE HELP

For a list of resources on children's health, see box on page 275.

German Measles (Rubella)

SIGNS AND SYMPTOMS

- Fever of 102 degrees or lower.
- Swollen glands, most often in the neck.
- By the second or third day, a rash that starts on the face and spreads to the chest and back, then the legs and arms. Rash can appear as tiny red or pink spots or as irregular blotches. It lasts only a few days.
- Painful, aching joints, especially in teens.

German measles, also known as rubella, is a mild viral illness that used to be one of the milestones of early childhood. Now that a vaccine exists, rubella is far less common than it was 10 years ago.

The virus spreads through the air when a person who has it coughs or sneezes. A child who catches it may feel no worse than he or she would with a simple cold. But an adult who catches it may feel much more sick. Rubella most often clears up on its own 5 to 7 days after the first symptoms appear.

The infection presents a serious threat to a growing fetus in early pregnancy. If a woman gets rubella in her first 3 months of pregnancy, her child has a 50 percent chance of being born with birth defects. These can include blindness, deafness, mental retardation, and heart problems.

WHAT YOU CAN DO NOW

- Keep your child quiet and provide lots of liquids.
- Give your child acetaminophen for discomfort. (Never give aspirin to a child under 12 who has rubella, a cold, chicken pox, flu, or any other illness you suspect of being caused by a virus; see box on **Reye's syndrome,** page 96.)
- If you think your child has rubella, keep him or her away from others, above all pregnant women. Rubella is contagious 2 days before and up to a week after the rash appears.

WHEN TO CALL THE DOCTOR

Call for advice:

- Whenever your child gets a rash. Most rashes are not serious, but they can be a sign of illness (see **children's rashes** chart, page 253).
- If you suspect your child has rubella.
- If your child has rubella or just had it and gets symptoms such as lethargy, a stiff neck, or severe headache. This could signal **meningitis** (see page 57), a very rare complication.
- If you are pregnant, even if you have been immunized in the past. You need to find out whether you are still immune.

HOW TO PREVENT IT

- Make sure your children get the MMR (measles, mumps, and rubella) vaccine, a routine part of early childhood immunizations (see **children's immunizations** chart, page 256).
- If you're a woman of childbearing age and you weren't immunized in childhood, and never had German measles, get the rubella vaccine. If you are not sure whether you had the disease or were immunized, ask your doctor to give you a test. The vaccine should never be given to a pregnant woman.

  You should have the shot at least 3 months before you get pregnant. Use birth control for 3 months after the shot to make sure you don't get pregnant while the vaccine is still present and could affect your baby.

FOR MORE HELP

For a list of resources on children's health, see box on page 275.

Hand, Foot, and Mouth Disease

SIGNS AND SYMPTOMS

- Painful small, raw, cankerlike sores on the tongue and insides of the cheeks.
- An itchy rash with red spots, bumps, and/or small blisters on the hands and feet, between the fingers and toes, sometimes on the buttocks.
- Fever under 102 degrees, or none.
- Tiredness.

Like many childhood illnesses, hand, foot, and mouth disease is caused by a virus. Most often spread by the feces-to-mouth route, the virus is also spread in the air. Once it takes hold, symptoms show up in 3 to 6 days.

Outbreaks of hand, foot, and mouth disease occur most often in the summer and fall, when the virus grows best. The disease most often clears up by itself within a week. There's no treatment, but you can help your child feel better at home.

WHAT YOU CAN DO NOW

- Don't give your child citrus fruits, spicy foods, or other foods that might make his or her mouth more sore. Serve liquids, such as chicken or vegetable broth, and soft foods, such as oatmeal or mashed banana, if solid foods are too painful for your child to chew.
- Saltwater rinses and gargles can soothe mouth sores. Mix ½ teaspoon salt in 1 cup (8 ounces) of warm water, and have your child rinse his or her mouth after eating. Be sure your child is old enough to rinse and then spit out rather than swallow the saltwater.
- Boil eating utensils (your dishwasher may have a hot cycle) or use disposable cups, forks, and spoons to avoid spreading the disease.
- Be sure your child drinks plenty of fluids. Water and juice (not citrus) are best. Popsicles and ice chips are also good choices. They can ease the pain and add fluids.
- If the rash is itchy, apply an over-the-counter anti-itch cream.
- To help relieve pain or reduce your child's fever, give acetaminophen. (Never give aspirin to a child under 12 who has hand, foot, and mouth disease, a cold, chicken pox, flu, or any other illness you suspect of being caused by a virus; see box on **Reye's syndrome,** page 96.)

WHEN TO CALL THE DOCTOR

Call for a prompt appointment:

- If your child has trouble swallowing.

Call for advice:

- Whenever your child gets a rash. Most rashes are not serious, but they can be a sign of illness (see **children's rashes** chart, page 253).

HOW TO PREVENT IT

- Make sure children wash their hands after using the toilet.
- See that children don't share glasses, silverware, or toys that have been in other children's mouths.
- Choose a babysitter or day care center with high standards of cleanliness. Check that the staff members wash their hands often, above all after they change children's diapers.

FOR MORE HELP

For a list of resources on children's health, see box on page 275.

Impetigo

SIGNS AND SYMPTOMS

- Small patches of red or pus-filled blisters, most often on the face, legs, or arms; blisters range from the size of a matchstick head to a quarter.
- After blisters pop: a sticky golden crust.
- Itching.

Impetigo is a skin infection most common in children because they're prone to scrapes, skinned knees, and other minor breaks in the skin that give bacteria a place to thrive. Children with colds or runny noses often get it because the skin around the mouth and nose becomes raw. Impetigo is very catching and spreads quickly over the body and from one person to others through touching or sharing towels.

The bacteria that cause it are harmless until they enter the skin through a cut, insect bite, or other break. Impetigo occurs most often in the summer, chiefly in hot, humid climates. It's also common in hospitals, day care centers, schools, and other crowded places.

Impetigo is ugly and uncomfortable but easy to treat.

WHAT YOU CAN DO NOW

- Gently wash away the crusty discharge with warm water and soap.
- Apply an over-the-counter antibiotic ointment to help clear up a minor case.
- It's catching: To protect other people, warn them not to touch your child's sores, towel, washcloth, or unwashed clothing. Change linens daily; wash them in hot water and detergent, with bleach.
- To limit its spread, do all you can to help your child avoid touching or scratching the blisters.
- To keep the bacteria from growing, expose blisters to air; don't bandage them.
- Give your child lukewarm baths, not hot ones (heat increases itching). Use an antibacterial soap.
- Dress your child in long-sleeved shirts and long pants to go to school or day care until the crusts are gone and the skin clears, which takes 7 to 10 days. This will lower the chance of spreading the ailment to others.

WHEN TO CALL THE DOCTOR

Call for a prompt appointment:

- If your child's urine turns red or dark brown. This signals a rare related kidney ailment.

Call for advice:

- Whenever your child gets a rash. Most rashes are not serious, but they can be a sign of illness (see **children's rashes** chart, page 253).
- If the impetigo covers a large area or keeps spreading after 3 days. The doctor may prescribe antibiotic cream or oral antibiotics.
- If your child gets a fever of more than 100 degrees or has a blister larger than 1 inch wide. This could mean a deeper skin infection.

HOW TO PREVENT IT

- Wash all cuts, scrapes, and wounds with antibacterial soap and water to prevent infection. Keep them clean and dry while they heal.
- Make sure children wash their hands often with soap and keep their nails trimmed. Remind them not to scratch insect bites, scabs, or other skin irritations.
- Don't have children share towels, washcloths, or bedding.
- Guard against **diaper rash** (see page 259) to protect your baby from impetigo.

FOR MORE HELP

For a list of resources on children's health, see box on page 275.

Lead Poisoning

SIGNS AND SYMPTOMS

Most children with low levels of lead poisoning show no distinct symptoms. Sometimes, though, they will have:

- Constipation.
- Vomiting.
- Loss of appetite.
- Fatigue.
- Learning disabilities and/or behavior problems.

Severe lead poisoning:

- Stomach pain.
- Headaches.
- Loss of coordination.
- Loss of recently learned skills.

One in 11 American children has a high level of lead in his or her blood. Lead poisoning is not confined to inner-city families trapped in poor housing; many children of middle- and upper-income families living in older houses (most often houses being repaired) are also at risk.

Almost three-quarters of the houses built before 1980 have lead paint either inside or outside. Most children are exposed through lead-based paint and paint dust. Lead may also be present in the water from your faucet, in the dishes in your cabinets, and in your backyard soil.

Children between the ages of 6 months and 6 years are at highest risk. They are more likely than older children and adults to put objects in their mouths and to play in places where lead collects in dirt, dust, and peeling paint. Lead can harm a fetus as well, so pregnant women should also avoid it.

Severe lead poisoning can cause mental retardation, intestinal problems, hearing loss, anemia, and even death. At low but chronic levels, it can result in learning disabilities, behavior problems, and reduced IQ.

The Centers for Disease Control and Prevention (CDC) advises parents to have their children's blood tested for lead by the time they are 1 year old.

WHAT YOU CAN DO NOW

- ➤ Ask your doctor to test your child's blood for lead. This is the only way to know your child's blood level.
- ➤ If test results show a high lead level—10 micrograms per deciliter or more—talk to your doctor about ways you can keep your child from being exposed further. Also, call your local health department. Many now have programs to prevent lead poisoning.
- ➤ For severe cases (45 to more than 69 micrograms per deciliter), a treatment called chelation therapy can help the body get rid of lead.

WHEN TO CALL THE DOCTOR

- ➤ If you believe your child has been exposed to lead—if your house paint is old and peeling or if work has recently been done on your house.

HOW TO PREVENT IT

Have the paint, water, and soil in and around your home tested. You may find you need to rid it of lead hazards. Other steps to take:

- ➤ If your house was built before 1980, keep it as clean and dust-free as you can. Note places where dust tends to gather, such as windowsills and baseboards. Damp-mop floors often, and damp-dust surfaces.
- ➤ If your house was built before 1980 and you plan to repaint or repair it, ask your local health department for a list of companies whose workers take care around lead hazards. Children and pregnant women should move out of the house while work is being done. If they can't, they should take extra care to avoid being exposed to lead.
- ➤ Have your tap water tested for lead. If any shows up, use bottled water or a water filter that removes lead from the water (get the maker's certification that it does). Use only cold water from the tap for drinking, cooking, and making baby formula.
- ➤ Wash children's toys, pacifiers, and bottle nipples often.
- ➤ Wash your hands before touching food,

and wash your child's face and hands before meals.

- Feed your child meals that include plenty of calcium and iron-rich foods; these can reduce lead absorption.
- Never eat foods canned in other countries. They may contain lead.
- Have painted toys and glazed dishes that were made outside the United States tested for lead, or get rid of them. Never use imported dishware to store foods.
- If you work with lead in your job, take off your work clothes and shower before going home.

FOR MORE HELP

Information line: National Safety Council's National Lead Information Center, 800-LEAD-FYI, 24-hour recording. 800-424-LEAD, M–F 8:30–5 EST. Staff answers questions.

Organization: Lead Poisoning Prevention Branch, Centers for Disease Control and Prevention, 4770 Buford Hwy. NE, Mail Stop F42, Atlanta, GA 30341. 770-488-7330, M–F 8–5 EST. Provides facts about lead hazards.

Organization: The Alliance to End Childhood Lead Poisoning, 227 Massachusetts Ave. NE, Suite 200, Washington, DC 20002. 202-543-1147, M–F 9–5:30 EST. Provides publications and referrals.

Book: *Lead Is a Silent Hazard,* by Richard Stapleton. Offers advice on how to avoid lead poisoning. Walker and Company, 1994, $11.95. **Web site:** *http://www.cdc.gov/diseases/e_health.html.* Click on *Programs of National Center for Environmental Health,* then on *Infants & Children* for facts about lead poisoning.

Web access: California Department of Health Services. After logging on to the Internet, type: *http://www.parentsplace.com/readroom/lead.* Offers pamphlets about the hazards of lead, a guide to poison prevention, and other resources.

Further resources: See box on page 275.

Measles

SIGNS AND SYMPTOMS

First 2 to 3 days:

- Fever (as high as 105 degrees).
- Coldlike symptoms that include a runny nose; dry cough; swollen glands; red, watery eyes sensitive to light; loss of appetite; and aching muscles.

A day or two later:

- Painless small gray or white bumps, like grains of salt, surrounded by red rings inside the mouth.

In another day or so:

- Red bumps that first show on the face and neck, then spread down the entire body.

Measles is a very contagious viral illness that can be quite severe. One to 2 weeks after your child has been exposed, coldlike symptoms show up. During this time, the disease is most catching, although it can be spread until the fever and rash are gone, about 5 to 8 days later. Infected children most often pass measles to others via coughing or sneezing.

Today, though, few children in the United States get measles, thanks to a vaccine given between ages 1 and 6.

There's no cure for measles, but you can help your child feel better. Rarely, measles can go on to become a more serious problem, such as a middle **ear infection** (see page 73) or **pneumonia** (see page 98), which can be treated with antibiotics. Very rarely, measles can trigger **encephalitis** (see page 57), an inflammation of the brain.

WHAT YOU CAN DO NOW

- Call your doctor for advice. Many other diseases have a rash and symptoms that look like measles (see **children's rashes** chart, page 253).
- Give your child lots of fluids to drink.
- Help your child rest in bed.

- ➤ Use a cool-mist humidifier in your child's bedroom (see **hints on humidifiers and vaporizers,** page 93).
- ➤ If your child's eyes are sensitive to light, darken the bedroom.
- ➤ If your child has minor aches or pains, give acetaminophen. (Never give aspirin to a child under 12 who has measles, a cold, chicken pox, flu, or any other illness you suspect of being caused by a virus; see box on **Reye's syndrome,** page 96.)
- ➤ Keep your child away from others.

WHEN TO CALL THE DOCTOR

Call 911 or go to an emergency room **right away:**

- ➤ If your child has a headache, can't stand bright light, and feels so drowsy that he or she is hard to wake up. These can be warning signs of encephalitis.

Call for a prompt appointment:

- ➤ If your child has a feeling of fullness in the ear, and maybe some pain. He or she may have an ear infection.
- ➤ If your child is short of breath while resting. He or she may also have chills, sweating, and chest pain. This can be a sign of pneumonia.
- ➤ If your child gets a fever of 102 or higher (100 or higher for infants 6 months or younger).

HOW TO PREVENT IT

- ➤ Make sure your child gets the MMR vaccine for measles, mumps, and rubella (see **children's immunizations** chart, page 256). The shot is most often given at 12 months, with a booster at 12 years.

FOR MORE HELP

Web access: Health Information Highway. After logging on to the Internet, type: *http://www.stayhealthy.com/hrd/DICOPr_CHDI_Mees.htm.* Offers brochures and fact sheets on measles from a number of sources.

Further resources: See box on page 275.

Mumps

SIGNS AND SYMPTOMS

- Low fever (100 to 101 degrees).
- Headache.
- Loss of appetite.
- Fatigue.
- Swollen glands in the neck below the ear near the jawbone, on one or both sides.
- Earache (sometimes).
- Nausea and vomiting (sometimes).
- In adults (sometimes), swelling in one or both testes in men; swelling of ovaries in women.

Mumps is a viral infection of the salivary glands that is most common in children between the ages of 2 and 12. But unvaccinated adults who have never had mumps can get it too. The virus is spread through the air when an infected person coughs or sneezes. It is only mildly catching. Mumps is uncomfortable but not often serious, and symptoms should go away within 7 to 10 days.

Infected adults are more likely to have a very painful symptom: inflamed testes in men and inflamed ovaries in women. Children can also have this: A boy may have pain in his testes, while a girl may feel pain in her lower abdomen. The symptom should pass within 4 days. It carries a slight risk of sterility, however, so check with your doctor if you have concerns.

Once a person has had mumps, she or he is immune and not likely to get it again.

WHAT YOU CAN DO NOW

- ➤ Call your doctor for advice if you suspect your child has mumps.
- ➤ Be sure your child gets lots of rest while he or she has a fever. That doesn't have to mean staying in bed—quiet play is okay.
- ➤ Provide plenty of liquids and a diet of soft foods, such as soups, cooked vegetables, and fruits. Don't offer sour fruits, foods,

or juices—they can make swollen salivary glands more sore.

- ➤ To soothe swollen places, try cold or warm packs—whichever feels best. Apply ice packs (a bag of frozen peas wrapped in a washcloth makes a good one), or warm cloths or heating pads.
- ➤ Give acetaminophen or ibuprofen to ease pain and reduce fever. (Never give aspirin to a child under 12 who has mumps, a cold, chicken pox, flu, or any other illness you suspect of being caused by a virus; see box on **Reye's syndrome,** page 96.)

WHEN TO CALL THE DOCTOR

Call for emergency advice (if you can't get anyone, call 911 or go to an emergency room):

- ➤ If your child has the symptoms of mumps and a severe headache or neck pain, is listless, or behaves oddly. This could mean **meningitis** (see page 57).

Call for a prompt appointment:

- ➤ If your child has mumps and feels severe abdominal pain or vomits. This could signal an inflamed pancreas.

HOW TO PREVENT IT

- ➤ Make sure your child gets the MMR vaccine for measles, mumps, and rubella (see **children's immunizations** chart, page 256). The shot is most often given at 12 months, with a booster at 4 years or 12 years.
- ➤ To prevent others from catching mumps, keep your child home from school or day care for 7 to 10 days after the swelling appears.

FOR MORE HELP

Web access: MedAccess. After logging on to the Internet, type: *http://www.medaccess.com/cdcimun/mumps/mum2_01a.htm.* Gives an overview of mumps and covers vaccination schedules.

Further resources: See box on page 275.

Rheumatic Fever

SIGNS AND SYMPTOMS

Early symptoms:

- ■ Sometimes a sore throat (usually 1 to 6 weeks before other symptoms appear), maybe with swollen glands in the neck.

Later:

- ■ Fever of 100 degrees or higher.
- ■ Very sore, swollen joints.
- ■ Fatigue and shortness of breath.
- ■ Loss of appetite.
- ■ Pale skin.
- ■ Rash on chest, back, and abdomen (sometimes).

Rheumatic fever is a rare but sometimes dangerous offshoot of a strep infection, most often **strep throat** (see page 271). It's most common in children between the ages of 5 and 15, although adults can also get it.

Rheumatic fever occurs as part of the body's immune response to strep. Antibodies made to destroy the bacteria instead attack the joints or, in some cases, the valves of the heart. If rheumatic fever follows a strep infection, symptoms most often appear 1 to 6 weeks later.

If treated promptly with antibiotics, rheumatic fever poses little threat and passes within 2 to 12 weeks. If the heart has been affected, symptoms may last as long as 6 months. Any damage to the heart valves may not show up until years later.

WHAT YOU CAN DO NOW

- ➤ Have your child rest in bed and drink plenty of liquids.
- ➤ When your doctor confirms rheumatic fever, he or she may advise aspirin for joint pain. That's all right, because this illness comes from bacteria. But never give aspirin to a child under 12 who has a cold, chicken pox, flu, or any other illness you suspect of being caused by a virus (see box on **Reye's syndrome,** page 96).

WHEN TO CALL THE DOCTOR

- If a child or an adult has just had strep and then shows symptoms of rheumatic fever.
- Whenever a child gets a rash. Most rashes are not serious, but can be a sign of illness (see **children's rashes** chart, page 253).
- If a child or an adult has a fever, sore throat, and swollen glands that last for 48 hours or more; these symptoms could signal a strep infection.
- If new symptoms appear after treatment has begun. This could be a reaction to a prescribed drug.

HOW TO PREVENT IT

- Get prompt tests and treatment for **strep throat** (see page 271) or any other strep infection.

FOR MORE HELP

For a list of resources on children's health, see box on page 275.

Roseola

SIGNS AND SYMPTOMS

Early symptoms:

- Sudden high fever (102 to as high as 105 degrees).
- Decreased appetite.
- Mild diarrhea.
- Slight cough.
- Runny nose.
- Mild irritability, drowsiness.
- Swollen glands (rarely).

In severe cases:

- Convulsions.

Later symptoms:

- Normal temperature after 3 to 6 days. At the same time, a spotty, slightly raised red rash appears on the torso.
- Rash may spread to the arms, neck, legs, and face. It disappears in a few hours to a few days.

Roseola is sometimes called "baby measles" because children get it most often between the ages of 6 months and 2 years. It often frightens parents because of its alarming symptoms: high fever followed by an abruptly blooming rash. In fact, this common viral ailment poses little risk, although sometimes children will have **fever seizures** from the high temperature (see box, page 260). These seizures are mostly harmless, but you should call your doctor right away.

The illness usually passes within a week of the first symptoms. As soon as the rash is gone, the child is no longer contagious and can return to school and playing with others.

WHAT YOU CAN DO NOW

- Give your child plenty of fluids.
- Have your child rest as long as he or she has a fever.
- Sponge a feverish child with lukewarm water—not cold water or alcohol.
- Ask your doctor if you should give acetaminophen to reduce fever. (Never give aspirin to a child under 12 who has roseola, a cold, chicken pox, flu, or any other illness you suspect of being caused by a virus; see box on **Reye's syndrome,** page 96.)

WHEN TO CALL THE DOCTOR

Call for a prompt appointment:

- If your child has a fever of 102 or higher.
- If your child has seizures.

Call for advice:

- If your child gets a rash. Most rashes are not serious, but can be a sign of illness (see **children's rashes** chart, page 253).

HOW TO PREVENT IT

- Don't let a child with roseola play with other children until the rash clears up.
- Make sure all family members wash their hands often—always before touching food and after using the bathroom.

FOR MORE HELP

For a list of resources on children's health, see box on page 275.

Scarlet Fever

SIGNS AND SYMPTOMS

Symptoms vary, but most go as follows:

- First day: fever from 101 to 104 degrees, red and sore throat, fuzzy tongue, white coating on tonsils, headache, swollen neck glands, vomiting (sometimes).
- By the second day: bright red rash that breaks out on face (except right around mouth) and in groin area.
- By the third day: rash, which feels like sandpaper to the touch and may itch, spreads to rest of body. Temperature falls, and tongue turns bright red.
- By the sixth day: rash fades and skin and tongue may peel, leaving raw, tender skin.

Scarlet fever is caused by strep bacteria. Children between the ages of 2 and 10 get it most often. It's a **strep throat** (see this page) with a rash, and it is contagious.

If not treated, scarlet fever can lead to abscesses on the tonsils or, rarely, **rheumatic fever** (see page 269), which may develop 2 to 3 weeks after the rash appears.

After treatment with antibiotics for 10 days or 1 shot of penicillin, the fever, sore throat, and headache disappear. The rash may linger. Prompt treatment most often results in full recovery.

WHAT YOU CAN DO NOW

- Call the doctor for advice whenever your child gets a rash with any other symptoms. Scarlet fever needs prompt treatment with antibiotics.
- Make sure your child gets plenty of rest and drinks lots of liquids. Give soft foods that won't hurt a raw throat.
- Your doctor may advise acetaminophen to reduce fever and relieve pain (see **pain relief,** page 317). Never give aspirin to a child under 12 who has a cold, chicken pox, flu, or any illness you suspect is caused by a virus (see box on **Reye's syndrome,** page 96).

WHEN TO CALL THE DOCTOR

Call for a prompt appointment:

- If your child has a fever of 102 or higher.
- If your child has a sore throat with a rash, or if he or she has other symptoms of strep throat or scarlet fever.

Call for advice:

- If symptoms don't improve with treatment.

HOW TO PREVENT IT

- Get prompt tests and treatment for strep throat or other strep illnesses.
- Keep your child away from anyone who has strep.
- Once your doctor confirms scarlet fever, make sure other family members are tested for strep if they develop a sore throat, with or without a rash.

FOR MORE HELP

For a list of resources on children's health, see box on page 275.

Strep Throat

SIGNS AND SYMPTOMS

Young children:

- Mild sore throat.
- Swollen glands in throat.
- Low fever (100 to 101 degrees).
- Irritability.
- Loss of appetite.

Older children and adults:

- Sudden severe sore throat.
- Swollen glands in throat.
- High fever (102 degrees or higher).
- White coating on tonsils or throat.

The streptococcus bacteria that cause strep throat are spread by contact or through the air when an infected person

Children's Health

coughs or sneezes. Strep throat is most common in 5- to 15-year-olds but it can affect adults. It's rare in children under 3.

If strep throat goes untreated, it can lead to **rheumatic fever** (see page 269), kidney problems, and other illnesses. It's easy to mistake strep symptoms for signs of a cold or flu. So if your child has a sore throat that lasts 48 hours or longer, you should call your doctor. A throat culture or strep test can tell whether it's strep.

Prompt treatment with antibiotics such as penicillin or erythromycin most often eases symptoms within a day or so.

WHAT YOU CAN DO NOW

- Your child should rest, drink liquids, and eat foods that won't hurt a raw throat.
- Give your child acetaminophen for pain relief. (Never give aspirin to a child under 12 who has a cold, chicken pox, flu, or any other illness you suspect of being caused by a virus; see box on **Reye's syndrome,** page 96.)
- For children 3 and older, gargling with warm saltwater can ease throat pain.
- Don't smoke or let others smoke in the room with a sick child.
- Over-the-counter throat lozenges may help. Some have a local painkiller—ask your doctor or pharmacist.
- Take all antibiotics as prescribed, even after the symptoms are gone.

WHEN TO CALL THE DOCTOR

- If a child or an adult has the symptoms listed or a sore throat that lasts 48 hours or longer.

HOW TO PREVENT IT

- Wash your child's hands and face often—and yours, too—with soap and warm water, mainly after being in public places.
- Stay away from people who are coughing and sneezing.
- To prevent your sick child from infecting others, wait until he or she has been on antibiotics for 48 hours before you send him or her back to school or day care.

FOR MORE HELP

For a list of resources on children's health, see box on page 275.

Teething

SIGNS AND SYMPTOMS

Sometime in the first year, baby teeth appear with:

- Fussy, clingy behavior, and nighttime crying.
- Lots of drooling.
- Chewing on fingers, teething rings, and other objects.
- Red, swollen, and inflamed gums.
- More demand for nursing or bottle-feeding, or child may refuse breast or bottle because sucking action hurts sore gums.
- Poor appetite.

Few parents forget their children's first teeth, and in most cases, the memories are as painful as they are sweet. New teeth pushing their way through tender gums can hurt. Your normally sunny toddler, who appears otherwise healthy, may suddenly be crabby and restless all night long.

Children teethe at different ages. The front teeth tend to appear during the child's first year, and the first and second molars appear between the ages of 1 and 3.

For most children, the front teeth cause less trouble, though some children fuss with each tooth. The first and second molars, which seem to cause more pain, often disrupt eating and sleeping routines. The pain is likely to last a few days with each new tooth.

WHAT YOU CAN DO NOW

- When your child seems to be in pain, rub his or her gums with a clean finger. A chilled (but not frozen) washcloth or teething ring can ease soreness and provide something to chew on.
- Wrap an ice cube in a soft cloth and rub it

CARING FOR THOSE FIRST TEETH

Here are some simple steps you can take to protect your baby's new teeth and ensure healthful habits later on:

- When the first teeth appear, make toothbrushing part of your child's daily routine. Use either a child's toothbrush with small, soft bristles or a gauze pad. Gently rub the teeth bottom to top, front and back.
- Never put your baby to bed with a bottle. Juice and milk contain sugars that if left in the mouth for long can lead to tooth decay.
- Try to limit the amount of sweets your child eats.
- Begin visits to the dentist when all 20 baby teeth have appeared (around age 3).

For more help:

- American Academy of Pediatric Dentistry, 211 E. Chicago Ave., Suite 700, Chicago, IL 70611. Send a business-size, self-addressed, stamped envelope for "The Pediatric Dentist" pamphlet.
- American Academy of Pediatrics, Box 927, Elk Grove Village, IL 60009-0927. Send a business-size, self-addressed, stamped envelope for the brochure "A Guide to Your Children's Dental Health."

gently on your child's gums to reduce inflammation. Keep the ice moving over the gums to avoid hurting tissue.

- ➤ Comfort and distract your child with holding, cuddling, and rocking.
- ➤ If the pain lasts, consult your doctor about using acetaminophen. (Never give aspirin to a child under 12 who has a cold, chicken pox, flu, or any other illness you suspect of being caused by a virus; see box on **Reye's syndrome,** page 96.)
- ➤ The drooling that comes with teething can cause a rash on the face, neck, and upper chest. Using an infant cream can help. Change wet clothing often, or use bibs.
- ➤ Never rub brandy or any other alcoholic drink on your child's gums (no matter what you might have heard). Alcohol, even in small amounts, is bad for children.

WHEN TO CALL THE DOCTOR

- ➤ If your child runs a fever that lasts more than 48 hours or is higher than 100 degrees, has diarrhea, or is lethargic. These symptoms may signal something more serious than teething.
- ➤ If your child has cold symptoms, a constant fever, trouble eating or sleeping, or grabs at the side of his or her face or tugs at the ears. This could signal an **ear infection** (see page 73).
- ➤ If your child has no teeth by 12 months of age. This could mean a harmless, inherited tendency to late teething, but it might mean delayed bone growth.

FOR MORE HELP

For a list of resources on children's health, see box on page 275.

Vomiting in Children

See **nausea and vomiting,** page 133.

Whooping Cough

SIGNS AND SYMPTOMS

First stage (lasts 1 to 2 weeks):

- Runny nose and sneezing.
- Dry cough.
- Low fever (100 to 101 degrees).

Second stage (lasts 2 to 10 weeks):

- Frequent, severe coughing spasms, sometimes followed by a whooping sound when breathing in (as air is forced over the swollen voice box). Babies may have repeated coughing fits without making the whooping sound.

- Red or blue face during coughing spells. If your child turns blue or stops breathing, call 911 and give CPR **right away.** (See page 18 or 19 for how to do **CPR.**)
- Vomiting may follow coughing fits.

Third stage (which may last months):

- Cough that slowly becomes less frequent and severe.

Whooping cough, also called pertussis, is one of the most serious of the classic childhood ailments. This highly catching bacterial infection attacks the throat and lungs and is spread through the air by coughing or sneezing. If untreated, it can cause pneumonia and lung damage.

Thanks to widespread immunization, whooping cough is now rare among children in the United States. Those who do get it are most often infants and children under 4 who haven't had shots to prevent it.

Teens and adults can also get whooping cough even though they've had their shots—the immunity wears off. In fact, experts have recently counted a surprising number of cases in adults who had their shots as children. The danger this poses is that adults may pass the illness to children. Adults don't make the whooping sound that children do, so they may think they simply have **bronchitis** (see page 91). If you have a cough for more than 2 weeks, call your doctor for advice.

An antibiotic can prevent the worst symptoms—the spasms of coughing—if given during the first stage of the illness, before the whooping type of cough begins. Once that cough starts, the antibiotic doesn't do much to get rid of it, but can make the illness less catching.

Infants may need to be taken to a hospital to get rid of mucus blocking the nose and airways. They may also need oxygen.

WHAT YOU CAN DO NOW

After diagnosis:

- Keep your child calm.
- Give plenty of liquids to prevent dehydration. Water and juice are good choices.
- Make sure a child gets enough to eat. Frequent small meals may reduce the chance of vomiting. Even though whooping cough can be tiring and a child may not feel like eating, it's important to keep him or her well nourished.
- To keep a baby from inhaling mucus while coughing, place the baby on his or her stomach with the head turned to the side. Older children may be able to breathe better if they sit up and lean forward.
- Don't give your child a cough suppressant, as it may prevent the clearing of mucus from blocked airways.
- Give acetaminophen for pain relief. (Just to be on the safe side, even though this illness comes from bacteria.) Never give aspirin to a child under 12 who has a cold, chicken pox, flu, or any other illness you suspect of being caused by a virus; see box on **Reye's syndrome,** page 96.

WHEN TO CALL THE DOCTOR

Call 911 **right away** and give CPR:

- If your child turns blue or stops breathing during or after coughing (see page 18 or 19 for how to do **CPR**).

Call for a prompt appointment:

- If your child's cough becomes more severe and frequent, or if he or she has been exposed to someone with whooping cough, even if your child has been immunized.

HOW TO PREVENT IT

- Starting at the age of 2 months, a child should get shots against whooping cough (see **children's immunizations** chart, page 256). The vaccine is about 80 percent effective after 3 doses.
- Your doctor may advise preventive antibiotics for family members or schoolmates of a child who has whooping cough, even those who have been immunized.
- Don't expose your child to anyone who has whooping cough.

FOR MORE HELP

For a list of resources on children's health, see the next page.

CHILDREN'S HEALTH RESOURCES

General Health

Organization: American Academy of Pediatrics, Box 927, Elk Grove Village, IL 60009-0927. Send a business-size, self-addressed, stamped envelope for the Parent Resource Guide, a listing of the AAP's publications and videos. **Web site:** *http://www.aap.org.*

Book: *The American Academy of Pediatrics, Caring for Your Baby and Young Child: Birth to Age 5,* edited by Steven P. Shelov, M.D. Bantam, 1993, $16.95.

Book: *The American Academy of Pediatrics, Caring for Your School-Age Child: Ages 5 to 12,* edited by Edward L. Schor, M.D. Bantam, 1995, $29.95.

Book: *What to Expect: The First Year,* by Arlene Eisenberg, Heidi Murkoff, and Sandee E. Hathaway. Workman Publishing, 1994, $12.95.

Book: *What to Expect: The Toddler Years,* by Arlene Eisenberg, Heidi Murkoff, and Sandee E. Hathaway. Workman Publishing, 1994, $15.95.

Book: *Your Baby and Child: From Birth to Age 5,* by Penelope Leach. Alfred A. Knopf, 1992, $19.95.

Book: *Dr. Spock's Baby and Child Care,* by Benjamin M. Spock, M.D. Revised edition of the child-care bible. Pocket Books, 1992, $7.99.

Book: *You and Your Adolescent: A Parents' Guide for Ages 10 to 20,* by Laurence Steinberg and Ann Levine. HarperPerennial, 1991, $14.

Web access: Johns Hopkins University. After logging on to the Internet, type: *http://www.med.jhu.edu/peds/neonatology/poi.html.* Click on *Organizations* or *Resources for Parents* for a good list of children's health resources and links to other sites.

Web access: ParentsPlace.com: Health Issues and Your Children. After logging on to the Internet, type: *http://www.parentsplace.com.* Offers articles, support groups for parents, and links to other sites.

Food and Health

Information line: Weight Information Network, 1 Win Way, Bethesda, MD 20892-3665. 301-570-2177 M–F 9–5 EST. Call or write for reports on childhood obesity.

Book: *The PDR Family Guide to Nutrition and Health.* A guide to healthy eating and fitness for all age groups. Medical Economics, 1995, $25.95.

Web access: Johns Hopkins University, Cardiovascular Health Promotion for Children. After logging on to the Internet, type: *http://www.jhbmc.jhu.edu/cardiology/partnership/kids/kids.html.* Includes heart-healthy tips for kids, research, and links.

Mental Health

Information line: Parents Anonymous, 909-621-6184 (collect), M–F 8–4:30 PST. Provides lists of free support groups for parents under stress.

Organization: National Clearinghouse on Family Support and Children's Mental Health. 800-628-1696, 24-hour recording. Sends reports on many emotional issues that children face.

Organization: Parents Leadership Institute, Box 50492, Palo Alto, CA 94303. 415-424-8687. Ask about parenting and listening skills workshops, videos, and publications. Brochure series "Listening to Children" includes Crying, Healing Children's Fears, Tantrums and Indignation, and Reaching for Your Angry Child.

Book: *Lonely, Sad, and Angry: A Parent's Guide to Depression in Children and Adolescents,* by Barbara D. Ingersoll, Ph.D., and Sam Goldstein, Ph.D. Doubleday, 1995, $11.95.

Web access: The American Academy of Child and Adolescent Psychiatry. After logging on to the Internet, type: *http://www.aacap.org.* Offers 54 fact sheets on a range of psychiatric issues affecting children.

Sensible Advice on Discipline

As a parent, you want more than anything else to keep your child healthy and safe—both physically and emotionally. One of the best ways to do this is to provide loving discipline that helps your child grow and learn with support and respect.

At home, you teach by example. No parent is perfect, of course; everyone flies off the handle or makes mistakes now and then. But if you treat your child with respect, honesty, and understanding—above all when you have to discipline—your child will likely find the self-esteem to give those qualities back to the world. And, he or she will learn self-discipline.

Here are some guidelines:

- **Set clear limits.** Mean what you say. If you make a rule for your child—say, going to bed at 8:30—you must be ready to follow through and enforce it. It's natural for kids to test limits, but children won't feel secure unless the limits are firm and consistent. You can change house rules and let your child argue for a new policy—but not when you are both upset. Talk the next day instead.
- **Remember to praise.** Show your child when you are pleased with hugs, smiles, and other signs of approval. (Don't reward acts you dislike, though; giving a whining child candy might get you more of the same.)
- **Criticize with care.** If you have to criticize, try to add some praise for balance. You might thank your children for putting your clothes back in the closet after playing dress-up, but remind them that they shouldn't pull out the clothes without asking you.
- **Keep the rules simple.** Save "don't" for the big rules, and try not to use it for small things: Unless your child is in danger, "Wait for me" is better than "Don't run."
- **Put love first.** Always make it clear that you don't think your child is a bad person, and that you're talking about his or her *actions*. Your children need to know that you love them even when you are upset with them. You can cut down on acts you don't like by letting your child know you love him or her. Many parents care deeply about their children but can't show that love. One way is simply to listen to your child with complete attention, rather than mumbling "Mm-hmmm" while thinking about something else.
- **Explain yourself.** When your child is old enough to understand, explain why you have set certain rules—above all if he or she challenges you on them. Young children don't need a long speech.
- **Admit it when you're wrong.** Your children will respect you for it, and you'll set a good example for them. The best apology is a short and simple one.
- **Never hit your child.** Today experts agree that hitting children harms them emotionally as well as physically, fosters rage and self-hate, and often does lasting damage to their sense of worth. It doesn't work as discipline and it tends to leave a child angry rather than sorry.

  Psychologists also point out that hitting children teaches them that might makes right, and that children whose parents hit them often grow up to be violent, abusive, or self-destructive adults themselves. If you are so angry that you feel you're about to hit your child, leave the room or call Parents Anonymous (see **children's health resources**, page 275).
- **Know what's going on at school.** If your child goes to a school that uses physical punishment, talk to the superintendent, the principal, and the teachers, and write a letter saying you do not want your child hit or physically punished in any way. Insist on it.
- **Never shake an infant.** Parents or caregivers at the end of their rope when trying to calm a crying baby should take a time-out. Put the baby in the crib and go into another room for a few minutes—or call someone for support. Frustrated, desperate parents sometimes shake a baby who won't stop crying—not knowing that be-

cause babies' necks are so weak and their brains so fragile, shaking them can cause severe damage, including blindness, seizures, and brain damage, even death.

➤ **Don't say cruel things.** Verbal abuse can hurt as much as physical abuse. Avoid lashing out in a moment of anger, telling your children they're lazy or stupid, or that you wish they had never been born: They might believe you.

Likewise, avoid sarcasm, name-calling, or other unkind asides; treat your children as you would like to be treated yourself. Rather than blaming, show your displeasure by saying how your child's actions make you feel. Instead of saying, "You never think of anybody but yourself," tell your child, "I don't want to clean up after you"; or say, "I can't stand all this squabbling," instead of "You're impossible!"

➤ **Build trust.** Keep your promises and be honest with your child. Avoid mixed messages. If you are upset, say so; don't pretend you're not. Children can read your body language and will feel insecure if your words don't match it.

➤ **Keep a cool head with teenagers.** They, too, need steady limits, but remember that rebellion is normal at their age. Try to listen rather than lecture, and don't take things personally or get too upset during conflicts. (To get to the deeper issues troubling your teenager, try asking over and over, "What else is on your mind?" or "Anything else?") No matter how distant or disdainful teenagers may seem, they still want and need your love and support.

General Problems

Anemia

SIGNS AND SYMPTOMS

Main symptoms:
- Feeling tired and weak.
- Pasty skin; pale gums, nail beds, and eyelid linings.
- Shortness of breath, dizziness, and fainting.
- Headaches and trouble focusing.

Iron deficiency anemia:
Main symptoms, plus:
- Brittle nails.
- Black or bloody stools from bleeding in the intestines.

Folic acid deficiency anemia:
Main symptoms, plus:
- Sore mouth and tongue.
- Loss of appetite.
- Swollen abdomen.
- Nausea and diarrhea.

Vitamin B12 deficiency anemia:
Main symptoms, plus:
- Sore mouth and tongue.
- Problems with walking and balance.
- Tingling in hands and feet.
- Memory loss and confusion.

If you are anemic, your blood has trouble carrying oxygen to your tissues and taking away carbon dioxide. You become anemic either because you don't have enough red blood cells or because your red blood cells lack a protein that allows them to carry oxygen. There are many kinds of anemia:

Women who have heavy menstrual flow, or who are pregnant or nursing, may get **iron deficiency anemia.** It is most often handled with iron supplements. On the other hand, if your anemia stems from ailments that cause blood loss, such as **ulcers** (see page 136) or stomach or **colon cancer** (see page 118), the problem behind it needs to be treated.

Lack of folic acid, a vitamin needed to make red blood cells, can cause **folic acid deficiency anemia.** Teens, pregnant women, smokers, alcoholics, and people who don't eat well are at risk.

Vitamin B12 deficiency anemia (the most common type is called pernicious anemia) may affect the brain, spinal cord, and mental functions for life. In the United States, B12 anemia is rarely caused by a lack of B12 in the diet. Instead, it most often comes on if you're unable to absorb the vitamin from food—a problem that can be in your genes.

A rare form, **aplastic anemia,** isn't related to diet; it can be caused by radiation, powerful medicines, or toxins such as benzene.

Anemia can also be a sign of leukemia, lymphoma (cancer in the lymph system), chronic kidney disease, or other chronic ailments.

WHAT YOU CAN DO NOW

If you think you have anemia, call your doctor. **Note:** Don't take over-the-counter iron pills. Too much iron can cause symptoms like anemia and make you feel worse, and may make it hard to tell what's really wrong.

Fever

The average body temperature is 98.6 degrees, but some people have higher or lower normal levels. Temperatures also tend to rise as the day goes on. In adults, a fever is a temperature of 100 or above. A temperature of 100.4 in infants under 3 months, 102 in children, and 104 in adults is reason to call your doctor for advice. Most of us try to detect a fever by feeling the forehead, but that isn't the best way. Use a thermometer—after shaking it down and rinsing it with cool water—and leave it under the tongue for 3 minutes. (See **how to take a temperature,** page 261, and **fever in children,** page 260.)

SYMPTOMS	WHAT IT MIGHT BE	WHAT YOU CAN DO
Fever after some hours in a hot place, no sweating, rapid heartbeat, confusion, loss of consciousness.	Heat stroke (see page 40).	Call 911 or go to emergency room **right away.**
Fever with very painful headache, pain when bending over, nausea, trouble seeing in bright light, drowsiness, confusion, red or purple rash.	Meningitis (see page 57).	Call 911 or go to emergency room **right away.**
Fever and stiff jaw, muscle spasms and pain, sweating, trouble swallowing.	Tetanus (sometimes called lockjaw)—bacterial infection from a wound.	Call 911 or go to emergency room **right away.**
Sudden, high fever; vomiting and diarrhea; red rash; fatigue; headache, confusion, and dizziness.	Toxic shock syndrome (see page 248).	Call 911 or go to emergency room **right away.**
In children: fever, sudden seizures; turning blue in face (maybe).	Fever seizure (see fever in children, page 260).	If seizure is severe or lasts more than a few minutes, call 911 or go to emergency room **right away.** Otherwise, lay child on side or stomach, away from sharp objects. Most often harmless.
Rapid onset of fever, chills, pounding heart, confusion, signs of infection.	Blood poisoning (see box on page 31).	Call doctor **right away;** if you can't get one, call 911 or go to emergency room.
Low fever, pain in lower right part of abdomen, nausea and vomiting.	Appendicitis (see page 26).	Call doctor for prompt appointment. Meanwhile, don't eat or take laxatives; surgery may be needed.

(continued)

Fever *(continued)*

SYMPTOMS	WHAT IT MIGHT BE	WHAT YOU CAN DO
Low fever at first, higher 1–3 weeks later; pain in lower pelvis; foul discharge from vagina; painful urination.	Pelvic inflammatory disease (see page 242).	Call doctor for prompt appointment.
Fever and cough with or without sputum; chest pain; shortness of breath; abdominal pain.	Pneumonia (see page 98).	Call doctor for prompt appointment.
Sudden onset of fever and sore throat with white coating on tonsils; bright red rash about 24 hours later.	Scarlet fever (see page 271).	Call doctor for prompt appointment.
Fevers, night sweats, swollen lymph nodes, repeat infections, weight loss, fatigue, diarrhea, sores.	HIV infection. • AIDS (see page 224).	Call doctor for advice and testing appointment.
Low fever, nausea or loss of appetite, yellowish skin or eyes (jaundice), dark urine, light-colored stools, fatigue.	Hepatitis (see page 284).	Call doctor for advice and appointment.
Fatigue lasting weeks or months, bad sore throat, fever, swollen lymph glands.	Mononucleosis—viral illness spread by close contact such as kissing; attacks breathing system, liver, spleen, and lymph glands; most common in teens and young adults.	Call doctor for advice and appointment. Getting well takes 10 days to 6 months. Go back to normal activities over time.
Low fever, heavy night sweats, weight loss, chest pain, coughing—sometimes with bloody sputum.	Tuberculosis (see page 105).	Call doctor for advice and appointment.
High fever (over 103), weakness, headache, chills, raw throat, dry cough, runny nose, aching muscles.	Flu (see page 96).	Call doctor for advice. In children, fever of 102 or higher may be risky.
In children: fever with dry cough, loud breathing, runny nose, red eyes, blisters, swelling, or rash.	Any of many childhood diseases (see children's health chapter, page 252).	See fever in children, page 260.

WHEN TO CALL THE DOCTOR

Call 911 or go to an emergency room **right away:**

- If, after taking iron pills, you get: bloody diarrhea, fever, fatigue, vomiting, or seizures. Too much iron in your system can be fatal.

Call for advice:

- If you have symptoms of anemia.
- If you are being treated for diet-related anemia and don't get better in 2 weeks.

HOW TO PREVENT IT

To get enough iron:

- Eat plenty of iron-rich foods, including potatoes, broccoli, raisins, dried beans, oatmeal, and blackstrap molasses.
- Include lean red meat, liver, and shellfish in your diet.
- Don't drink coffee or tea with meals. They contain a substance that makes it hard for your body to absorb iron.

To get enough folic acid:

- Eat plenty of citrus fruits (oranges, grapefruit), dried beans, and green vegetables.
- Include liver, eggs, and milk in your diet.
- If you drink alcohol, drink just a little—no more than 2 drinks a day for men, 1 for women. A drink is a 1.5-ounce jigger of hard liquor, a 12-ounce can of beer, or a 5-ounce glass of wine. Alcohol can affect how well your body absorbs folic acid.
- If you're pregnant or nursing, or if you have very heavy periods, discuss your diet with your doctor.

To get enough vitamin B12:

- Include meat, chicken, fish, and/or dairy products in your diet. Buy cereals with added B12.

FOR MORE HELP

Information line: National Heart, Lung, and Blood Institute Information Center, 301-251-1222, M–F 8:30–5 EST. Staff answers questions and sends facts about anemia.

Book: *Dr. Susan Lark's Heavy Menstrual Flow & Anemia Self-Help Book,* by Susan Lark, M.D. Celestial Arts, 1996, $16.95.

Chronic Fatigue Syndrome

SIGNS AND SYMPTOMS

- Flulike symptoms; fatigue not caused by work or exercise that lasts longer than 6 months.
- Weakness and fatigue that last for more than 24 hours after mild exercise (sometimes fatigue occurs 1 or 2 days later).
- Sore throat.
- Low fever (temperature up to 101 degrees) or chills.
- Painful lymph nodes.
- Headaches that don't feel the same as those you've had in the past.
- Pains that spread to joints without causing redness or swelling.
- Short-term blind spots and trouble looking at light.
- Trouble thinking or staying focused; forgetting things, being moody and confused.
- Trouble sleeping.

Little is known about chronic fatigue syndrome (CFS). Its causes are unclear, and it is diagnosed by ruling out other diseases. CFS strikes people of all ages and races, and of both sexes, although 75 percent of those who have it are women. There's no proof that you can catch it from other people.

The pain, fatigue, and thinking problems that mark the ailment often keep people out of work or school. This can lead to depression. The symptoms sometimes ease up or go away on their own after a number of months or years, but often they come and go for any amount of time. Treatment stresses plenty of rest, a healthful diet, and gentle exercise. Drugs such as antidepressants and over-the-counter pain relievers can help ease some symptoms.

WHAT YOU CAN DO NOW

- Take over-the-counter painkillers, such as ibuprofen, for muscle aches and headaches (see **pain relief,** page 317).
- Stay active, but don't become overtired.
- Join a support group for those with chronic pain or depression.

WHEN TO CALL THE DOCTOR

- If you have fatigue that won't go away and other symptoms of CFS.
- If you feel new symptoms after you are diagnosed.

HOW TO PREVENT IT

There is no known way to prevent chronic fatigue syndrome.

FOR MORE HELP

Information line: Centers for Disease Control and Prevention, 404-332-4555, 24-hour recording. Offers data on current research and treatments for chronic fatigue syndrome, by phone or fax. **Web site:** *http://www.cdc.gov/ncidod/publications/cfs/cfshome.htm.* Answers common questions about chronic fatigue syndrome.

Information line: Chronic Fatigue and Immune Dysfunction Syndrome Association of America, 800-442-3437, 24-hour recording. Sends information, a newsletter, notices of forums for patients, and a list of local support groups. **Web site:** *http://www.YBI.com/cfids/index.html.*

Information line: American Chronic Pain Association, 916-632-0922, 24-hour line. Ask for information and a list of support groups run by and for those with chronic pain.

Book: *Osler's Web,* by Hillary Johnson. Explores the history of chronic fatigue syndrome; charges the medical world with ignoring the ailment. Crown Publishers, 1996, $30.

Book: *Running on Empty,* by Katrina Berne, Ph.D. A guide to chronic fatigue syndrome symptoms and coping skills. Hunter House, 1995, $14.95.

FIBROMYALGIA

Fibromyalgia may come with chronic fatigue syndrome and is sometimes confused with it. Symptoms include pain and fatigue in muscles, tendons, and ligaments (though not in joints), and sleep problems. Unlike chronic fatigue syndrome, fibromyalgia can be spotted with the "18 Tender Points" test that applies pressure to 18 body parts. Tenderness in at least 11 often means fibromyalgia.

Fibromyalgia tends to affect women between the ages of 20 and 50. It may be present all the time or run in 3- or 4-day cycles. Symptoms are treated with antidepressants, painkillers, and muscle relaxants. Exercising often may also relieve pain.

For more help: Fibromyalgia Network, 800-853-2929, M–F 8–5 PST. Call for advice, names of doctors, a list of support groups in your area, and a newsletter.

Diabetes

SIGNS AND SYMPTOMS

- Extreme thirst.
- Need to urinate often, sometimes every hour.
- Loss of weight for no known reason.
- Blurred vision.
- Lasting tiredness.
- In women: frequent yeast and bladder infections, sometimes missed menstrual periods.

Diabetes mellitus affects about 16 million people in the United States, yet perhaps only half know they have it. *Mellitus,* from the Latin for "sweetened with honey," refers to having too much unused sugar in the blood.

People with the most common type, which

tends to show up in older adults, often think their symptoms are a result of aging or being overweight. As a result, they don't get the treatment they need. Untreated diabetes can cause severe problems, including stroke and heart attack, blindness, kidney trouble, nerve damage, and loss of limbs due to circulatory problems.

The two main types of diabetes are Type I and Type II. Type I most often starts in childhood when the pancreas fails to make insulin, a hormone that converts sugar in the muscles to energy. People with Type I diabetes need daily insulin shots.

About 90 percent of diabetes is Type II: The muscles fail to take up insulin even though the body may be making enough of it. People with Type II may not need insulin shots.

Type II is also called adult-onset diabetes because it mostly comes on after age 40. You're at greater risk if someone in your family has Type II diabetes. A high-fat diet, lack of exercise, and being overweight also raise the risk.

Some women get a kind of high blood sugar called gestational diabetes when they are pregnant. In most cases, it goes away once the baby is born.

While neither Type I nor Type II diabetes can be cured, you can manage either one quite well by watching your blood sugar levels and combining medicine, exercise, and a healthful diet.

DANGER IN THE MEDICINE CABINET

Some drugs can affect blood sugar levels, which people with diabetes need to track closely.

- Aspirin can lower blood sugar if taken in large amounts over a long period of time.
- Phenylephrine, epinephrine, and ephedrine—in some asthma and cold medicines, and even herbal teas—can raise blood sugar and blood pressure.
- Fish oil, which some people take to lower their cholesterol, may raise blood sugar.
- Caffeine, found in coffee, sodas, hunger suppressants, some headache drugs, "pep" pills, and diuretics, may also raise blood sugar.

WHAT YOU CAN DO NOW

- If you know you have diabetes, follow your doctor's advice about diet, exercise, and tracking your blood sugar levels.
- Keep a log to help manage your diabetes. For a month, record your blood sugar level many times each day, always at the same times (use a home glucose monitor). Also record when and what you eat at each meal; the type of exercise you do and for how long; your times of low and high energy. Take this record to your doctor.
- Practice good foot care. Check your feet often for cuts and sores. Call your doctor if you think you have an infection.
- Get eye exams often.
- Eat a low-fat, low-cholesterol diet to keep your blood sugar and your weight in check.
- Exercise often to help balance your blood sugar, control your weight, and cut your risk of heart disease. Ask your doctor how that works, and about the right way to balance your blood sugar with medicines.
- Wear a medical alert tag. Make sure the tag says the type of diabetes you have.
- Stay in touch with your doctor and schedule visits with him or her often.
- If your blood sugar level drops too low, you may notice symptoms of hypoglycemia: feeling confused, dizzy, or weak, sweating, shaking, hunger, headache, and blurred vision. As soon as you can, eat one of these: 4 ounces of fruit juice or a sugared drink; some candy, such as 6 or 7 jelly beans; 3 large marshmallows; or half a tube of Glutose (80 gram size). If you don't feel better in a few minutes, eat one more portion. (Don't eat chocolate for quick sugar—the fat in it slows the rate at which sugar gets into your bloodstream.)
- If your blood sugar level rises too high, you may have hyperglycemia. Symptoms include blurred vision, thirst, hunger, and the need to urinate. Test your blood sugar

level with your monitor. If it is much higher than your normal reading, call your doctor promptly.

WHEN TO CALL THE DOCTOR

Call 911 or go to an emergency room **right away:**

- If your stomach hurts, you are tired and nauseated, you are breathing quickly and urinating very often, and your breath is very sweet. Ketoacidosis, a sometimes fatal ailment, may be the problem.
- If you are extremely thirsty, tired, weak, and confused. You may have very high blood sugar levels that could lead to coma.
- If a person known to have diabetes loses consciousness.

Call for a prompt appointment:

- If you have symptoms of diabetes, or your child does.
- If you have diabetes and you get the flu. Flu and some other illnesses can make your blood sugar levels go out of control.
- If you have any problems with your vision.
- If you notice swelling that is not normal, often in the legs.
- If you have painful urination or feel the urge to urinate often.

HOW TO PREVENT IT

There is no way to prevent Type I diabetes. To prevent Type II diabetes:

- Keep your weight within the healthy range for your age, height, and build.
- Exercise often. This is vital for preventing diabetes or managing it once it occurs.
- If you are over 40 and overweight, or have a family history of diabetes, get screened for diabetes every 1 to 3 years.

FOR MORE HELP

Organization: American Diabetes Association, 800-342-2383, M–F 8:30–8 EST. Offers facts on how to manage diabetes, other brochures, and a list of local diabetes groups. **Web site:** *http://diabetes.org.* Select your state to access news and facts.

Organization: Juvenile Diabetes Foundation, 800-533-2873, M–F 9–5 EST. Offers names of local chapters that have free materials, a list of support groups, and names of local doctors.

Organization: National Diabetes Information Clearinghouse, 1 Information Way, Bethesda, MD 20892-3560. 301-654-3327, M–F 9–5 EST. Offers free brochures.

Book: *Diabetes, Type II: Living a Long, Healthy Life Through Blood Sugar Normalization,* by Richard K. Bernstein, M.D. A fine resource for the treatment of diabetes Types I and II. Although the book is out of print, a photocopy can be ordered from Dr. Bernstein's practice at 914-698-7500 for $75. Or borrow it from your local library.

Book: *50 Essential Things to Do When the Doctor Says It's Diabetes,* by Diana Tonnessen. Simple guide to taking charge of your illness. Plume Books, 1996, $10.95.

Video: *Diabetes at Time of Diagnosis.* Clear overview of causes and treatments, with 4 reports—Understanding the Diagnosis, What Happens Next?, Treatment and Management, and Issues and Answers. Time Life Medical, 1996, $19.95. Sold in many pharmacies; for one near you, call 800-588-9959.

Hepatitis

SIGNS AND SYMPTOMS

Note: Some forms of hepatitis produce no symptoms.

First symptoms are flulike:

- Fever and fatigue.
- Nausea, vomiting, lost appetite.
- Abdominal pain.

Other, less common symptoms:

- Dark urine; clay-colored stools.
- Jaundice—yellow eyes and skin.

Hepatitis means "inflammation of the liver." A group of viruses that target the liver are most often the cause. But it can be brought on—or made worse—by other diseases, poisons, and long-term alcohol or drug abuse.

Viral hepatitis, a worldwide health prob-

FIVE KINDS OF VIRAL HEPATITIS					
Type of hepatitis	**How transmitted**	**People at risk**	**Incidence in United States**	**Risks**	**Vaccine available**
A	Food, water, feces, sex.	Those exposed to poor sanitation.	32% of acute hepatitis cases.	Few long-term effects.	Yes.
B	IV drug use, sex, blood, body fluids.	IV drug users, people with multiple sex partners, health workers.	43% of acute hepatitis cases.	Can be chronic; increases risk of liver cancer.	Yes.
C	IV drug use, blood, maybe sex.	IV drug users, health workers.	21% of acute hepatitis cases.	High risk of chronic liver disease, cancer.	No.
D	Found only with B.	Same as B.	Not common.	May become chronic.	B vaccine prevents D as well.
E	Food, feces, water.	Travelers to Asia and Africa, where it's common.	Very rare.	High death rate for pregnant women.	No.

lem, is highly contagious. Symptoms can be mild or can lead to liver failure and death. It comes in 2 basic forms—oral and blood-borne—with several subtypes:

Oral—hepatitis types A and E. These are spread through feces, tainted food and water, or sex. They are common in places with poor water and toilet facilities. Hepatitis E, rare in the United States, is found mostly in India and Africa, but A is common in the United States—1 in 3 Americans has had it.

These types come on quickly, and may feel like a mild flu or make you very sick. Nearly everyone with A gets better and is then immune to it. The vaccine for A is advised for those who travel or live in areas with poor sanitation. Hepatitis E can be fatal to pregnant women.

Blood-borne—hepatitis types B, C, and D. These are spread through body fluids much the same way that HIV (the human immunodeficiency virus that causes AIDS) is—by intravenous needles, blood, and sex. As in HIV, few or no symptoms may show up when you are first infected, but these hepatitis types can lead to lifelong problems or death. Most people remain able to pass the illness along for the rest of their lives, even if they have no symptoms.

Hundreds of millions of people worldwide carry hepatitis. Many get better, but a large number who get hepatitis B and more than 70 percent who get C have chronic illness. C alone accounts for more than a third of liver transplants today. Hepatitis D infects only those who already have B, and makes it worse.

A vaccine against B also protects against D. A vaccine for C is under study.

WHAT YOU CAN DO NOW

➤ Don't drink alcohol. Alcohol can damage a *healthy* liver—and it's much worse for one that's sick.

- Rest as much as you need to.
- Eat frequent small meals.
- Drink at least 8 glasses of water each day.
- Don't take aspirin or acetaminophen. Ask your doctor about pain relief, and see box on page 317.
- Urge those close to you to be vaccinated. Tell sex partners you have hepatitis, and practice **safe sex** (see box on page 227).
- If you have chronic B or C, join a support group.

WHEN TO CALL THE DOCTOR

- If you have any of the less common symptoms listed on page 284.
- If you have been exposed to hepatitis.
- If you have had hepatitis and you start to have symptoms again.

HOW TO PREVENT IT

- Don't drink alcohol, or don't drink much: for men, no more than 2 drinks per day; for women, no more than 1 (a drink is 1.5 ounces of hard liquor, a 12-ounce can of beer, or a 5-ounce glass of wine).
- If you have a drinking problem or are an alcoholic, get help right away (see **alcohol abuse,** page 206).
- Hepatitis A and E:
  - Get a vaccination for hepatitis A if you plan to travel to a place where it is widespread or that has poor water or toilet facilities. It takes 2 to 4 weeks for the vaccine to take effect, but you can get faster-acting short-term shots.
  - While in areas with poor sanitation, drink only boiled or bottled fluids. Don't eat unpeeled or uncooked foods or shellfish, and don't use ice cubes.
  - Wash your hands with soap and water after using the toilet and before touching food.
  - If you are infected with A or E, don't prepare or touch other people's food. Take extra care to wash hands, clothing, and bedding.
- Hepatitis B, C, and D:
  - Get a vaccination for B if you are a teenager, have more than one sex partner, work in a health field, travel widely, or live with anyone who has B or who is from Asia (where it is widespread). Hepatitis B vaccine is now given at birth. It also protects against type D.
  - Use the same safeguards as for HIV: Practice safe sex. Don't share IV needles, manicuring tools, razors, toothbrushes, or other items that can collect or hold blood (see **AIDS,** page 224).
  - Insist on sterile needles for acupuncture, body or ear piercing, or tattoos.
  - If you are infected, take care not to spread hepatitis to others through your blood or body fluids. Tell sex partners about your illness, and practice safe sex.

FOR MORE HELP

Hotline: National STD Hotline, Centers for Disease Control and Prevention, 800-227-8922, M–F 8AM–11PM EST. Ask for reports on hepatitis and lists of clinics.

Information line: American Liver Foundation, 800-223-0179, M–Th 9–6:30, F 9–5 EST. Staff answers questions and sends brochures on hepatitis. **Web site:** *http://sadieo.ucsf.edu/alf/alffinal/homepagealf.html.*

Organization: Hepatitis B Foundation, 101 Greenwood Ave., Suite 570, Jenkintown, PA 19046. 215-884-8786, M–F 9–5 EST. Staff answers questions, suggests HBV support groups, and sends a quarterly newsletter ($35 donation). **Web site:** *http://www.libertynet.org/~hep-b.*

Web access: The Hepatitis Information Network. After logging on to the Internet, type: *http://www.wp.com/hepatitis.* Offers reports on all types of hepatitis, answers to common questions, and other links on the Web.

Infections

SIGNS AND SYMPTOMS

Main symptoms:

- Fever higher than 100 degrees (oral thermometer reading) and/or chills and sweating.
- Headache.

- ■ Muscle aches or soreness.
- ■ Fatigue.
- ■ Swollen lymph nodes (sometimes).

Intestinal infection:

- ■ Diarrhea.
- ■ Nausea and vomiting.
- ■ Abdominal cramps or gas pains.
- ■ Dehydration.

Respiratory infection:

- ■ Coughing and sneezing.
- ■ Sinus or chest pain, sore throat, congestion, and excess mucus.
- ■ Watery eyes.

Bladder infection:

- ■ Burning pain when you urinate; need to urinate often.
- ■ Bloody urine.

Infection of the mouth, ears, or eyes:

- ■ Pain or irritation in the affected area.
- ■ Swelling, tenderness, and/or redness that is not normal.

Joint infection:

- ■ Tenderness, redness, or pain and swelling in the joints, often in only one part of the body.

Germs get into our bodies in a number of ways: through torn skin, sex, the air we breathe, the food we eat, and the water we drink. Whether a germ is a bacterium, virus, or fungus, it tries to survive once it's inside your body. Viruses invade living cells and multiply. They may weaken the body's defenses for a time against more dire bacterial infections.

You feel sick in part because of your body's response. When your body senses an attack, your immune system releases antibodies and white blood cells to fight off the invaders. The white blood cells make chemical triggers; these cause the fevers that often come with infection. Some germs release toxins and steal nutrients from healthy cells. This assault also makes you feel sick.

In most cases, all your immune system needs to fight infection is for you to rest and maintain a healthy diet. For more stubborn infections, germ-destroying drugs will help. Sometimes, your body will recall an earlier bout with an ailment, such as measles, mumps, or chicken pox. If your body meets the same germ again, it is quite often able to ward off a new attack. This is what gives you immunity. Vaccines can also offer immunity to some infections.

For infected wounds, see **cuts, scrapes, and wounds,** page 30.

WHAT YOU CAN DO NOW

- ➤ If you are in good health, let a low fever run its course. A fever under 104 degrees (oral thermometer reading) in adults, 102 in children, and 100.4 in infants under 3 months is seldom risky and may even speed recovery from the infection.
- ➤ Give your body a chance to get better. Rest, drink lots of water, and eat well. Don't smoke or drink alcohol.

WHEN TO CALL THE DOCTOR

Call for advice and an appointment:

- ➤ If you are over 65 and in poor health, and have symptoms of an infection.
- ➤ If your temperature rises to 104 or higher, or goes over 101 with joint pain; if a child's rises to 102 or higher; or an infant's to 100.4 or higher.
- ➤ If you have symptoms of severe infection, such as problems speaking, seeing, swallowing, or breathing, or if you have trouble moving.
- ➤ If your skin has been broken by a human or animal bite.
- ➤ If your throat is sore, or if you're vomiting or have diarrhea that doesn't go away after a few days.

HOW TO PREVENT IT

- ➤ Keep your immune system strong:
  - Eat well. Drink plenty of fluids.
  - Exercise often.
  - Get enough sleep.
  - Don't smoke or use drugs.
  - If you drink alcohol, do so lightly (no more than two 1.5-ounce drinks of hard liquor, 2 12-ounce cans of beer, or two 5-ounce glasses of wine a day for men, one for women).
  - Take steps to reduce stress in your life;

Sudden Weight Gain or Loss

Your weight changes slightly from day to day even when you eat normal amounts of food. Dieting or overeating can, of course, cause greater weight changes. But not all changes come from gains or losses of fat. You might lose several pounds of fluid in a single day from sweating if you're doing hard work. Changes in hormone levels during the menstrual cycle, or eating a lot of salty food, can make your body hold fluids (often signaled by puffy hands and ankles) and may cause you to gain several pounds in a short time. Many medicines can cause loss of appetite and loss of weight. So can depression. But weight gain or loss for no known reason can be a sign of a hidden disease—such as those listed here. If you gain or lose more than 10 to 15 pounds in a month and you don't know why, call your doctor for advice and an appointment.

WEIGHT GAIN

SYMPTOMS	WHAT IT MIGHT BE	WHAT YOU CAN DO
Rapid weight gain with swelling in legs, ankles, and midriff; fatigue; yellow skin; easy bruising and bleeding; impotence; dark urine; black or bloody stools; blood in vomit.	Cirrhosis—liver damage. May be caused by alcohol abuse, hepatitis (see page 284), or a disease passed on in your genes.	If you vomit blood, call 911 or go to emergency room **right away.** Otherwise, call doctor for prompt appointment.
Rapid weight gain with swelling in legs, ankles, and midriff; shortness of breath; fatigue; heart flutters; need to urinate often; loss of appetite.	Congestive heart failure (see page 111). • Kidney disease.	If you have severe chest pain or shortness of breath, call 911 or go to emergency room **right away.** Otherwise, call doctor for prompt appointment.
Slow weight gain, with swollen face, fat on torso and upper back; fatigue; acne; reddish skin; trouble sleeping. In men: impotence, breast growth. In women: facial hair, periods that slow or stop.	Cushing's syndrome—adrenal glands make too much of hormone that affects connective tissue. Most often caused by taking corticosteroids for rheumatoid arthritis, asthma, or other illnesses.	Call doctor for advice.
Slow weight gain, fatigue, dry skin, goiter (swelling in neck).	Underactive thyroid gland (see thyroid problems, page 294).	Call doctor for advice.

Sudden Weight Gain or Loss

WEIGHT LOSS

SYMPTOMS	WHAT IT MIGHT BE	WHAT YOU CAN DO
Rapid weight loss despite increased appetite, anxiety, sweating, rapid heartbeat, goiter (swelling in neck).	Overactive thyroid gland (see thyroid problems, page 294).	Call doctor for prompt appointment.
Weight loss, fatigue, vomiting, diarrhea, brownish skin, hair loss, feeling cold, big mood changes (confusion, aggression, or depression).	Addison's disease—adrenal glands make too little of hormones that control metabolism and responses to stress. Very rare.	Call doctor for prompt appointment.
Slow weight loss, fevers, night sweats, swollen lymph nodes, repeat infections, fatigue, diarrhea, sores.	HIV infection. • AIDS (see page 224).	Call doctor for advice and testing appointment.
Weight loss with changes or lumps in skin, bleeding that is not normal, digestive problems, changes in bowel or bladder habits.	Cancer—unchecked growth of cells. Symptoms vary with type of cancer.	Call doctor for advice and appointment.
Rapid weight loss, fatigue, extreme thirst, frequent urination, infections in vagina.	Diabetes (see page 282).	Call doctor for advice and appointment.
Weight loss and diarrhea; fatigue; gas and stomach pains; large, very bad-smelling stools.	Malabsorption—intestines fail to absorb one or more nutrients from food.	Call doctor for advice and appointment if symptoms last longer than a few days.
Extreme weight loss from not eating, compulsive exercising, periods that slow or stop, increase in facial hair, depression (in anorexia). Extreme weight loss from binge eating and vomiting (in bulimia).	Eating disorder.	See eating disorders, page 218.

stress weakens the immune system. Try meditation, yoga, or deep breathing.
- Get a flu shot before each flu season.
- Ask your doctor about getting immunized against pneumonia.
- Have your children vaccinated against childhood diseases (see **children's immunization** chart, page 256).
- Wash your hands very often, and avoid putting your fingers in your mouth or rubbing your eyes.
- Practice **safe sex** (see box on page 227).
- Women who have their periods should change tampons at least every 6 hours to keep harmful bacteria from growing. (See **toxic shock syndrome,** page 248.)
- Keep an eye out for changes in your body—from swelling around nicks and cuts to a runny nose or genital discharge. Attend to symptoms right away.

Lupus

SIGNS AND SYMPTOMS

- Butterfly-shaped rash across the nose and cheeks.
- Aching, swollen joints.
- Fever over 100 degrees.
- Long-lasting fatigue.
- Sores in the nose, mouth, or throat.
- Bleeding or bruising that is not normal.
- Numbness in the fingers and toes.
- Swollen abdomen and ankles (sometimes).
- Dark urine.
- Chest pain when breathing deeply.
- Sensitivity to sunlight; a rash that results after time spent in the sun.
- Mental or personality changes, including depression.

When you have lupus, your body's immune system attacks proteins in your tissues as if they were invaders. This war in your body causes swelling and pain, most often in the joints. It may also inflame the kidneys, skin, and lining of the lungs, heart, and brain, and it may damage white blood cells. When it is severe and untreated, lupus can lead to kidney failure. A person with lupus may also become depressed.

The disease is chronic—you may have it for the rest of your life, with symptoms that come and go—but it may lie low for a long time between flare-ups.

Why the body attacks itself in this way is unknown. It is known that lupus can be triggered by infections, ultraviolet or fluorescent light, and certain drugs, such as some used to treat heart flutters or high blood pressure.

Lupus most often strikes people between 35 and 45, women almost 10 times more often than men. It's most common among African Americans, Asians, and Native Americans. It also runs in families.

The long-term outlook for people with lupus has improved in recent years. Now 80 to 90 percent can expect to have long and healthy lives with early treatment, including drugs to ease symptoms, as well as changes in diet, exercise, and mental outlook.

WHAT YOU CAN DO NOW

- Get lots of rest if you're tired. Take naps when you're having a flare-up.
- When the disease is low-level and not causing you pain, and you feel well, start an exercise program. Swimming is one good way for people with lupus to keep their muscles in shape.
- Put warm compresses on achy joints.
- For pain, take aspirin or ibuprofen—with meals to avoid stomach upset (see **pain relief,** page 317).
- Sunlight alone can cause a flare-up in some people. Avoid the sun during the middle of the day. Half an hour before leaving home each day, apply a sunscreen with an SPF of at least 15.
- Eat well—stick to a diet that's low in fat and salt, high in complex carbohydrates and calcium.
- Protect your hands from anything that may cause pain by wearing gloves.
- Avoid alcohol, tobacco, and caffeine.

WHEN TO CALL THE DOCTOR

Call for emergency advice (if you can't get any, call 911 or go to an emergency room):

- If you have symptoms of kidney disease: need to urinate often; swollen ankles; shortness of breath; nausea and vomiting; chest and bone pain; itching, bruising, or bleeding; confusion; loss of consciousness.

Call for advice:

- If you have symptoms of lupus.
- If you know that you have lupus and your symptoms get worse or change.

FOR MORE HELP

Information line: National Institute of Arthritis and Musculoskeletal and Skin Diseases Information Clearinghouse, 301-495-4484, M–F 8:30–5 EST. Request a packet of recent articles on lupus.

Organization: Lupus Foundation of America, 800-558-0121, 24-hour recording. Sends a packet with brochures on lupus and a listing of Lupus Foundation chapters with support groups near you.

Book: *The Lupus Handbook for Women*, by Robin Dibner, M.D., and Carol Colman. Fireside, 1994, $11.

Web access: Hamline University. After logging on to the Internet, type: *http ://www.hamline.edu/lupus/index.html.* Offers reports on lupus, clinical trials, conferences, and other sources of help.

Lyme Disease

SIGNS AND SYMPTOMS

- Rash in a bull's-eye shape with pale center, from a tick bite 2 days to a month before. The rash may last 2 to 4 weeks or longer. (Some people don't recall having a rash.)
- Within a month, aching joints and muscles, weakness, fever, chills, sore throat, headache.
- After a few weeks or a few months, paralysis of the face, stiff neck, sensitivity to light, uneven heartbeats, and fainting.
- Joint pain and swelling.

Lyme disease, a bacterial infection spread by tick bites, can be a long illness. More than 10,000 people get it each year.

The ticks pick up the bacteria from mice, deer, and other animals. The tick, often as small as a poppy seed, must remain attached to a person for 36 to 48 hours to transmit the bacteria, which can then invade the skin, nervous system, heart, and joints.

Lyme disease can be hard to diagnose. It has vague symptoms that seem like those of other illnesses, and the blood test can't always be counted on. If untreated, the infection can lead to nerve problems, a type of arthritis, and heart troubles such as uneven heartbeats.

The good news is that the illness can be prevented, responds well to treatment in the early stages, and sometimes goes away by itself. Treatments include antibiotics and, if arthritis develops, corticosteroids for inflamed and painful joints.

WHAT YOU CAN DO NOW

After a walk in the woods or through dense grass, check your clothing and skin for ticks. If you find one:

- Get rid of it right away. Using tweezers, grab it as near to your skin as you can. Then pull up with slow, even pressure to remove the entire tick. Avoid squeezing or twisting the tick's body, since this may spread bacteria into your skin or blood (see **tick bites,** page 47).
- Drop the tick in a jar of rubbing alcohol to save it for tests.
- Clean the bite with alcohol. Wash your hands in soap and water.
- Don't try to dislodge a tick with kerosene, petroleum jelly, or a lighted cigarette or match. None of these methods work.

WHEN TO CALL THE DOCTOR

- If you've been in tick country or you've

been bitten by a tick, and you have symptoms of Lyme disease.

➤ If your symptoms return after treatment.

HOW TO PREVENT IT

➤ Wear light-colored clothes in grassy or wooded areas to make ticks easy to spot. Wear shoes (not sandals), long pants, and long-sleeved shirts. Pull your socks up over your pant legs.

➤ Use an insect spray with DEET on clothing. Use just a little on skin.

➤ Check your skin, hair, and clothing for ticks after an outing. Also check your pets for ticks.

➤ Fit your pet with a tick-repellent collar.

➤ Clear away brush near your home that might attract ticks. Stack your firewood away from the house (woodpiles attract mice, which carry ticks).

FOR MORE HELP

Information line: American Lyme Disease Foundation, 800-876-5963, 24-hour recording. 914-277-6970, M–F 9–5 EST. Offers a list of doctors and free brochures on Lyme disease and how to control ticks.

Organization: Arthritis Foundation, 1330 W. Peachtree, Atlanta, GA 30309. 404-872-7100, M–F 9–5 EST. Offers a free brochure on Lyme disease and a list of local arthritis support groups.

Book: *Coping With Lyme Disease,* by Denise Lang and Derrick DeSilva, Jr., M.D. Offers advice on how to live with Lyme disease, explores treatment, and lists support groups nationwide. Henry Holt, 1993, $12.95.

Web access: Lyme Disease Information Resource. After logging on to the Internet, type: *http://www.sky.net/~dporter/lyme1.html.* Offers basic facts, research findings, lists of support groups, and links to other sites on the Web.

Sleep Disorders

SIGNS AND SYMPTOMS

Insomnia:

- Trouble falling asleep.
- Waking often during the night.
- Early waking.
- Being sleepy often during the day.
- Trouble staying focused.

Obstructive sleep apnea:

- Loud bursts of snoring and snorting that jerk the sleeper (and anyone nearby) awake.
- Morning headaches.
- Daytime sleepiness with trouble staying focused.
- Short temper, bad moods.

Narcolepsy:

- Falling asleep all of a sudden and with no control in the daytime.
- Sudden loss of muscle control triggered by strong emotion or fatigue.
- Vivid dreams or visions when falling asleep or waking up.
- Fatigue.

Restless legs syndrome:

- Creepy, crawly, or sometimes painful feelings in the legs, most often at night when trying to fall asleep, or during sleep.
- Constant urge to move the feet and legs.
- Jerking of legs (and sometimes arms) that you can't control.

Sleep disorders range from mild insomnia caused by jet lag to severe cases of sleep apnea. They affect as many as 70 million Americans.

Short-term insomnia is chiefly caused by stress, emotional upset, or a change in schedule. Long-term trouble with sleep may be a sign of a medical problem, such as **thyroid problems** (see page 294), **chronic bronchitis** or **emphysema** (see page 92), **Parkinson's disease** (see page 59), **Alzheimer's disease** (see page 50), **alcohol abuse** (see page 206), or **drug abuse** (see page 215). Another major cause is **depression** (see page 213). Treating the basic ailment, and creating restful bedtime routines, can often help.

Obstructive sleep apnea is most common among overweight men who sleep on their backs. The muscles in the throat sag, briefly closing off the airway. The effort to catch a breath wakes the sleeper. The process goes on all night long. People with sleep apnea don't get enough deep sleep and feel tired during the day. Obstructive sleep apnea can cause serious health problems over time, including heart disease. People deprived of sleep may become depressed or have other personality changes.

People with **narcolepsy** may fall deeply asleep just about anywhere, anytime during the day. Not much is known about the ailment, but it seems to run in families. It can be treated with stimulants and antidepressants your doctor can prescribe.

Those with **restless legs syndrome** are bothered by odd feelings, most often in the legs, at night when they are still awake or trying to fall asleep, or even after they've been asleep for a while. People with this ailment may feel tired the next day, above all if they can't get back to sleep or if they get out of bed and walk around to relieve discomfort. No one knows what causes restless legs syndrome, but it, too, seems to run in families.

CATCHING UP TO JET LAG

When you change time zones quickly, your sleeping patterns are out of sync with the local time. Jet lag can leave you drowsy and confused.

If you will be staying more than 2 days in a new place, you can avoid many of the symptoms. (It's hard to adjust on trips of 2 days or less.) Here's what to do:

- A few days to a week before leaving, adjust your schedule to the new time zone. Get up and go to bed as if you were already there.
- If you arrive in the daytime, spend some time outdoors. The sunlight helps reset your inner clock.
- Avoid alcohol, caffeine, rich and sweet foods, and too much talking before bed. All can keep you awake.
- Bring earplugs and a blindfold to block out noises and lights when sleeping.
- Wake up at the right local time, even if you don't have to.

WHAT YOU CAN DO NOW

Insomnia:

- Follow a calming bedtime routine: Drink warm milk, listen to soothing music, or read a book.
- Use your bed only for sleep or sex, not for working or watching TV.
- Don't toss and turn. If you can't fall asleep, get up and read until you feel sleepy.

Obstructive sleep apnea:

- Sew a tennis ball into the back of your pajamas so you don't sleep on your back.
- For mild snoring, try an over-the-counter nasal strip, which widens your nostrils and eases breathing.
- For severe snoring, ask your dentist about a retainerlike device that moves your tongue and lower jaw forward. Or ask your doctor about a special device called CPAP (continuous positive airway pressure) that pumps air to you through a mask. Another option is surgery: One type removes parts of the soft palate at the back of the mouth. Another removes the uvula, the fleshy cone that hangs down from the soft palate at the back of the throat.

Narcolepsy:

- Schedule one or more daytime naps at regular times.

Restless legs:

- For restless legs syndrome, your doctor can prescribe a drug that may relieve the twitching and discomfort and help you get some sleep.

WHEN TO CALL THE DOCTOR

- If you have symptoms of obstructive sleep apnea or narcolepsy, above all if you feel sleepy all the time.
- If you have had insomnia for more than 2 weeks.

- If you are taking prescription drugs. They can cause insomnia.

HOW TO PREVENT IT

- Avoid drinks with caffeine for at least 6 hours before bedtime.
- Don't drink alcohol or smoke for at least 2 hours before bedtime.
- Exercise often, but not within 3 hours of bedtime.
- If you have sleep apnea and are overweight, lose the extra pounds.
- Make sure your bedroom is quiet and dark and has plenty of air.
- Don't take a nap in the late afternoon or early evening.
- Get up each day at the same time. When you go to sleep doesn't matter.

FOR MORE HELP

Organization: National Sleep Foundation, 1367 Connecticut Ave. NW, Suite 200, Washington, DC 20036. Write for free brochures on sleep and sleep disorders.

Organization: Narcolepsy Network, Box 424601, Cincinnati, OH 45242. 513-891-3522, M–F 9–5 EST. Fax: 512-891-9936. Request a brochure and a newsletter.

Organization: Restless Legs Syndrome Foundation, 514 Daniel St., Raleigh, NC 27605. Send a stamped, self-addressed envelope for a brochure on RLS. **Web site:** *http://www.rls.org*.

Booklet: National Heart, Lung, and Blood Institute Information Center, Box 30105, Bethesda, MD 20824-0105. 800-575-WELL, 24-hour recording. Request "Breathing Disorders During Sleep."

Book: *No More Sleepless Nights,* by Peter Hauri, Ph.D., and Shirley Linde, Ph.D. Revised edition of the classic sleep guide. Wiley, 1996, $14.95.

Book: *How to Get a Good Night's Sleep,* by Richard Graber and Paul Gouin, M.D. Offers more than 100 useful tips for sleeping through the night. Chronimed Publishing, 1995, $10.95.

Web access: The Sleep Medicine Home Page. After logging on to the Internet, type: *http://www.cloud9.net:80/~thorpy*. Offers a wide range of links to other sites (including Sleepnet), research centers, and support groups.

Video: *Insomnia at Time of Diagnosis*. Clear overview of causes and treatments, with 4 reports—Understanding the Diagnosis, What Happens Next?, Treatment and Management, and Issues and Answers. Time Life Medical, 1996, $19.95. Sold in many pharmacies; for one near you, call 800-588-9959.

Thyroid Problems

SIGNS AND SYMPTOMS

Hyperthyroidism:

- Losing weight even though you want to eat more than ever.
- Trembling hands.
- Higher-than-normal blood pressure, faster heartbeat, anxiety, sweating.
- Bulging, watery eyes.
- Frequent bowel movements.
- Lighter and less frequent menstrual periods.
- Sometimes a goiter—swelling in the front of the neck.

Hypothyroidism:

- Low energy, slower pace of thinking than normal.
- Weight gain for no reason.
- Feeling cold too easily; hands and fingers numb or tingling.
- Dry, thick, flaky skin and hair loss.
- Constipation.
- Heavier, longer menstrual periods.
- Sometimes a goiter—swelling in the front of the neck.

Thyroiditis:

- Pain in the front of the neck, either mild or sharp.
- Pain when swallowing or turning the head.
- Fever.

Your thyroid gland makes hormones that control how fast your body absorbs food and turns it into energy.

People with **hyperthyroidism** have a thyroid that makes too large a supply of hormones. One result is that some of their body's processes speed up. Graves' disease, the most common form, is sometimes brought on by severe stress. Hyperthyroidism is 5 times more likely to strike women than men, and is most common in people between 20 and 40.

People with **hypothyroidism** have a shortage of the hormones. Most people with this ailment—mainly women over 50—don't know they have it. Hypothyroidism can be caused by some drugs, or it can follow treatment for hyperthyroidism.

In **thyroiditis,** the body's own immune system attacks the thyroid, causing it to produce too much or too little of the hormones. Thyroiditis can follow a viral illness or pregnancy.

Most of these conditions can give rise to a goiter, which is a swelling of the thyroid gland. The goiter goes away with treatment.

Most thyroid problems can be treated. Some hyperthyroidism responds to drugs; sometimes doctors cut back hormones either with radioactive iodine or by removing part of the gland. Hypothyroidism is treated with hormone supplements. Thyroiditis often goes away on its own or after treatment with medications, including hormones.

WHAT YOU CAN DO NOW

- If you suspect you have a thyroid problem but aren't sure, think about whether you're taking an over-the-counter cold medicine or getting a lot of caffeine—for instance, drinking 10 cups of coffee a day, or lots of sodas with caffeine. Either one can cause some of the symptoms of hyperthyroidism, except weight loss. If you stop the medicine or caffeine and still have symptoms, call your doctor.
- For thyroiditis, try aspirin and other over-the-counter pain relievers to ease pain (see **pain relief,** page 317).

WHEN TO CALL THE DOCTOR

- If you feel nervous, tremble (above all in your hands), lose weight, and have a rapid pulse. You could have an overactive thyroid gland.
- If you feel cold, drowsy, and low on energy more and more, and you gain weight. You could have an underactive thyroid gland.
- If you have symptoms of thyroiditis.
- If someone in your family has had a thyroid problem, tell your doctor when you have your next checkup.

HOW TO PREVENT IT

There is no known way to prevent thyroid problems.

FOR MORE HELP

Organization: Thyroid Foundation of America, Ruth Sleeper Hall–RSL 350, 40 Parkman St., Boston, MA 02114-2698. Send a stamped, self-addressed envelope with your questions about thyroid problems. Members receive a newsletter.

Book: *Your Thyroid: A Home Reference,* by Lawrence C. Wood, M.D., et al. A guide to thyroid problems, causes, and treatments. Ballantine, 1995, $5.99.

Video: *Thyroid Disorders at Time of Diagnosis.* Clear overview of causes and treatments, with 4 reports—Understanding the Diagnosis, What Happens Next?, Treatment and Management, and Issues and Answers. Time Life Medical, 1996, $19.95. Sold in many pharmacies; for one near you, call 800-588-9959.

Staying Healthy

Doing all the things you're supposed to do to stay healthy isn't easy. How many of us really get up and move around briskly for 30 minutes, 5 or more days a week, every week? Who wants to pass up every ice cream sundae that comes along?

One reason it's hard to follow all the rules for staying healthy is that so many of them take a while—sometimes a long while—to show big results like not getting heart disease. But there's more to life than trying to defend yourself against heart attacks, diabetes, and other ailments. There is also living well.

This section of the *Self-Care Advisor* gives you the blueprint:

Eight Ways to Feel Your Best lays out a clear, complete plan of action for lifelong good health, based on the latest research.

Helping Your Doctor Help You offers tactics for making sure that you and your doctor are full partners in your health care.

Your Personal Health Record shows how to set up a family health tree and keep track of the things you should know about, from ailments that run in the family to self-tests, checkups, and immunizations.

Medicines: Playing It Safe shows, at a glance, medications you shouldn't mix, as well as foods to avoid when you're taking certain drugs.

You'll likely see a number of things you're doing now. And whatever else you choose to add from this feast of expert advice will only improve your chances of feeling your best.

Eight Ways to Feel Your Best

You get the most out of life when you're healthy, fit, and full of energy. It's easier to pull off than you might think. For all its complexity, the human body needs little special care. Of course, there are some obvious don'ts: Don't live on potato chips. Don't drink and drive. Don't let a plugged-in hair dryer drop into the tub while you bathe. But the key to feeling your best is to take charge of what you do every day—how much you move, what you eat, how you deal with stress. Experts can always argue over details (butter or margarine? mammograms starting at 40 or 50?), but the basics are well known and simple, and even the experts agree on them. If you follow these 8 proven steps, you'll not only enhance your prospects of a long and healthy life, you'll add spring to your step right now.

1. Get some exercise.
2. Maintain a healthy weight.
3. Eat well.
4. Put out the smoke.
5. Be careful out there.
6. Stay involved.
7. Relax.
8. Take care of your teeth.

1
Get Some Exercise

Our bodies were made to move—to walk and run, to climb and carry. Movement builds our bones and muscles and keeps us feeling our best. Among the rewards of exercise:

More energy and a stronger heart. When you raise your heart rate often, you improve your body's ability to deliver oxygen to cells. This not only determines how much pep you have day to day, it also cuts your risk of heart disease.

A stronger immune system. In one study, women who began a program of brisk walking 45 minutes a day, 5 days a week, cut their risk of colds and flu in half. In another, women who had been active through their 20s and 30s, four hours weekly, had a 60 percent lower risk of breast cancer than women who hadn't been active.

Less stress. More than a hundred studies have shown that regular doses of rhythmic exercise—walking, running, or swimming, for example—cut anxiety. And after 10 weeks of workouts, these studies show, the calmer feeling starts to last from one day to the next.

Greater strength. Any kind of exercise can maintain and even build muscle mass. Weight-bearing exercise such as walking, running, or weight training also helps build and preserve strong bones. This is important for women at risk of thinning bones (osteoporosis). One study found that men and women in their 80s doubled their strength after 10 weeks of workouts. Many got better at climbing stairs, and a few even replaced their walkers with canes.

Weight control. The more calories you burn with exercise, the fewer you store as fat. And as you replace fat with new muscle, you ratchet up the calories your body burns even while you're just sitting around. (Muscle burns more calories to maintain itself than fat does.)

A sharper mind. An active life preserves blood supply to the brain and boosts the brain chemicals we need to learn and remember. Active older people score better on tests of thinking skills than inactive older people.

But how much exercise, and what *kinds*, offer these glowing benefits? If you're out of shape, even a little bit helps—neighborhood strolls, weeding in the garden, taking the stairs instead of the elevator. The chart below can help you figure out how to build such life-giving spurts into your day-to-day life.

But for the *most* rewards, you'll need to do more. (See the next page for more details on how much exercise you need to get which benefits.) Start with a program of at least three 20-minute workouts a week, then build from there. Work hard enough to get your heart beating faster and feel your breathing quicken. Brisk walking, jogging, bicycling, swimming, or using a stair-climbing machine are good choices. For added stress-reducing benefits, repeat a calming word, phrase, or even a prayer as you go.

Twice-a-week strength training sessions might be the best exercise of all, say some experts. That's because they not only build new muscle, they help you develop the balance, endurance, and confidence you need to keep active into old age. Work all the major muscle groups—back, chest, shoulders, arms, hips, thighs, and abdomen—either by using the weight machines you'll find in most gyms or by lifting hand and ankle weights at home. Do 2 sets of 10 to 12 repetitions. How much weight is enough? Use about half the weight you can lift just once.

HOW TO EXTEND YOUR LIFE—WITHOUT WORKOUTS

You know the slightly winded feeling you get when you're rushing to catch a train or scrubbing a tough stain on the floor? That feeling means you're exercising hard enough to enjoy real health benefits—in numerical terms, burning 4.5 or more calories a minute if you weigh about 130 pounds or 6 calories a minute if you weigh about 180. (The heavier you are, the more calories an activity burns.)

Burn about 200 calories a day beyond your normal output by doing things like weeding or biking to work: You'll cut your risk of disease and live longer—without ever going near the gym. Not all household tasks qualify, though. Changing bed linens or putting on makeup, for instance, burns but 2.5 calories a minute; doing the dishes, just 2.3. Walking around the office (3.5) won't cut it either. The important thing is to get your heart rate up and breathe a little harder. When you vacuum, it won't count unless you're a whirling dervish. When you walk the dog, make sure the dog is trotting after *you*.

Here are the calories burned by 20 common activities.

Calories Burned (10 minutes)*	Women	Men
Walking fast	45	60
Painting	45	60
Weeding	45	60
Passionate sex	45	60
Washing car	45	60
Playing tag with a child	50	67
Cleaning gutters	50	67
Pushing a lawn mower	55	73
Square-dancing	55	73
Scrubbing floors	55	73
Hiking off-trail	60	80
Biking to work	60	80
Shoveling snow	60	80
Moving furniture	60	80
Walking upstairs	70	93
Cross-country skiing	80	106
Backpacking	80	106
Carrying a two-year-old upstairs	80	106
Running to catch a plane	115	153
Running upstairs	150	200

**Figures are for a 132-pound woman and a 176-pound man.*

Exercise: What You Get for What You Do

How much exercise do you need? It all depends on what you want. To cut the risk of heart disease, stroke, diabetes, and even cancer, you barely need to work up a sweat. But if you want to do more—for instance, trim a few pounds and tighten up your torso—get ready to push harder. Here's what the latest studies say exercise has to offer—and what it takes to get there.

A Longer Life

Every hour you're active, the experts say, adds one and a half hours to your life. But to ward off most of the major killers and perhaps osteoporosis, you don't have to kill yourself.

What it takes: Move around enough each day to burn at least 200 calories beyond your usual output—all told, about 30 minutes—by walking, gardening, climbing stairs, playing with the kids, lifting groceries, or formal exercise. Don't worry about how hard you're working; what matters in Exercise Lite is making it a part of your daily life.

What to expect: Nothing right away. The payoff—reduced risk of heart attack and many chronic diseases—doesn't come until later in life. Don't expect to see extra pounds melt away quickly. Over time you may slim down, but it will happen gradually.

Better Health Now

When you commit to working out, you start getting more benefits more quickly—a boost in energy, a more robust immune system, a more relaxed outlook, lower blood pressure, and lower cholesterol levels.

What it takes: To notice quick health gains, you need to get your heart thumping hard enough so you're winded for at least 20 minutes at a stretch 3 times a week. Brisk walking, aerobics classes, fast dancing, running, swimming, or any other aerobic exercise will do the job.

What to expect: Fewer colds and bouts of flu. A better ratio of good to bad cholesterol. For people with high blood pressure, an average drop of as much as 10 points. Most important, you'll look better and feel better, and you'll feel better about yourself.

Ready-for-Anything Fitness

More vigorous exercise will help maintain strength and vitality well into old age.

What it takes: Twenty minutes to an hour of walking, running, swimming, biking, or other aerobic activity 3 to 5 times a week. You need to drive your heart rate up to at least 60 percent of its maximum (220 minus your age). Add to that a twice-weekly program of floor exercises or strength training, plus stretching or yoga, to put your arms, abdomen, and legs through their paces.

What to expect: Greater strength, balance, flexibility, and endurance. Improved sports performance with fewer injuries and less soreness. The beginnings of a better body. And, for those who stay this fit for their whole lives, a slower decline in the immune system—the body's defense against invaders—which could further help ward off infection and even cancer.

A Sleeker Physique

A weight-loss program that works must include both exercise and healthy eating. But if the formula sounds simple—cut the calories you take in and increase the calories you burn—in truth, it's hard to do.

What it takes: Set a goal of 60 minutes total of brisk walking, running, swimming, biking, or other exercise 5 days a week. The more calories you burn, the better, so go for things you can stick with. Then, to tighten muscles, put your body through a full round of floor exercises, weight lifting, and stretching 3 times a week.

What to expect: Exercise builds muscle, which is denser than fat. That's why you may gain weight at first, even as you lose inches off your waist. But by adding muscle, you'll speed up your metabolism, making weight loss easier. Keep at it, eat right, and weight loss will follow.

2

Maintain a Healthy Weight

In the past 20 years, we've become fatter—8 pounds fatter, in fact. Now at least 1 of every 4 people in the United States is overweight. (For how you're doing, see the box on the next page.) Hauling around that extra weight does more than keep us from being as active as we want to be. It also can kill us. When you weigh too much, you have a much higher risk of heart disease, high blood pressure, stroke, diabetes, gallbladder disease, and some cancers.

But how do you determine *your* healthy weight? And what's the best way to stay at that weight for life? Here's what the experts advise.

Be realistic. Many diets fail because people shoot for a fantasy weight they can't maintain. To know whether your weight-loss goal makes sense for you, ask yourself: What is the least I've weighed as an adult for at least a year? What weight was I able to reach and stay at during previous diets without feeling a lot of hunger pangs? Those weights are good places to start when you set your goal for weight loss. And remember: Losing as little as 5 percent of your current weight will help you feel and look better.

Start by exercising. In one study, 90 percent of people who lost weight and kept it off made a habit of staying active. A brisk half-hour walk burns about 150 calories—roughly as much as you'd get in a scoop of ice cream. Exercise is vital when you're dieting. That's because cutting back on calories tends to decrease muscle mass; the exercise will help you *increase* it.

Cut calories. When you take in fewer calories than you burn, you can't help dropping some weight. The best way to cut calories, oddly, is to eat *more* of some kinds of food—such as fresh fruit, vegetables, and grains. These are full of the nutrients we need for good health, yet they carry less than half the calories in the same amounts of fatty foods. An example: Half a cup of tomato sauce weighs in at 35 calories. Exactly the same amount of cheese sauce, which is high in fat, packs 230 calories. See page 303 for more tips on how to choose tasty, healthful, slimming foods over foods that make you fat.

Don't deprive yourself. Instead of giving up all the fat-filled foods you love, just eat less of them. Treat yourself to 1 cookie instead of 4—and savor every bite.

Give yourself time. Any program that promises fast weight loss is almost certain to fail. When you set out to lose weight, think in terms of a year or more. The more gradually you lose weight, the more likely you'll keep it off. Remember: The healthful changes in

HOW TO KEEP YOURSELF FROM QUITTING

Starting an exercise program is easy. Staying with it is the challenge. Here's what fitness experts suggest:

Slow down. When they start off, many exercisers walk, run, or swim too hard (or, with strength training, they heft too much weight). Then they quit after a few workouts because they dread the pain. Sure, you should feel tired after a workout, but an hour later you should feel full of energy. If not, you're doing too much, too soon.

Find a partner. Working out with someone doubles the chance that you'll stick with it.

Write up a contract. Set sensible goals for yourself and write them down. Tell friends and family members so they can support you.

Chart your progress. Keep a training log. Reward yourself along the way when you meet clear-cut goals, such as pedaling that extra mile or lifting twice a week for a month straight.

Be patient. The first 3 to 6 months on a new exercise program are the hardest. If you make it to 6 months, the experts say, odds are good you'll still be working out a year later.

your exercise and eating habits will make you look and feel better in ways that don't show up on the bathroom scale. So stick with them even if the pounds are slow to budge.

IS YOUR WEIGHT HEALTHY?

The weight chart below will help you get an idea of where you stand. But don't take it as the final word. You should also think about:

Your fitness level. If you land in the moderately overweight zone, your weight is less likely to be a health risk—*if* you're in good shape.

Your family history. Overweight people with a family history of heart disease, high blood pressure, or diabetes should make weight loss a top priority.

Your body type. People with a "pear" shape (fat in the thighs, hips, and buttocks) seem to have a far lower risk of weight-related diseases than those with an "apple" shape (fat around the abdomen), so they can worry less about being moderately overweight.

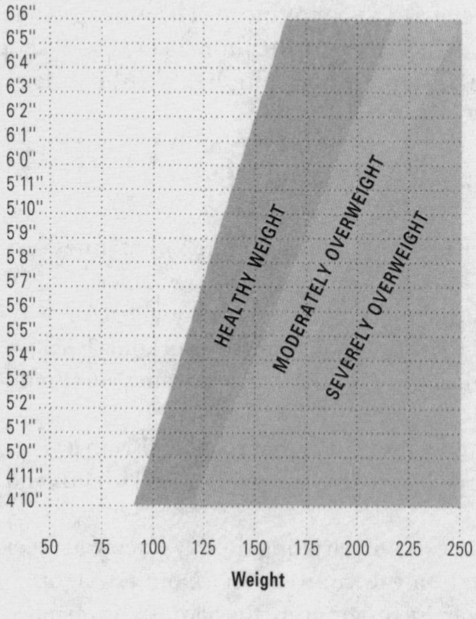

Source: U.S. Department of Agriculture

3
Eat Well: Tips for Creating Healthy Meals

The only way to keep your health, Mark Twain once quipped, is to "eat what you don't want, drink what you don't like, and do what you'd druther not." For once, Twain was wrong. That's because the hallmark of healthful eating is in fact good taste and variety. Even the best diets have room for sweets, meats, and other treats when you:

Eat plenty of fruits, vegetables, and grains. High in fiber, plant-based foods fill you up with nutrients without loading you down with fat and cholesterol. And the fiber in fruits, vegetables, and grains helps speed toxins out of the body. Plants also contain a wealth of active compounds, called phytochemicals—*phyto* for plant—that boost the body's cancer-fighting defenses. The more of these foods you eat, the better your health.

Cut back on saturated fat. All of us know we should eat less fat—especially the big culprit, the saturated kind found in fatty meats, whole milk, ice cream, and cheese. This fat raises cholesterol levels and increases heart disease risk. Reach for nonfat or low-fat milk. And help yourself to 3-ounce portions (the size of a deck of cards) of lean beef, pork, poultry, or fish. On your pasta, try a light tomato sauce instead of a heavy cream sauce. Instead of a rich dessert, reach for a piece of fruit.

Go easy on smoked, salt-cured, and charbroiled foods. All contain high levels of nitrates, which have been linked to several forms of cancer. Enjoy them only now and then, if at all.

If you drink, go easy. A little alcohol—1 drink a day for women, 2 a day for men—may have some health benefits. As a group, moderate drinkers have less risk of heart disease and seem to live longer than nondrinkers. But if you don't drink now, that's no reason to start. You'd be much better off eating less saturated fat than adding alcohol.

What's 1 drink? A bottle of beer (12 ounces), a glass of wine (5 ounces), or a jigger of liquor (1.5 ounces).

The Mediterranean Diet

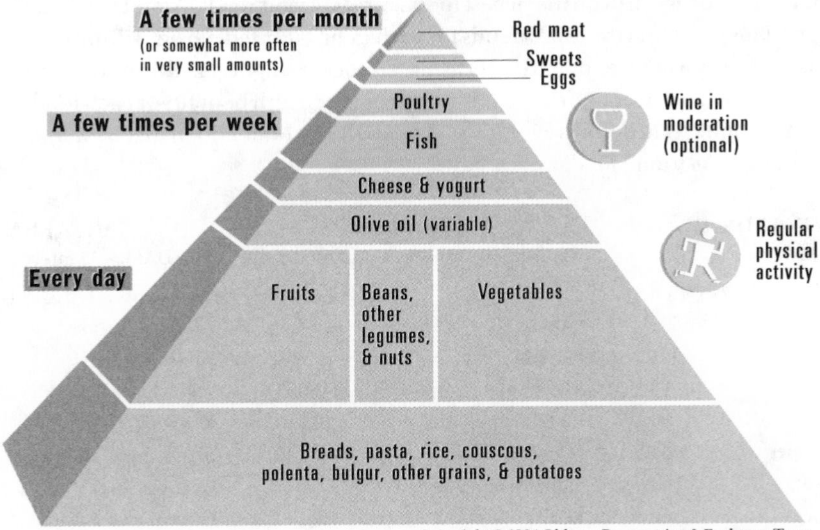

Eat this way. For the ideal mix of foods, some experts favor a change from the well-known U.S. Department of Agriculture Food Pyramid. It's the Traditional Healthy Mediterranean Diet Pyramid, developed in 1994 by researchers at the Harvard School of Public Health and endorsed by the Oldways Preservation & Exchange Trust. Based on the eating habits of southern Italy and Greece—where people tend to live long, healthy lives—it calls for big helpings of starches and other carbohydrates every day in the form of bread and grains, fresh fruits, beans, potatoes, and other vegetables, along with protein from small portions of cheese or yogurt. Modest amounts of fish and poultry are okay, but not every day. Red meat is only a once-in-a-while treat.

EASY EXCHANGES: TRUSTY LOW-FAT SUBSTITUTES

Cutting back on fat doesn't mean going hungry. The swap chart below offers some low-fat alternatives to common foods. (Portions are average serving sizes.)

INSTEAD OF	fat grams	GO FOR	fat grams
Corn muffin	5	English muffin and jam	1
Granola	12	Nonfat yogurt sprinkled with granola	2
Bacon and eggs	37	Pancakes with syrup	6
Tuna salad sandwich	16	Turkey breast sandwich with mustard	7
Cheeseburger	30	Bagel with lox and low-fat cream cheese	10
French fries	20	Oven-fried potatoes	8
Cream-of-chicken soup	18	Chicken noodle soup	6
Potato chips	18	Pretzels	2
Bean dip	4	Salsa	0
Alfredo sauce	10	Tomato sauce	1
Sautéed vegetables	14	Steamed vegetables	0
Ranch-style dressing	18	Vinaigrette	8
Ice cream	18	Sorbet	0
Apple pie	16	4 Fig bars	4

The Nutrition Top Ten

Here's a handy chart to fill you in on the richest food sources of vitamins C, A, and E, folic acid, calcium, iron, and fiber. This chart lists the top 10 foods for each item. Granted, no one sitting down for a meal eats 3½ ounces—nearly a quarter pound—of Parmesan cheese (highest in calcium) or parsley (rich in vitamin C, vitamin A, and iron). But as you think about the health benefits of each food on the lists, keep this point in mind: A little goes a long way. The RDA (recommended dietary allowance) figure shows you the minimum to aim for daily.

VITAMIN C

RDA: 60 milligrams

	mg per 3½ ounces
Red bell peppers	190
Parsley	133
Kiwifruit	98
Broccoli	93
Green bell peppers	89
Brussels sprouts	62
Edible-pod peas	60
Strawberries	57
Red cabbage	57
Oranges	53

VITAMIN A

RDA: 4,000–5,000 international units

	IU per 3½ ounces
Carrots	28,129
Pumpkin, canned	22,056
Sweet potatoes	20,063
Red chile peppers	10,750
Apricots, dried	7,240
Spinach	6,715
Red bell peppers	5,700
Parsley	5,200
Watercress	4,700
Squash, winter	4,060

VITAMIN E

RDA: 12–15 international units

	IU per 3½ ounces
Wheat germ oil	178
Sunflower seeds	74
Vegetable oils	12–73
Almonds	41
Margarine	19
Wheat germ	17
Peanuts, dry-roasted	11
Peanut butter	9
Butter	3
Asparagus	3

FOLIC ACID

RDA: 180–200 micrograms

	mcg per 3½ ounces
Fortified breakfast cereal	353
Wheat germ, toasted	352
Spinach	194
Lentils, cooked	181
Pinto beans, cooked	172
Peanuts, dry-roasted	145
Romaine lettuce	136
Peanut butter	92
Hummus (garbanzo puree)	65
Peas	59

CALCIUM

RDA: 800 milligrams*

	mg per 3½ ounces
Parmesan cheese	1,376
Mozzarella cheese, part skim	646
Ricotta cheese, part skim	272
Almonds	266
Tofu	250
Salmon, canned, with bones	213
Plain low-fat yogurt	183
Collard greens	156
Orange juice with added calcium	131
Skim milk	123

IRON

RDA: 10–15 milligrams

	mg per 3½ ounces
Clams	14–28
Fortified breakfast cereal	12–28
Oysters	4–12
Tofu, firm	10
Liver	7
Cashews, dry-roasted	6
Parsley	6
Apricots, dried	5
Lean beef	4
Spinach	3

FIBER

Suggested daily total: 20–35 grams

	g per 3½ ounces
High-fiber breakfast cereal	35–46
Bran flakes	18
Rye crisp crackers	16
Popcorn, air-popped	15
Wheat germ, toasted	13
Granola	11
High-fiber bread	11
Pinto beans, cooked	10
Mixed nuts	9
Whole-wheat bread	9

TOP TEN MOST NUTRITIOUS VEGETABLES

Broccoli
Spinach
Brussels sprouts
Lima beans
Peas
Asparagus
Artichokes
Cauliflower
Sweet potatoes
Carrots

*Up to 1,500 mg for women after menopause; 1,000 mg for younger women taking hormone replacement therapy.

Sources: U.S. Department of Agriculture *Handbook 8; The Vitamin E Fact Book*

Some heavily fortified breakfast cereals, designed to provide most or all of the RDAs, have been omitted from this ranking.

4

Put Out the Smoke

Smoking kills. Period. Cigarettes are the nation's top cause of preventable death—they kill more than 350,000 people a year and ruin the health of millions more. If you don't smoke, don't start. If you do, quit.

Nicotine is one of the most addictive drugs around, so many people find they have to try over and over before they give up smoking for good. Even if you've tried and failed, don't give up. There are many strategies for kicking the habit. These range from nicotine patches to support groups. And the body quickly mends itself once you do quit. Within 2 days of quitting, carbon monoxide levels in the blood return to normal. Within 3 months, lung function improves by as much as 30 percent.

For more about smoking and a list of resources that can help you kick this deadly habit, see **smoking and illness,** page 220.

5

Be Careful Out There

Accidents are the top reason Americans land in the emergency room. In fact, for people under the age of 45, accident—not disease—is the leading cause of death. More than half of all these deaths involve motor vehicles or firearms. Guns kill more than 38,000 Americans a year and wound hundreds of thousands more—and the numbers keep climbing. Half a million people a year are hurt riding bicycles. Nearly 20 million a year have an accident at home that sends them to a doctor or limits what they can do for at least

VITAMIN AND MINERAL BASICS

Pills can't replace a healthy diet. But if you don't always eat as well as you should, vitamin and mineral supplements can help ensure that you get all the nutrients you need.

Be careful about getting too much of some vitamins. Vitamin A is toxic in doses above 50,000 international units (IU). Supplements are usually safe to about 10,000 IU daily. During pregnancy, high doses can cause birth defects. Vitamin B6 in high doses (100 milligrams a day for several months) can cause nerve damage. Very high doses of vitamin D (5,000 IU every day) can cause kidney and heart problems.

A few tips:

Skip fancy pills loaded with vitamins C and E. Instead, choose a basic formula that provides the recommended dietary allowance (RDA) of a broad range of vitamins and minerals.

If you want extra vitamins C and E, buy them separately. For C, take 25 to 500 milligrams (mg) once a day. For E, choose a capsule with 100 to 400 international units—a lot more than the RDA.

Folic acid cuts the risk of birth defects in the spine, so pregnant women should eat foods rich in it—leafy green vegetables, beans, cereals, and whole-grain breads. Many doctors suggest 400 micrograms (mcg) daily before and during pregnancy.

Calcium can protect against osteoporosis (thinning of the bones). Milk, yogurt, and leafy green vegetables have plenty. But if you don't feel you're getting enough in your food, take a supplement. Choose one that contains vitamin D if you don't eat dairy products (you need some D to help use calcium). Common antacids are also good calcium sources. Take no more than 1,500 mg of calcium a day, since too much can cause nausea, constipation, or even kidney stones in some people.

For iron, the RDA of around 15 mg for women and 10 mg for men is plenty. Pregnant women—especially those who eat little red meat—are often advised to take 30- to 60-mg supplements. But don't go higher than that. More than 100 mg a day can cause heart and liver problems.

SUN LOVERS: ARE YOU IN THE DARK?

Close to 1 million Americans will find out they have skin cancer this year (see color illustration, page 166). The next step isn't pretty. At best, the cut-away tumor will leave a scar. At worst, it'll turn out to be melanoma, which kills 7,000 people a year. But most skin cancers can be avoided. All we have to do is protect our skin from sunlight. Did you know, for instance, that men get lip cancer far more often than women? It may be that ordinary lipstick protects the lips as well as light-duty sunscreen. Still, what gives true protection? Do your sunscreen habits measure up? Take this quiz: Are these statements true or false?

1. **A light tan is fine, as long as I don't get a sunburn.** T F
2. **A T-shirt will protect my shoulders from sun damage.** T F
3. **I'm safe driving around with my windows rolled up.** T F
4. **I'm more likely to get too much sun when I'm swimming than when I'm sunbathing.** T F
5. **Growing my hair long is the best way to protect my ears and scalp.** T F
6. **For best blockage, I should put on sunscreen just before I go outside.** T F
7. **The higher my sunscreen's sun protection factor (SPF) rating, the better protected I am.** T F

---

1. False. Some always-tan people—those who work outside for at least 40 hours a week—do have lower rates of melanoma. That could be because tan skin protects against the sunburns linked to the cancer. But if you don't work as a park ranger, you raise your odds for getting skin cancer each time you burn or tan. That's because the damage that causes most cancers adds up; ultraviolet light causes cells in the skin to reproduce faster, at the same time holding down the body's immune response to this growth. After decades, the result can be a reddish patch, shiny bump, or open sore—a tumor.

2. True. A boldly colored T-shirt might have a sun protection factor, or SPF, of 15. That means someone who might burn in 15 minutes is protected for 15 times as long—about 4 hours—before starting to color. But one study did find that wearing a very light-colored or loosely knit shirt let through too much light: A plain white T-shirt has an SPF of 9 at most. Hold a layer of fabric up to a window. If you can see outlines through it, think about changing your shirt.

3. True. Glass windows block the most harmful ultraviolet rays, UVB. But if your car has a sunroof, you're being exposed to UVA rays, which shine through horizontal (but not slanted) panes of glass.

4. False. Whether you're playing in the water or lounging on a beach chair, the exposure to the sun is the same. But you should use a waterproof sunblock and put on more after your dip.

5. False. A full head of hair—it doesn't matter which color—does shield against tumors on the scalp and ears. (Cancer on the tops of the ears is a special risk for people with short hair). But the best defense isn't hair, which can leave many parts of your head exposed. It's a wide-brimmed hat.

6. False. Put on sunscreen (SPF 15 or higher) 30 minutes before leaving the house. That's how long it takes for sunscreen to bond to the outer layer of your skin.

7. True. For most people, SPF 15 lotion or moisturizer blocks the sun. But watch your skin. If you see signs of sunburn despite being covered with SPF 15, switch to a stronger sunscreen—say, SPF 30. And use plenty. It takes at least 2 tablespoons to cover most bodies, but in one study beachgoers put on just a third that much.

half a day. Many people each year get sunburns, and sunburn can lead to skin cancer.

To increase safety on the road:

- Always wear seat belts in the car.
- Use child safety seats for kids under 4.
- Wear a helmet when you ride a bike or inline skates (it should meet the ANSI or Snell standard) or motorcycle (U.S. Department of Transportation—DOT—standard).
- Never drink and drive—or ride with anyone who has been drinking.
- Keep a flashlight in the car for emergencies and for walking through unlit parking areas after dark.

To accident-proof your home or office:

- Install smoke detectors.
- Keep a fire extinguisher in the kitchen.
- Plan escape routes in case of fire.
- Buy antiscald devices for showerheads or faucets, or keep your water heater set at 120 degrees or lower to protect children from scalding.
- Store drugs and toxic chemicals out of the reach of children.
- Post poison control and other emergency numbers near the phone.

To prevent falls:

- Have a sturdy stepladder handy for reaching high shelves.
- Install nonslip pads and mats in showers and bathtubs.
- Don't use loose throw rugs.
- Be sure stairways are well lighted.
- Use night-lights in bathrooms and halls.
- Never leave objects on stairs.

To protect yourself outdoors:

- Wear a sunscreen with an SPF of at least 15 and a wide-brimmed hat when in the sun.
- Use bug spray with 10 to 15 percent DEET to keep ticks and mosquitoes at bay.

6
Stay Involved

How would you describe the healthiest person you know? Perhaps as someone who is alert and curious. Excited about new possibilities. Good at love and friendship. Passionate about life's simple pleasures. Well, experts couldn't agree more. They've found

SHOULD YOU REACH OUT?

There's no magic recipe for social support that works for everyone. A loner might need just one close confidant, while a "people person" may feel lost without an army of friends. This quiz is based on one given by Carnegie Mellon psychologist Sheldon Cohen to gauge whether a person has the right mix of connections to stay healthy. Circle the statements as true or false for you.

1. **If I needed a loan of $100, there is someone I could get it from.** T F
2. **There is someone who takes pride in my accomplishments.** T F
3. **I often meet or talk with family or friends.** T F
4. **Most people I know think highly of me.** T F
5. **If I needed an early morning ride to the airport, there's no one I would feel comfortable asking to take me.** T F
6. **I feel there is no one with whom I can share my most private worries and fears.** T F
7. **Most of my friends are more successful at making changes in their lives than I am.** T F
8. **I would have a hard time finding someone to go with me on a day trip to the beach or country.** T F

For your score, add your number of true answers to questions 1 to 4 to the false answers you gave to questions 5 through 8.

If that score is 4 or above, you have enough support to protect your health, even if your safety net has a few holes. During tough times people need connections to draw on or the confidence to ask for help; you have one or both.

If your score is 3 or below, you may need to reach out. If you're not a group person, make an effort to become close to a trusted relative, friend, or neighbor. If closeness isn't your strength, join a social or religious group or sign up for a class.

IS STRESS PUTTING YOUR HEALTH AT RISK?

Each of us reacts in unique ways to life's challenges. Faced with a long line at the bank, most of us will get heated up for a few seconds before we shrug and move on. But for others—the 1 in 5 of us whom the experts call hot reactors—such moments are an assault on good health. That's why rating your stress requires you both to tally your life's stressors (part one) and to figure out whether you are prone to stress (part two).

Part One
The Stress in Your Life

How often are the following stressful situations a part of your daily life?

1 Never 2 Rarely 3 Sometimes
4 Often 5 All the time

I work long hours 1 2 3 4 5

There are signs my job isn't secure 1 2 3 4 5

Doing a good job goes unnoticed 1 2 3 4 5

It takes all my energy just to make it through the day 1 2 3 4 5

There are severe arguments at home 1 2 3 4 5

A family member is seriously ill 1 2 3 4 5

I'm having problems with child care 1 2 3 4 5

I don't have enough time for fun 1 2 3 4 5

I'm on a diet 1 2 3 4 5

My family and friends count on me to solve their problems . . 1 2 3 4 5

I'm expected to keep up a certain standard of living 1 2 3 4 5

My neighborhood is crowded or dangerous 1 2 3 4 5

My home is a mess 1 2 3 4 5

I can't pay my bills on time 1 2 3 4 5

I'm not saving money 1 2 3 4 5

Your total score . . . .

Below 38: You have a lower-stress life.

38 and above: You have a high-stress life.

Part Two
Your Stress Susceptibility

Think how you would react in these situations.

You've been waiting 20 minutes for a table in a crowded restaurant, and the host seats a party that arrived after you. You feel your anger rise as your face gets hot and your heart beats faster. **T F**

Your sister calls out of the blue and starts to tell you how much you mean to her. Uncomfortable, you change the subject without telling her what you feel. **T F**

You come home to find the kitchen looking like a disaster area and your spouse lounging in front of the TV. You tense up and can't seem to shake your anger. **T F**

Faced with a public speaking event, you get keyed up and lose sleep for a day or more, fretting about how you'll do. **T F**

On Thursday your repair shop promises to fix your car in time for a weekend trip. As the hours go by, you become more and more worried that something will go wrong and your trip will be ruined. **T F**

Two or Fewer True: You're a cool reactor, someone who tends to roll with the punches when a situation is out of your control.

Three or More True: Sorry, you're a hot reactor, someone who responds to mild stress with a "fight-or-flight" adrenaline rush that drives up blood pressure and can lead to a host pf problems such as heart rhythm troubles, accelerated clotting (which can cause strokes and heart attacks), and damaged blood vessel linings. Some hot reactors can seem cool as a cucumber on the outside, but inside their bodies are silently killing them.

What Your Scores Mean

Combine the results from parts one and two to get your total stress rating.

Lower-Stress Life — Cool Reactor

Whatever your problems, stress isn't one of them. Even when stressful events do occur—and they will—your health is not likely to suffer.

Lower-Stress Life — Hot Reactor

You're not under stress—at least for now. Though you tend to overreact to problems, you've wisely managed your life to avoid the big stressors. Before you honk at the guy who cuts you off in rush hour traffic, keep in mind that getting angry can destroy thousands of heart muscle cells within minutes.

High-Stress Life — Cool Reactor

You're under stress, but only you know if it's hurting. Even if you normally thrive with a full plate of challenges, now you might be biting off more than you can chew. Note any increase in headaches, backaches, or insomnia; that's your body telling you to lighten your load. If your job is the main source of stress, think about reducing your hours. If that's not possible, find a way to make your job more enjoyable, and stress will become manageable.

High-Stress Life — Hot Reactor

You're in the danger zone. Make an extra effort to exercise, get enough sleep, and keep your family and friends close. It's too bad, but even being physically fit does little to protect you if your body is always in stress mode. To survive, you may need to make major changes—walking away from a life-destroying job or relationship, perhaps—and you may need to work out a whole new approach to life's hourly obstacles. Such effort will pay off. In one experiment, 77 percent of hot reactors were able to cool down—lower their blood pressure and cholesterol levels—by training themselves to stay calm.

that healthy people tend to stay enthusiastic about life as they age. They suggest you:

Be an optimist. Studies show that people who most often look on the bright side remain healthier than pessimists, perhaps because their immune systems are stronger.

Join a group. Even among retired people, those who remain active in volunteer work or church and social groups have better health and sharper minds than those who shut themselves in.

Challenge yourself. The more we challenge our bodies and minds, the more vital they remain. Studies show that the act of learning something new increases the links between brain cells and makes the brain more robust.

Cherish your friends and loved ones. In one study, single people who didn't feel they had anyone to share their feelings with were 3 times more likely to die over the next 5 years than those who had someone close to talk to. Indeed, social isolation can be as bad for your health as smoking or high cholesterol.

Stay active. A lifetime of exercise helps preserve blood supply to the brain, because it keeps the heart, lungs, and blood vessels in top shape. Exercise also seems to boost chemicals in the brain that strengthen memory and help us think. The bottom line: Active and fit older people not only live longer, they also have faster reaction times and score better on tests of thinking power than do inactive older people.

7
Relax

These days, most of us lead busy, crowded lives. And most of the time we cope smoothly with the pressures we face. But sometimes life's strains and letdowns become too much and our bodies react. Blood pressure rises, heart rate quickens, and the stress hormone adrenaline surges through the bloodstream. Stress can lead to everything from colds, headaches, and back pain to allergies, asthma, arthritis, infertility, insomnia, depression, and heart disease.

Luckily, you can do a lot to reduce stress and cut your risk of health problems. In one

HOW WELL DO YOU KNOW YOUR TEETH?

Of course we're supposed to brush every day. But how many of us know why? Take this test to find out if you're truly treating your teeth well.

❶ You can catch gum disease from
a. kissing
b. sharing a toothbrush
c. both
d. neither

❷ Toothbrushing prevents
a. detached gums
b. root decay
c. stained teeth
d. none of the above

❸ You're least likely to get cavities from eating
a. raisins
b. pure sugar
c. an English muffin

❹ Who's most at risk of getting gum disease?
a. pregnant women
b. menopausal women
c. teetotalers

❺ If you can't brush your teeth after a meal, what's the best thing to do?
a. eat a banana
b. chew gum
c. use a toothpick

❻ Thorough toothbrushing takes at least
a. one minute
b. three minutes
c. four minutes

❼ Which will relieve toothache pain fastest?
a. aspirin
b. clove oil
c. salt water

Answers

1. c By age 35, three in four Americans have at least the beginnings of gum disease, an infection below the gum line caused by certain bacteria in dental plaque. But sometimes bacteria passed in the saliva of someone with gum disease can bring on the condition in someone who doesn't even have plaque. So if your partner isn't taking care of his or her teeth, take the problem seriously. Your own gums may be at risk.

2. d Toothbrushing removes plaque and prevents cavities above the gum line, but not below. When plaque isn't cleaned out, the gums fall away, allowing germs to get at your roots and even at the bone anchoring the teeth. Gum disease is the nation's leading cause of tooth loss. To prevent it, you have to floss.

3. b Sugary foods, such as candy and chocolate, are cleared from the mouth more quickly than starchy foods. Raisins are a special case because they stick like glue between the teeth.

4. a Nearly all pregnant women get some signs of gum disease because hormone changes during pregnancy increase swelling, bleeding, and tiny infections in the gums. There's an old saw: Lose a tooth for every child. To keep it from coming true, brush after every meal, floss daily, and see a dentist at the beginning of your pregnancy.

5. b We make more saliva when we chew gum, and saliva's chemicals neutralize tooth-decaying acids. Pop in a piece when you finish a meal. Sugarless gum works much better than regular, and gum containing xylitol works best of all, reducing tooth decay by as much as 85 percent. (The sweetener keeps bacteria from multiplying.) This gum is sold mostly in health food stores.

6. b To make this task seem less daunting, divide your mouth into 10 sections. (Include a section each for the roof of your mouth, your tongue, and the insides of your right and left cheeks, all places where bacteria gather.) Then count to 20 alligators as you brush each section. The average American spends about 30 seconds brushing.

7. b If your dentist can't see you right away for a painful tooth, saturate a cotton ball in oil of clove (sold at many pharmacies) and put it on the aching tooth. The pain-killing oil should ease the ache in a couple of seconds.

study, students who used simple relaxation techniques at exam time were much less likely to show a slump in their immune systems than other students. Here are several simple ways to calm frazzled nerves:

Take a 15-minute breather. When things get hectic, go for a walk, listen to music you like, browse through a magazine, or soak in a hot bath. Any pleasant "time-out" from the day's pressures can calm you down.

Practice relaxation techniques, such as deep breathing, meditation, or simply sitting with your eyes closed. All have been shown to reverse the symptoms of stress. Studies have shown that meditation lowers levels of a chemical linked to tension. Meditation also protects the body from the harmful effects of adrenaline—exactly what the leading blood-pressure-lowering drugs do. Here are a couple of simple methods:

- Deep breathing: 10 minutes. Lie on a comfortable surface with your arms at your sides and a book on your stomach. Inhale slowly through your nose. Expand your belly so the book rises. Then slowly exhale through pursed lips. Let the book sink back. Repeat 15 times.
- Body scan: 20 minutes. Find a quiet place to lie down. Now relax, one body part at a time. Begin with your toes and work slowly up to the top of your head. Focus on each part as you go. You might start with the toes of your left foot. Note how each one feels. Don't do anything: Just observe them. Then move on—slowly—to the top of your foot, to your ankle, your lower leg, your hip. Go to the toes on your other foot, and repeat. Move slowly up through your body. Don't hurry.

  It helps to think of breathing in and out through each part as you focus on it. Or you can imagine it getting heavy. If your mind wanders, bring it back gently. You may fall asleep before you finish. Don't worry—letting go is the goal.

  For more help, see **stress,** page 222.

Use your imagination. Positive mental images can have a strong calming effect on the body. If you feel your stress level spiking, close your eyes and take 5 minutes to picture yourself in a quiet, peaceful, pleasant setting—say, you and a friend on a clean, sunny beach lapped by gentle waves, or a green mountainside meadow.

Move around. Doing a favorite form of exercise—one that leaves you slightly winded—will ease your anxiety and help you feel more in control of your life.

Laugh it off. Laughter really *is* one of the best medicines. A good laugh eases tension and boosts levels of anti-stress brain chemicals. Read a book that makes you laugh, or sit down to watch a favorite comedy show or film. Another good bet: Meet some friends for a lighthearted conversation.

8

Take Care of Your Teeth

Cavities used to be the big deal in dental care. While people still get them, the new frontier is gum disease—a bacterial infection that works below the gum line to ravage the bone and ligaments holding your teeth in place. So, as they say, "Clean only the teeth you want to keep." Here's what to do:

Brush *and* floss at least twice a day, in the morning and before bed. It doesn't matter whether you floss first or brush first—just be thorough. (See **tips on tooth and gum care,** page 84.) The nighttime cleaning amounts to a preemptive strike—knocking down the bacteria before you lie there all night asleep, letting the fluids in your mouth stagnate. The morning cleaning knocks them down again when their numbers have peaked.

Dentists want you to have your teeth cleaned at least once every 6 months to keep ahead of any damage that might creep in despite your best efforts.

If you can follow all 8 steps, great. If you can't, try 7, or 6. The point is not just to live longer, though you very well might. The real reward is feeling better and enjoying life.

Helping Your Doctor Help You

To get the most from your health professionals, you'll need to meet them halfway. Here's how. ❀ **Learn how to stay well.** It may seem obvious, but the better you take care of yourself, the less likely you are to get sick in the first place—and the more quickly you'll get well if you do get sick. ❀ **Know as much as you can.** Learn about your body and how it works. If you start feeling sick, pay close attention to your symptoms. If you have an illness, study up on it. When it comes to your health, knowledge really is power. ❀ **Be active on your own behalf.** When you visit the doctor, take an interest, listen closely, and ask questions. Here are 10 ways to help your doctor help you, plus tips on how to find out what you need to know.

1 **Talk first about what worries you most.** Don't save your biggest concern for last—or you may not have time to ask about it.

2 **Be specific.** Saying, "I feel hot and I've had a sharp pain in the right side of my stomach since last night," is more helpful than saying, "I feel rotten." Bring up all the changes you've noticed, even if you don't think they're important. (See **when you're sick** box, page 316.)

3 **Tell the truth.** Be honest about what you eat, how much you exercise, and whether you smoke or use drugs or alcohol. Your doctor needs to know.

You should also tell your doctor about any nonmedical or family remedies you've been using—going to a chiropractor, for instance, or taking big doses of vitamins. Even if you feel shy talking about sexual habits or problems, be sure to mention them.

Bring up any big life changes or stresses you may be under, such as the recent death of a loved one or working a double shift—and even good news, such as getting married.

4 **Ask questions.** Some doctors welcome questions from patients, and some don't. But many say they are surprised by how few questions patients ask, given that the patient's health is at stake.

Clear up things you don't understand during your visit. If you're the least bit puzzled, ask your doctor to show you a diagram or even to draw a picture. Ask for brochures and other sources of information.

Depending on your illness, ask what you can do to keep it from coming back.

If your doctor can't answer all your questions in one visit, ask for time to talk at the next appointment. Or ask when to call, if you can get the answer by phone. If a question is crucial, ask—politely but firmly—for an answer before you leave.

5 **Ask for translations.** If your doctor speaks in terms you can't follow, ask for a simpler approach. If information comes at you too fast, ask the doctor to slow down. To make sure you understand, say, "Now, let me see if I've got that straight," and repeat what you heard.

6 **Find out more about referrals and tests.** If your doctor suggests that you see a specialist, ask why (and also check to see if that doctor is on your health plan). If you're scheduled for a test, make sure you know:

Why it's necessary.
How accurate and reliable it is.
How you should prepare for it.
Whether it's painful.
How the results will affect treatment.
When and how you'll get the results.
Whether it's covered by your health plan.
Whether your health plan has to okay it first.
How much it will cost you.

If you learn you have something serious, you might face hard choices about treatment. Ask your doctor to explain all your options. Make sure you learn about the benefits and risks of each choice—as well as the pros and cons of doing nothing. You can also ask about other sources of information or how to get a second opinion.

Once you are fully informed, you and your doctor can pick the best course. Before deciding, though, give yourself time to think about these issues:

How much pain am I willing to endure?
How much risk am I willing to take?
How much cost am I willing to bear?

7 **Speak up.** If you want medication to relieve your symptoms, say so. If you're worried you can't afford a certain drug and wonder if a generic version might be cheaper, ask. If you want a certain test, say so. If you don't speak up, you may walk away frustrated—and still worried. If you need reassurance, be open about it—your doctor might be able to help you regain peace of mind. Don't forget: You have to say what's bothering you. Doctors are often rushed, and medical schools don't teach mind reading.

8 **If you can't follow a doctor's orders, say so.** There may be times when you just don't think you can do what your doctor advises—whether it's getting more sleep, cutting out fried foods, exercising every day, or taking a certain drug. Maybe your schedule's too irregular or you just tend to forget. But don't walk out feeling discouraged, thinking you'll just ignore it all. Instead, explain your concerns; together, you may be able to work out ideas for other treatment plans.

Don't be afraid to negotiate. For instance, if your doctor suggests a drug or treatment that has side effects that you would find hard to accept, try saying, "That's going to be hard to live with. Is there another option I could try?"

9 **Bring along your own ideas.** If you read or hear about a treatment or medicine you'd like to try, bring the information along. Ask your doctor if it could work for you. That way you can make informed choices about your own care.

10 **Don't leave what you've learned at the office.** It's tough to recall everything a doctor tells you, above all when you're nervous. You may want to take notes. (See **getting ready for a regular visit,** page 315.)

Before you leave the office, know what you should do once you get home. Be sure you have prescriptions for drugs you need, and be sure you know how you should take them, how you should handle any side effects, and what changes to make in your diet or activities. Ask your doctor to write down the key points. Find out whom to call and when to call if you run into any problems. Ask if a follow-up visit is needed. Again, you may want to take notes.

If for any reason you know you will find it hard to follow or remember what your doctor tells you, take along a tape recorder, or ask a trusted friend or relative to come with you to take notes and help clarify information.

CRITICAL INFORMATION

Don't wait until there's an emergency to look up your doctor's phone number or other important information. Take a minute to fill out the following. Make 2 copies. Carry one with you and put the other near your telephone.

Doctor's name ____________________

Address ____________________

Telephone ____________________

Number where your doctor can be reached in an emergency (ask your doctor) ____________________

Local emergency number ____________________

Your insurer or health maintenance organization telephone number ____________________

Your insurance or HMO identification number ____________________

Reminders for Recovery

Even if your doctor pinpoints your problem and comes up with a treatment plan that works, you won't get all the benefits unless you do your share of the work. Here are some ways to speed recovery:

Find out how long your recovery should take. If you know what to expect—how long it will take before you can go back to your walking routine, for example—you'll have a better idea about when to check in with the doctor. If you're taking longer to heal than you think you should, call and say so.

Stay in touch. Call for an appointment right away if your illness takes a turn for the worse or if you get new symptoms.

Take all medication exactly as prescribed—even if you start to feel better. This is very important if you're taking antibiotics, which kill bacteria. If you stop taking antibiotics too early, your infection may linger because some germs have survived. Be sure to call your doctor at once to report any new or extreme side effects. (See **medicines: playing it safe**, page 322.)

Find a care partner. If you are sick and feeling overwhelmed, ask for help. A friend, neighbor, or relative might serve as a care partner. He or she can help you stay on top of your medications, drive you to the doctor's office, and give you support. If you're facing a long illness, loneliness can be one of your worst enemies. Surround yourself with people who are cheerful and helpful. Ask your doctor if there is a support group for people with your problem.

View your health as a long-term project. Getting well and staying well isn't just a matter of taking a drug and then neglecting yourself. It's best to make good self-care a part of your life—for the rest of your life.

For More Help

A wealth of information is waiting for anyone who wants to seek it out. For a specific health concern, see the For More Help listing at the end of most entries in this book. Here are some other sources:

Your own health maintenance organization or hospital. Many HMOs offer resource centers stocked with pamphlets, books, and videos on health subjects—from

GETTING READY FOR A REGULAR VISIT

Routine visits can help you and your doctor catch any problems early, perhaps before you notice symptoms. If caught in time, many ailments can be treated successfully. Your doctor will suggest a schedule of exams based on your needs.

Before you go, make a list. Know ahead of time what you'd like to talk about—both broad concerns and specific questions. Putting your thoughts on paper can help you focus; list anything that's been worrying you and any questions you want to ask. Here's a way to organize your thoughts:

My major concerns:	Doctor's comments and advice:
1 ______	______
2 ______	______
3 ______	______
My minor concerns:	
1 ______	______
2 ______	______
3 ______	______

Things to talk about on the next visit:

______

______

Write down your own health history. If you're visiting for the first time, your doctor will need to gather the facts about you—chronic ailments you may have, such as asthma or high blood pressure, and any serious illnesses or injuries you've had in the past, including hospitalizations, surgeries, and accidents.

Know your family health history. Your doctor will want some health background on your parents, siblings, and grandparents, such as chronic illnesses and causes of death, because some patterns show up in families—heart disease and cancer, for example, or living to a very old age. Your doctor will write down your history on his or her own form, but you can help out by being prepared. (See **your family health tree,** page 319.)

Brown-bag all your medications and take them to your appointment. Round up all the bottles of pills and capsules. Include vitamin supplements and all your other nonprescription items, such as drugs for allergies, colds, and the like. Your doctor needs to know what prescription and over-the-counter drugs you're taking, including those you got from other physicians. That way he or she can protect you from taking too many drugs or mixing drugs in a harmful way. (See **drug combinations to avoid** chart, page 323.)

coping with Alzheimer's disease to losing weight. Many HMOs also have health educators, as well as support groups, lectures, and classes. These range from Lamaze sessions for expectant parents to programs for smokers who want to quit. If your HMO doesn't have a resource center, check with a local hospital to see if it has a library that patients and the public can use.

Many hospitals also offer classes, seminars, and support groups.

Libraries and computer networks. Both public and college libraries have health sections. Some libraries also have a computer database, such as Infotrac or MEDLINE, which can help you find health information.

The National Network of Libraries of Medicine will connect you to a medical library in your area. Call 800-338-7657, 24-hour recording.

The Planetree Health Resource Centers is a useful network of consumer health libraries. For the location of the center nearest you and for information about its services, call the national offices at 415-956-4215, M–F 9–5 PST.

The National Institutes of Health offers information on allergies and infectious diseases (including AIDS), mental health, aging, cancer, diabetes, and digestive diseases. For details on specific topics, call the NIH Office of Communications, at 301-496-4000, 24-hour line.

The National Health Information Center is a free service; if you have specific health or medical questions, the people there can direct you to national organizations. You can also order publications from the NHIC list for a fee. Call 800-336-4797, M–F 1–5 EST. **Web site:** *http://nhic-nt.health.org.*

Web access. Thrive@Health is a self-help resource that offers basic health information on a wide range of conditions, including resources and links to other sites. After logging on to the Internet, type: *http://pathfinder.com/thrive/health/health.resources.html.* Scroll to the topic you want and click on it.

Support groups. National organizations often have local support groups. Two major ones, the American Cancer Society and the American Heart Association, list local chapters in the phone book. If you don't find them, call the national office of the **American Cancer Society** at 800-227-2345, M–F 9–5 your time; or the **American Heart Association** at 800-242-8721, M–F 8–5 your time.

For referral to AIDS support groups, call the **National HIV and AIDS Hotline** at 800-342-AIDS, 24-hour line.

Videos. The *...at Time of Diagnosis* videotapes introduced by C. Everett Koop, M.D., the former U.S. surgeon general, cover 30 conditions, from Alcoholism to Ulcers. Each runs about half an hour and provides a clear overview of causes and treatments, with 4 reports—Understanding the Diagnosis, What Happens Next?, Treatment and Management, and Issues and Answers. Time Life Medical, 1996, $19.95. Sold in many pharmacies; for one near you, call 800-588-9959.

WHEN YOU'RE SICK

When you go to the doctor, give as much information as you can. Try to cover these :

- Every change you've noticed since you started feeling sick.
- When the symptoms began.
- The time of day they occur.
- Whether you've had them before.
- What makes them better or worse.
- If you've done anything unusual lately, such as camping out or playing softball for the first time in 5 years, that might be affecting how you feel.
- If you've eaten anything unusual lately, or if you've started taking any new over-the-counter or prescription drugs.
- If any unusual events have occurred recently in your family, such as the sudden death of a relative. Include anything else you can think of that might have a bearing on your illness.
- Any mood changes or changes in your sleep patterns.
- Activities that seem to make you feel better or worse.

PAIN RELIEF: THE BIG FOUR

In this era of high-tech medicine, over-the-counter pain relievers still rank as wonder drugs. They ease pain and reduce fever and are almost always harmless when used as they should be. You can get 3 of the basic 4—aspirin, acetaminophen, and ibuprofen—just about everywhere as generics, identical to name brands.

Of course, you should use any drug with care (check the **drug combinations to avoid** chart, page 323).

Some cautions:

- Pregnant women should ask their doctor before taking any medicine.
- Don't take any of these together, or along with other painkillers.
- Ask your doctor before taking any of these with other drugs. Be sure to read the labels.
- Ask your doctor before taking any of these with an anticoagulant or with an antacid or acid blocker. Some combinations can cause bleeding.

Acetaminophen (common brand name: Tylenol). For fever and pain but not for inflammation. It's the only one of the 4 that doesn't prolong bleeding and that can be taken with acid blockers (such as Tagamet) or antacids (Mylanta, Maalox). It's advised for people having dental work or other treatment that causes bleeding, and for those with ulcers, frequent nosebleeds, or other bleeding problems. It's safest for children because it isn't linked with **Reye's syndrome** (see box on page 96). **Cautions:** Taking larger-than-advised doses for several weeks or with alcohol can cause liver damage. Daily use for several months may damage the kidneys.

Aspirin (common brand names: Bayer, Bufferin, Anacin). For fever, pain, and inflammation. Many take an aspirin every day to guard against heart attack, stroke, and colon cancer. **Cautions:** Aspirin can cause stomach upset—take it with meals or try buffered or coated types. Don't take it with stomach-acid drugs.

More than the other 3, aspirin makes blood less able to clot: As a result, it makes bleeding harder to stop. Don't take it if you have ulcers or other bleeding problems, or for about 5 days before oral or other surgery. (If you take aspirin every day, ask your doctor if it's okay to quit.) Aspirin can also trigger asthma attacks. It's linked with **Reye's syndrome** (see box on page 96): Never give aspirin to a child under 12 who might have an illness caused by a virus.

Ibuprofen (common brand names: Advil, Motrin, Nuprin). For pain, inflammation, and fever. Very good for menstrual and other cramps, arthritis, and muscle aches. **Cautions:** Ibuprofen can cause bleeding in people with ulcers if taken for more than 2 weeks or with stomach-acid drugs. Like aspirin, it can cause stomach upset (take it with meals or milk), and may trigger asthma attacks. Also, it may cause fluid buildup. Daily use for several months can cause kidney problems.

Naproxen sodium (common brand name: Aleve). For fever, minor aches and pains, muscle pain, arthritis, and menstrual cramps. Naproxen works longer than the other 3 painkillers. For chronic pain, that's important, but for most pain naproxen may be more than you need. **Cautions:** Follow dose limits carefully. Don't give it to children under age 12. Don't use it in the last 3 months of pregnancy. Don't take naproxen if you've had a severe allergic reaction with any other painkiller. Naproxen can cause mild heartburn or stomach upset (drink an 8-ounce glass of water with each dose).

Your Personal Health Record

You can do a lot to improve your chances of staying well: Learn all you can about your family's health history. Do regular self-exams. Get regular checkups. Keep your shots up to date. It costs a lot less to prevent an illness than to treat it, and it hurts less. And the earlier you detect any problem, the easier it will be to treat. Here are the basic things to know about keeping track of your health.

A Family Tree

To get a clear look at your family's health history, make a family health tree—a genogram.

A genogram shows at a glance the names of family members, how they are related, their dates of birth, their health problems, and the dates and causes of their deaths. Making a genogram allows you to see patterns in your family's health history. It's a tool you and your doctor can use to judge your risks for some of the more than 3,000 ailments believed to run in families—including heart disease, cancer, diabetes, Alzheimer's disease, thyroid disease, certain birth defects, alcoholism, depression, and schizophrenia.

Illnesses that have occurred in family members before the age of 55 may particularly interest you and your doctor—because you may want to take extra steps to avoid them. If you know your risks, you can often decrease them by changing your health habits or by spotting an ailment early so it can be treated.

- To make your own genogram, start with yourself and work back through time. Use circles for women, squares for men.
- Write in your name, date of birth, and any serious health problems or operations you've had.
- To the side of your own information, add the names of your sisters and brothers. Include notes about their health.
- Add your parents and any aunts or uncles on the 2 branches above you. Above them, your 4 grandparents, each with date of birth and a list of any known ailments.
- For people who have died, include the date of death and the cause of death, if you know it. For example:

  Jane Smith: b. 4-1-1890, d. 6-14-1960. Tuberculosis, angina, high blood pressure. Died of stroke.

You may need to call some of your relatives or check family records to find out all you need to know. Then, update the genogram every year or so, and keep it with your other health records.

The sample on the next page can help you get started. Copy the form and make a chart for yourself. If you have children, make a chart for their other parent; then combine that chart with yours to make a single two-parent chart for your children. If your family is large, you will need to extend the chart.

Your Family Health Tree

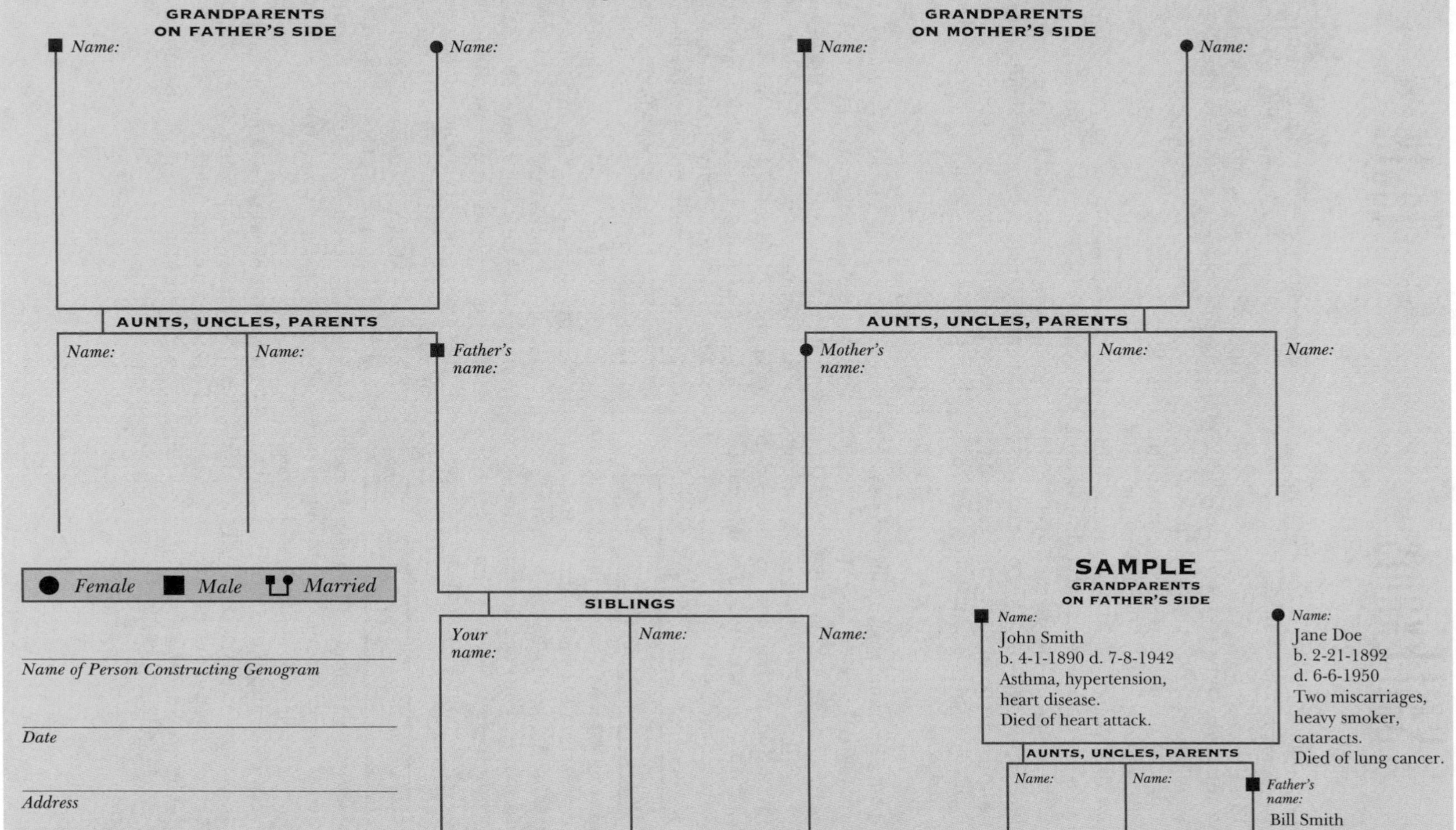

Self-Exams

Most doctors advise these self-exams:

Skin checkup. Once a month, look yourself over—more often if you have fair skin or a lot of moles, or if you spend a lot of time in the sun. Examine yourself fully. Use a mirror for hard-to-see places, or ask a partner to look. Keep an eye out for unusual scaliness, oozing, bleeding, or changes in freckles or moles. Report any changes to your doctor. (See **simple steps to save your skin,** page 181.) Once a year, see your doctor for a professional exam.

Weighing in. Maintain a healthy weight. It's vital for good health. (See page 302 for healthy weight ranges.) If your clothes start to feel too tight or too loose, step on a scale. Tell your doctor about any strange weight gain or loss. (Also see **sudden weight gain or loss** chart, page 288.)

FOR WOMEN

Breast self-exam (once a month). Check your breasts at the same time each month. You'll have a good chance of finding any lump that may need a doctor's attention. (For how to do it, see box, page 245.) Tell your doctor right away about any changes.

FOR MEN

Testicular exam (once a month). Though testicular cancer amounts to only 1 percent of all cancers, it is the leading cancer in men age 20 to 35. Finding it early can lead to a complete cure. Every month, roll each testicle between your thumb and forefinger, feeling for lumps. Report any new lump or swelling to your doctor.

Tests

The following tests require a visit to a doctor or clinic. Depending on your age and physical condition, your doctor may advise you to have checkups more often or less often.

Blood pressure (once a year for most adults; more often if your doctor advises it). Normal blood pressure is around 120 over 80. If yours is higher than that (see **high blood pressure,** page 112), your doctor may suggest exercise, diet changes, or medication.

Cholesterol (at least once every 5 years for most adults). High levels of cholesterol in your blood increase your risk of heart disease and stroke. One form of cholesterol—low-density lipoproteins, or LDL—has been nicknamed "bad cholesterol" because it can clog your arteries. There is also "good cholesterol"—high-density lipoproteins, or HDL—which actually helps remove bad cholesterol (see **artery disease,** page 106, and **eat well,** page 302).

One blood test measures total cholesterol. A reading of less than 200 (milligrams per deciliter) is good. A reading of 200 to 240 is borderline. A reading above 240 means a higher chance of heart disease. People with high readings should get a lipoprotein analysis, which will give LDL and HDL readings. To help guard against artery disease, your level of HDL should be at least 25 percent of your total cholesterol. An HDL reading above 60 gives good protection.

Colon: digital rectal exam (once a year after age 40). A doctor inserts a rubber-gloved finger into the rectum to check for rectal growths and, in men, signs of prostate cancer.

Colon: sigmoidoscopy (every 3 to 5 years after age 50). By guiding a flexible, lighted tube into the rectum and lower intestine, a doctor can look for colon cancer or polyps that may become cancer.

Fecal occult blood test (once a year after age 50). A stool sample is checked for traces of blood, which might mean colon cancer.

Dental checkup (every 6 months to a year for an exam and cleaning). If you go regularly, your dentist will be able to spot tooth decay or signs of gum disease early enough for effective treatment. Regular cleaning by a pro can help prevent gum disease.

FOR WOMEN

Breast exam by a doctor (every 3 years for women in their 20s and 30s, every year after age 40). Even if you do monthly breast exams yourself, get regular exams from your doctor as well.

Pap smear and pelvic exam (once a year for women 18 and over and for younger women who are sexually active). Cells gently scraped from the cervix can show changes that signal problems.

Mammogram (once a year for women 50 and over; some doctors recommend 40 and over—especially if there is a family history of breast cancer). An X-ray of the breast can spot cancer in its early stages by finding lumps too small to feel.

FOR MEN

PSA blood test for prostate cancer (some doctors suggest once a year for men 50 and over). The prostate-specific antigen test (PSA) can pick up early signs of prostate cancer, the most common cancer in American men. There is some debate about this test: It is not always reliable, and experts don't agree on how useful it is. Ask your doctor for advice.

Immunizations

Immunizations are a shot of prevention against many health problems, including polio, hepatitis, diphtheria, tetanus, and whooping cough.

They work by exposing the body to a killed or weakened form of a virus or other infectious agent. This makes the body's immune system strengthen its defenses. Most doctors advise the following:

CHILDREN AND TEENAGERS

See **children's immunizations** chart, page 256.

ADULTS

Tetanus-diphtheria (Td) booster. Once every 10 years for adults from age 19 to 64.

Influenza vaccine. Yearly for people age 65 and over and for those at high risk for flu, including adults with diabetes, kidney disease, cancer, chronic heart and respiratory conditions, or anemia; people with weakened immune systems; and adults who work with people at risk.

Pneumococcal vaccine. Once in a lifetime (or more, depending on your doctor's advice) for adults at high risk of pneumonia—including those age 65 and over, those who have had organ transplants, and those with diabetes, alcoholism, cirrhosis (liver damage), congestive heart failure, kidney failure, chronic pulmonary disease, or weakened immune systems.

Hepatitis B vaccine. A single series, once in a lifetime, for those at high risk—including health care workers, people who have contact with dirty needles, people with hemophilia who have frequent blood transfusions, and intravenous drug users (see **hepatitis,** page 284).

Medicines: Playing It Safe

If you're like most people, you've taken prescription drugs. And you've probably taken more than one kind at the same time. Most likely you also take over-the-counter drugs now and then—painkillers, for instance, or allergy medicines. Yet many drugs, whether over-the-counter or prescription, can have serious side effects when they bump up against each other. Other drugs are dangerous when combined with alcohol, nicotine, caffeine, some vitamins or minerals, or certain foods. Also, some drugs cancel out each other's usefulness if you take them together. (Older people are at higher risk of harmful drug combinations because their systems don't handle drugs as well as younger people's, and because they often take more than one prescription medicine at a time.)

Medication Safety Tips

To protect yourself, follow these suggestions:

- Tell *each* doctor you see about all the medications you are taking—both prescription and over-the-counter.
- Mention any vitamins as well, and whether you drink alcohol or use tobacco.
- If you're taking a number of medications, bring the containers with you to show the doctor; have them recorded in your file.
- Be sure all your doctor's directions about a drug make sense to you. Always read the label and follow the instructions exactly.
- Also ask your doctor:
  - What time should I take the medication? Should I take it with food or an hour or two before or after eating?
  - Should I avoid any foods, prescription medicines, or over-the-counter drugs while taking this? Should I avoid vitamins or other supplements? Is it safe to drink alcohol while I'm taking it? Will it affect my driving? What about caffeine, tobacco, or exposure to sunlight?
  - What side effects, if any, might I have?
  - What should I do if they occur?
- Your pharmacist is an excellent source of information. Fill all your prescriptions at the same pharmacy. That way your pharmacist will have a computerized record of your medications and can alert you to any problems.
- Always take the full course of medication prescribed for you. But call your doctor at once if you notice any new or strange symptoms. These include confusion, depression, insomnia, or memory loss. Dizziness as you get up, vomiting, diarrhea, constipation, or abdominal pain may also be side effects of certain drugs.
- Store medications as the label directs; some, for instance, should be refrigerated.
- Don't share medications.
- Don't buy a medicine if the packaging is broken or looks as though someone has tampered with it.
- Always take medications in good light—never in the dark. You need to see what you're swallowing or applying.
- Throw out leftover medicine if the package date shows it has expired. That makes it less likely that you—or someone else—will take it by mistake.

Drug Combinations to Avoid

This chart lists some dangerous drug combinations. Some drugs react badly with each other; others shouldn't be combined with alcohol or certain foods or vitamins. This is by no means a complete list of all harmful drug interactions. (To learn about others, see **for more help,** page 314.) Nor is the chart meant to replace medical advice. Be sure to tell each of your health care providers about every prescription medicine and over-the-counter drug you're taking. Never start or stop taking any medication without talking to your doctor first.

IF YOU'RE TAKING	DON'T MIX WITH	WHAT CAN HAPPEN	RECOMMENDATION
Antibiotic—ciprofloxacin (Cipro).	Antacids (Mylanta, Maalox, others).	The antibiotic may not work as well.	Don't combine these drugs without asking your doctor.
Antibiotics—ciprofloxacin (Cipro), erythromycin, others.	Theophylline (Theo-Dur, Slo-bid, Bronkaid, others), used to treat asthma.	High levels of theophylline in blood. Symptoms include nausea, vomiting, palpitations, seizures.	Make sure your doctor knows you are taking both. Ask for advice about checking theophylline levels in your blood.
Antibiotics—metronidazole (Flagyl, Femizole, others).	Alcohol (beer, wine, hard liquor).	Low blood pressure, vomiting, confusion, rapid heartbeat.	Don't combine these drugs with alcohol.
Antibiotics—quinolones, including ciprofloxacin (Cipro) and norfloxacin (Noroxin).	Iron—including supplements and iron-laden tonics.	The antibiotic may not work as well.	Check with your doctor or pharmacist before combining this antibiotic with iron.
Antibiotics—tetracycline, quinolone antibiotics (Cipro, Noroxin, others).	Calcium (dairy products) and calcium found in antacids (such as Tums); or aluminum and magnesium antacids (such as Mylanta or Maalox).	Much lower absorption of tetracycline or quinolones, so they don't work as well.	Wait 2 hours after eating dairy products to take medication. Do not take antacids with these medications without your doctor's approval. Then take the antacids only 6 hours before or 4 hours after taking the antibiotic.
Anticoagulants (oral)—including warfarin (Panwarfin, Coumadin, others), used to help prevent blood clots.	Aspirin, ibuprofen (Advil, Motrin), naproxen (Aleve), acetaminophen (Tylenol); stomach acid blockers (Tagamet, Zantac, Pepcid).	Bleeding, particularly in stomach. Symptoms include black stools, blood in urine.	Ask your doctor before taking *any* other drug—including over-the-counter drugs.
Anticoagulants—(oral)—including warfarin (Panwarfin, Coumadin, others).	Vitamin K–rich foods and drinks (broccoli, cabbage, green tea, lentils, soybeans, spinach, others); antacids (Mylanta, Maalox).	Reduce effect of anticoagulant.	Check with your doctor about combining drug with foods rich in vitamin K, or with any other drugs.

(continued)

Drug Combinations to Avoid *(continued)*

IF YOU'RE TAKING	DON'T MIX WITH	WHAT CAN HAPPEN	RECOMMENDATION
Antidepressants—selective serotonin re-uptake inhibitors, such as Fluoxetine (Prozac), sertraline (Zoloft), paroxetine (Paxil).	Monoamine oxidase (MAO) inhibitors (Marplan, Nardil, Parnate, others, used to treat depression); and Eldepryl, used for Parkinson's disease.	Confusion, muscle twitches, sweating, shivering, agitation; in very rare cases, can be fatal.	Don't take these antidepressants with an MAO inhibitor, or for 2 weeks after quitting an MAO. Wait 5 weeks after going off these drugs to start an MAO.
Antidepressants—monoamine oxidase (MAO) inhibitors (Marplan, Nardil, Parnate, others).	Over-the-counter cold medicines, decongestants, or diet pills with phenylpropanolamine (Allerest, Dexatrim, others); phenylephrine (Dristan Decongestant, others); and pseudoephedrine (Sudafed, others).	Rapid heartbeat; light-headedness; headache; sudden, rise in blood pressure; could lead to a fatal stroke.	Don't take these cold medicines with an MAO inhibitor, or for 2 weeks after quitting an MAO.
Antidepressants—MAO inhibitors (Marplan, Nardil, Parnate, others).	Alcoholic drinks containing tyramine (including red wines). Also foods with tyramine (aged cheeses; liver; yeast concentrates; broad beans; salted, smoked, or pickled fish; others).	Dramatic rise in blood pressure, dizziness, nausea; in rare cases, bleeding around brain and death.	Avoid alcoholic drinks and foods rich in tyramine if you're taking an MAO inhibitor.
Antidepressants—tricyclic medications (Elavil, Sinequan, others).	Antidepressants—MAO inhibitors (Marplan, Nardil, Parnate, others).	Confusion, fever, dizziness, seizures, overexcitement, coma.	These drugs should be combined only if prescribed to be taken together.
Antihistamines—terfenadine (Seldane) and astemizole (Hismanal). Nonsedating antihistamines, used to treat allergies.	Antifungal drugs—ketoconazole (Nizoral) and itraconazole (Sporanox); and certain antibiotics—including erythromycin (EryPed, others).	Changes in liver function. Symptoms include irregular heartbeat, chest pain, shortness of breath. Possibly lethal.	Don't combine these drugs.
Calcium channel blockers—(Plendil, Procardia, Adalat, others). Used to treat high blood pressure and angina.	Grapefruit juice (contains flavonoids, including naringenin).	Hazardous increase in the level of medication in blood. Symptoms include headaches and light-headedness.	Do not take these drugs with grapefruit juice.
Gastrointestinal drugs—acid blockers (Tagamet, Zantac, Pepcid) and antacids (Mylanta, Maalox, others) for heartburn and ulcers.	NSAIDs (aspirin, ibuprofen, naproxen); anticoagulants; some heart, antifungal, antibiotic, or other drugs.	Taken with NSAIDs, can mask ulcer symptoms. May change effects of many other drugs.	Read drug warnings carefully or ask your doctor or pharmacist before you mix these with other drugs.

Drug Combinations to Avoid

IF YOU'RE TAKING	DON'T MIX WITH	WHAT CAN HAPPEN	RECOMMENDATION
Gastrointestinal drugs—cisapride (Propulsid), for night-time heartburn.	Antifungal drugs and some antibiotics.	Irregular heartbeat, heart attack.	Don't combine these drugs.
Heart drugs—digoxin (Lanoxin).	Antacids (Mylanta, Maalox).	Heart drug won't work as well.	Don't combine these drugs.
Heart drugs—digoxin (Lanoxin).	Quinidine, diuretics, verapamil, and others.	Abnormal heartbeat, nausea, loss of appetite, vision changes.	Ask your doctor before mixing this with other drugs.
Hormonal drugs—estrogen-containing birth control pills (Demulen, Ortho Novum, others).	Tobacco (all forms) and nicotine patches, gum, or other products.	Increased risk of stroke, heart attack, blood clots.	Never smoke or use other nicotine products if you take birth control pills.
Hormonal drugs—estrogen-containing birth control pills (Demulen, Ortho Novum, others).	Some antibiotics (including ampicillin, penicillin, rifampin, tetracycline); barbiturates; tranquilizers.	Birth control pills may not work well while you take these and other drugs.	Talk to your doctor about using other birth control methods while taking any medications.
Pain relievers, NSAID-type—aspirin, ibuprofen (Advil, Motrin), naproxen (Aleve).	Anticoagulants; antacids and acid blockers; alcoholic drinks.	Irritation of stomach lining; greater risk of ulcers and bleeding.	Consult your doctor about mixing these drugs.
Pain relievers—acetaminophen (Tylenol, Panadol, others).	Alcohol (beer, wine, hard liquor); anticoagulants.	Possibility of liver damage; stomach bleeding.	Consult your doctor about mixing these drugs.
Tranquilizers and sleeping pills—benzodiazepines, including diazepam (Valium), chlordiazepoxide (Librium), others.	Alcohol (beer, wine, hard liquor).	With high amounts, dizziness, severe drowsiness, impaired reactions (in driving, operating machinery), coma.	Don't take these drugs with alcohol.

FOR MORE HELP

Organization: United States Pharmacopeia, 12601 Twinbrook Pkwy., Rockville, MD 20852. 301-881-0666, M–F 7:30–5 EST. Call to order free booklets on understanding your medications, using medicines properly, recognizing drug tampering, and preventing medication errors. **Web site:** *http://www.usp.org.*

Book: *The Customer's Guide to Drug Interactions,* by Jeffrey R. Schein and Philip Hansten, Pharm. D., Collier Books, 1993, $15.

Book: *The People's Guide to Deadly Drug Interactions,* by Joe Graedon and Teresa Graedon, Ph.D., St. Martin's Press, 1995, $25.95.

Index

Note: Page numbers in **bold** refer to the main discussion of a topic and to charts. Page numbers in *italic* refer to illustrations. Drugs named in the text are listed under *Drugs* on page 332.

A

Index

C

D

E

Index

F

G

H

I

J

K

L

M

N

O

P

Index

S

T

U

V

W

Y

The Self-Care Advisor

Editor
John Poppy

Art Director
Charli Ornett

Managing Editor
Karin Evans

Senior Editors
Diana Hembree, Judith Horstman, Eric Olsen, Colleen Paretty

Production Director
Linda K. Smith

Consulting Editor
Susan West

Writers
Barbara Boughton, Ingfei Chen, Jeanie Puleston Fleming, Deborah Franklin, Katherine Griffin, Sarah Henry, Peter Jaret, Katherine Kam, Susan LaCroix, Lisa Margonelli, Constance Matthiessen, Clark Norton, Mary Purpura, Laurie Udesky, Rob Waters

Copy Editors
Ann Bartz, Antonia Moore, Catharine Norton, Katherine Wright, O'Brien Young

Researchers
Mitzi Baker, Catherine Guthrie, Laird Harrison, Carol Levine, Joy Rothke, Jessica Shattuck, Christie Uhrowczik

Project Coordinators
Adrienne DeAngelo, Cassandra Wrightson, Colby Zintl

Indexer
Karen Hollister

Associate Art Directors
Kimberle Nogay, Bruce Purdy

Designers
Cici Kinsman, Philip Krayna, Marsha Levine, Judith Levinson, Mario Reyes, Emma Rybakova, Glen Shannon, Jerald Volpe, M. Elizabeth Williamson

Photo Editors
Nona Jones, Mary Schoenthaler

Production Coordinator
Michael A. Nealy

Senior Medical Review
Karen Jubanyik, M.D.

Medical Illustration
Many of the color images on pages 161–176 are taken from 3-D digital computer animation and graphics in the Time Life Medical *At Time of Diagnosis* video programs.

Senior Vice President, Executive Art Director
Jane Hurd

Art Director
Neil Lavey

Illustrators
Donna DeSmet, Brian Evans, Maura Flynn, Craig Foster, Neil Hardy, Rong-Zeng Li

Graphics Producers
Matthew Canton, Amy Lisewski

Graphics Coordinator
Kristin Ellington

3-D computer graphics produced in association with
Sonalysts Studios
Waterford, Connecticut

SONALYSTS STUDIOS
THE NEW ENGLAND FILM STUDIOS

Sonalysts Inc.

Time Inc Health

President and CEO
Eric W. Schrier

General Manager
Martha Lorini

Editor
Barbara Paulsen

Executive Editor
Sheridan Warrick

Managing Editor
Bruce K. Kelley

Time Life Medical
Patient Education Media, Inc.

President and CEO
J. Keith Green

Medical Director
C. Everett Koop, M.D.

Deputy Medical Director
Florence Comite, M.D.

President and COO, Consumer Products Division
James B. Arnold

Executive Vice President, Product Development
Nan-Kirsten Weinstock Forté

Print Production Manager
Sheldon Lazansky

Black and white illustrations: Neil Hardy: pages 66, 75, 203, 204. Jeffrey Smith: 15, 16, 17, 18, 20, 21, 22, 25, 34, 38, 100, 125, 140, 191, 193, 245.

Color Photographs, page 167: Moles A, B, and D: Custom Medical Stock Photo. Mole C: Biophoto Associates/PhotoResearchers, Inc.

Cover Photographs: Mother and son: Mugshots/Stock Market. Couple: Anthony Edgeworth/Stock Market. Father and daughter: Janeart/Image Bank. Child: Stephanie Rausser. Family: Brian Smith. Hands: Paul Clancy/Graphistock. Laughing woman: Michael Johnson. Runner: Michael Kevin Daly. Swimmer: Michael Douglas/The Image Works.

Acknowledgments

This book would not be as helpful and accurate as it is without the assistance of health professionals in every part of the United States—men and women who answered hundreds of questions, offered guidance and resources, and repeatedly displayed their commitment to improving information about health care. We owe them our sincerest thanks.

Emergency & First Aid
Sheldon Clark, M.D.
R. Scott Jacobs, M.D.
Eric A. Weiss, M.D.

Head & Nervous System
Seymour Diamond, M.D.
Robert G. Feldman, M.D.
R. Michael Gallagher, D.O.
Howard Gruetzner, M.Ed.
W. Michael Scheld, M.D.
Mark Spitz, M.D.
Cathi Thomas, R.N., M.S.

Eyes
Ronald M. Burde, M.D.
Monica L. Monica, M.D., Ph.D.

Ears
Richard Goode,M.D.
Michael Seidman, M.D.

Mouth
Bruce Bagley, M.D.
Donald Collins, D.D.S., M.P.H.
Jon Richter, D.M.D., Ph.D.
Thomas Weida, M.D.

Nose, Throat, Lungs, & Chest
Stephen Astor, M.D.
Robert Breiman, M.D.
James Cook, M.D.
Donald Donovan, M.D.
Dominick Iacuzio, Ph.D.
Clayton Kersting, M.D.
Barry Make, M.D.
Harold Nelson, M.D.
Carol Reid, M.D.
Nathan Schultz, M.D.

Heart & Circulation
Ralph S. Paffenbarger, Jr., M.D., Dr.P.H.
Rodman D. Starke, M.D.
Katharine Weiser, M.D.

Stomach, Abdomen, & Digestive System
Quan-Yang Duh, M.D.
Johannes Koch, M.D.
Peter McNally, D.O.
Stephen Pardys, M.D.
Theodore R. Schrock, M.D.
Marvin Schuster, M.D.

Skin, Scalp, & Nails
Deborah Allen, M.D.
William Epstein, M.D.
Glenn B. Gastwirth, D.P.M.
Richard Glogau, M.D.
Michael Heffernan, M.D.
Robert Jackson, M.D.
Mark Lebwohl, M.D.
Jerome Z. Litt, M.D.
Alan R. Shalita, M.D.
David Taplin
Stephen Tyring, M.D., Ph.D.

Muscles, Bones, & Joints
Daniel Benson, M.D.
Stanley Bigos, M.D.
Doyt Conn, M.D.
Scott Dye, M.D.
James Garrick, M.D.
David Kell, M.D.
Nancy Liu, M.D.
John Rugh, Ph.D.
Cody Wasner, M.D.

Behavior & Emotions
Robert Bailey, M.D.
Herbert Freudenberger, Ph.D.
Nancy Kennedy, Dr. P.H.
Vivian Hanson Meehan, R.N., B.A., D.Sc.
Robert Sapolsky, Ph.D.
Rick Seymour, M.A.
Joe Takamine, M.D.
Scott Thomas, Ph.D.

Sexual, Men's, & Women's Health
Stanley Althof, Ph.D.
Sondra Lynne Carter, M.D.
Stuart Howards, M.D.
Tom F. Lue, M.D.
Joseph E. Oesterling, M.D.
Michael Spence, M.D., M.P.H.
Paul Stumpf, M.D.

Children's Health
David Batts
Armando Correa, M.D.
Robert Prentice, M.D.
S. Norman Sherry, M.D.
Donald Shifrin, M.D.

General Problems
Grover Bagby, Jr., M.D.
Kathleen Bliese, M.D.
Alan Blum, M.D.
Robert Katz, M.D.
Rick Kellerman, M.D.
Clete Kushida, M.D., Ph.D.
Emmanuel Mignot, M.D., Ph.D.

Helping Your Doctor Help You
Pamela Stitzlein Davies, R.N., M.S.
Rachel Naomi Remen, M.D.
John Stoeckle, M.D.
David Stutz, M.D.
Mary Wade

Your Personal Health Record
Bruce Gollub, M.D.
Stirling Puck, M.D.
Robert Rakel, M.D.
Ssu Weng, M.D.

Medicines: Playing It Safe
Hemlata Chopra, Pharm.D.
Ron Finley, R.Ph.
Frederic J. Zucchero, M.A., R.Ph.

If I'd known I was going to live this long,
I'd have taken better care of myself.

~James Herbert (Eubie) Blake, age 100